Contact Lenses

Scrivener Publishing
100 Cummings Center, Suite 541J
Beverly, MA 01915-6106

Publishers at Scrivener
Martin Scrivener (martin@scrivenerpublishing.com)
Phillip Carmical (pcarmical@scrivenerpublishing.com)

Contact Lenses

Materials, Chemicals, Methods and Applications

Johannes Karl Fink
Montanuniversität Leoben, Austria

Scrivener Publishing

WILEY

This edition first published 2022 by John Wiley & Sons, Inc., 111 River Street, Hoboken, NJ 07030, USA and Scrivener Publishing LLC, 100 Cummings Center, Suite 541J, Beverly, MA 01915, USA

For more information about Scrivener publications please visit www.scrivenerpublishing.com.

Wiley Global Headquarters
111 River Street, Hoboken, NJ 07030, USA

For details of our global editorial offices, customer services, and more information about Wiley products visit us at www.wiley.com.

Library of Congress Cataloging-in-Publication Data

ISBN 978-1-119-85735-8

Cover image: Pixabay.com
Cover design by Russell Richardson

Set in size of 11pt and Minion Pro by Manila Typesetting Company, Makati, Philippines

Printed in the USA

10 9 8 7 6 5 4 3 2 1

Contents

Preface

This book focuses on the chemistry and properties of contact lenses and their fabrication methods.

The text starts with a chapter in which a detailed history of contact lenses spanning over almost 500 years is presented

Next, common materials that are used for the fabrication of contact lenses are listed and explained, including both the monomers and polymers that are used in their production. Special issues regarding soft lenses, clear contact lenses, and functional contact lenses are also discussed.

Functional contact lenses can be used for remote health monitoring and ocular drug delivery systems. Besides the materials used here, these issues are detailed in further separate chapters. Also, special fabrication methods are discussed, e.g., the fabrication of multifocal contact lenses and the fabrication of ultrathin coatings.

There is also an important discussion on additives that can be used, e.g., for oxygen-permeable materials or anti-biofouling materials.

The chapter ends with a discussion of simulation methods for contact lenes, such asocular topography parameters, gas-permeable lenses, and computerized videokeratography.

In the second chapter, several common fabrication methods for contact lenses are discussed. Here, computer-aided contact lens design, methods for the fabrication of colored contact lenses, and the fabrication of decentered contact lenses are detailed.

Also, special processes are reviewed, including mold processes, reactive ion etching, electrospinning and others.

Another chapter discusses the properties of contact lenses and methods of measurement. Here, a lot of standard methods are discussed. Besides standard methods, other issues are discussed such as the assessment of cytotoxic effects, the Schirmer tear test and others.

A chapter is devoted to drug delivery of contact lenses, a comparatively new issue.

Finally, a chapter details the possible medical problems related to contact lenses and how to avoid them. These are eye diseases, allergic and toxic reactions. Also, disinfection agents that can be used and methods for the medical treatment of such problems are detailed.

The text focuses on the literature of the past decade. Beyond education, this book will serve the needs of industry engineers and specialists who have only a passing knowledge of the plastics and composites industries but need to know more.

How to Use This Book

Utmost care has been taken to present reliable data. Because of the vast variety of material presented here, however, the text cannot be complete in all aspects, and it is recommended that the reader study the original literature for more complete information.

The reader should be aware that mostly US patents have been cited where available, but not the corresponding equivalent patents in other countries. For this reason, the author cannot assume responsibility for the completeness, validity or consequences of the use of the material presented herein. Every attempt has been made to identify trademarks; however, there were some that the author was unable to locate.

Index

There are three indices: an index of acronyms, an index ofchemicals, and a general index.

In the index of chemicals, compounds that occur extensively, e.g., "acetone," are not included at every occurrence, but rather when they appear in an important context.

Acknowledgements

I am indebted to our university librarians, Dr. Christian Hasenhüttl, Margit Keshmiri, Friedrich Scheer, Christian Slamenik, Renate Tschabuschnig, and Elisabeth Groß for their support in literature acquisition. I also want to express my gratitude to all the scientists who have carefully published their results concerning the topics dealt with herein. This book could not have been otherwise compiled.

In addition, I am very grateful to the ophthalmologists Dr. Anna Schlanitz-Bolldorf and Dr. Ferdinand Schlanitz, who inspired me to write this text. Last, but not least, I want to thank the publisher, Martin Scrivener, for his abiding interest and help in the preparation of the text. In addition, my thanks go to Jean Markovic, who made the final copyedit with utmost care.

Johannes Fink
Leoben, December 2, 2021

1

Types of Lenses

1.1 History of Contact Lenses

A history of contact lenses spanning over almost 500 years has been detailed (1, 2). It is based on historical works, scientific papers and journal articles and looks at both the modern disposable lens as well as the hard and soft lenses that came before. Some important events are collected in Table 1.1.

Table 1.1 History of contact lenses (2).

Year	Inventor	Issue
1508	Leonardo da Vinci	Corneal neutralization
1637	René Descartes	Fluid-filled tube
1685	Philippe de La Hire	Neutralization of cornea
1801	Thomas Young	Three color theory of perception
1827	George Biddell	Theory of astigmatism
1845	Sir John F. W. Herschel	Convex lenses
1846	Carl Zeiss	Optical instruments
1851	Johann Nepomuk Czermak	Water-filled goggle
1887	Adolf Eugen Fick	First successful contact lens
1961	Otto Wichterle	Soft contact lenses
1979	Kyoichi Tanaka	Silicone hydrogel materials

In 1508, Leonardo da Vinci first had the idea of placing a corrective lens directly onto the surface of the eye (3–5). In 1637, René Descartes proposed another idea in which a glass tube filled with liquid is placed in direct contact with the cornea.

In 1887, Adolf Eugen Fick, a German physiologist, created the first successful contact lens (6). Glass-blown scleral lenses remained the only form of contact lens until 1938, when poly(methyl methacrylate) (PMMA) was developed, and Mullen and Obring used the plastic to manufacture scleral lenses. Obring developed the Plexiglass series in New York in 1940 (4).

In 1961, the Czech chemist Otto Wichterle invented soft contact lenses (7, 8). In 1970, rigid gas-permeable contact lenses were developed, and widely accepted for the advantages of small diameter (about 9 *mm*) and gas permeability. Silicone hydrogel materials were developed in 1979 (9). In 1999, an important development was the launch of the first silicone hydrogels onto the market. These new materials showed an extremely high oxygen permeability with comfort performance (4).

The factors that influenced the development of special materials have been reported (10). Accounts of early attempts to improve vision by use of a lens contacting the eye are limited to a few isolated observations (11). Practical success was not realized until techniques for fabrication of lenses from glass were sufficiently developed (12). PMMA replaced glass in the late 1930s. This material is more durable, more readily fabricated and was claimed by some authors to show a better ocular compatibility (13). During the same broad period of time, there was also a change in emphasis from scleral to corneal contact lenses, which placed different demands on material design and development.

More is demanded from ophthalmic treatments using contact lenses, which are currently used by over 125 million people around the world (14). Improving the material of contact lenses is currently a rapidly evolving discipline (10).

A search has been performed of the titles of papers in the Scopus database to identify contact lens-related articles published this century (15). The ten most highly cited papers were determined from the total list of 4,164 papers found. Rank-order lists by count were assembled for the *top 25* in each of four categories: authors, institutions, countries and journals. A 20-year subject-specific contact lens h-index was derived for each author, institution, country and journal to serve as a measure of impact in the field. The top 10 constituents (of the top 25) of each category were ranked and tabulated (15).

1.2 Materials

Contact lens materials (10) are typically based on polymer- or silicone-hydrogel, with additional manufacturing technologies employed to produce the final lens. These processes are simply not enough to meet the increasing demands for contact lenses and the ever-increasing number of contact lens users (14).

An advanced perspective on contact lens materials has been presented, with an emphasis on materials science employed in developing new contact lenses (14, 16). The future trends for contact lens materials are to graft, incapsulate, or modify the classic contact lens material structure to provide new or improved functionality. Also, some of the fundamental material properties are discussed, and the outlook for related emerging biomaterials is presented.

Contact lens materials and lens types, treatment for contact lens and tear film complications, and myopia correction and contact lenses for abnormal ocular conditions have been detailed (17). Current topics in this field are miniscleral lenses, keratoconus, corneal crosslinking, and pediatric, cosmetic and prosthetic contact lenses. Furthermore, simulation programs for scleral lens fitting, sagittal values, soft toric mislocation, front vertex power, orthokeratology and rigid lens design are discussed.

1.3 Monomers

The monomers that can be used for contact lenses, which are described in the following sections and in both tables and references, are collected in Table 1.2.

These issues will be detailed in the following sections of this chapter.

1.3.1 Monomers for Block Copolymers

A block copolymer that contains both hydrophobic and hydrophilic blocks with amino acid groups has been described (18).

The principal monomers for such block copolymers are a combination of two monomers capable of forming a hydrogel; such monomers are collected in Table 1.3.

Table 1.2 Monomers for contact lenses.

Monomers and monomer types	Usage	References
2-Hydroxyethyl methyacrylate *N*-Vinyl-2-pyrrolidone Methyl methacrylate Isobornyl methacrylate *tert*-Butylcyclohexyl methacrylate	Soft lenses	(19)
Hydrophobic monomers	Strengthening agents	Table 1.8
Hydrophilic monomers		Table 1.8
Hydrophilic monomers	Hydrogels	Table 1.10
Azlactones	Surface treatment	Table 1.12
Acrylamide *N*-Hydroxyethyl acrylamide *N*-Isopropyl acrylamide 2-Acrylamido-2-methylpropanesulfonic acid 2-Hydroxyethyl methacrylate 2-Hydroxyethyl acrylate	Macromers	(20)
Acryl monomers	Water absorbable	Table 1.16
Poly(siloxane)	Water absorbable	Table 1.17
4-(Phenyldiazenyl) phenyl methacrylate	Blue-light blocking	(21)
Acrylates	UV-blocking	Table 1.22
Silicone hydrogel	Multifocal lenses	Table 1.23
Acrylates	Non-silicone hydrogel	Table 1.25
Crosslinking agents	Non-silicone hydrogel	Table Table 1.26
Oxyperm	Oxygen permeable	Table 1.32
Ionoperm	Oxygen permeable	Table 1.32

Table 1.3 Monomers (18).

Monomer	Monomer
2-Ethylphenoxy acrylate	2-Ethylphenoxy methacrylate
2-Ethylthiophenyl acrylate	2-Ethylthiophenyl methacrylate
2-Ethylaminophenyl acrylate	2-Ethylaminophenyl methacrylate
Phenyl acrylate	Phenyl methacrylate
Benzyl acrylate	Benzyl methacrylate
2-Phenylethyl acrylate	2-Phenylethyl methacrylate
3-Phenylpropyl acrylate	3-Phenylpropyl methacrylate
3-Propylphenoxy acrylate	3-Propylphenoxy methacrylate
4-Butylphenoxy acrylate	4-Butylphenoxy methacrylate
4-Phenylbutyl acrylate	4-Phenylbutyl methacrylate

Side-chain-linked amino acids are collected in Table 1.4. Some of these compounds are shown in Figure 1.1.

Table 1.4 Side-chain-linked amino acids (18).

Monomer	Monomer
Acryloyl-*L*-lysine	Acryloyl-*L*-serine
Acryloyl-*L*-threonine	Acryloyl-*L*-tyrosine
Acryloyl-*L*-amino-phenylalanine	Acryloyl-*L*-cysteine
Acryloyl-*L*-oxy-proline	Nϵ-acryloyl-Nα-Oelityl-L-Lysine

The synthesis of a variety of such monomers has been detailed (18). For example, the synthesis of (*S*)-6-acrylamido-2-aminohexanoic acid monomers is performed via a copper complex (18):

Preparation 1–1: L-lysine (14.62 *g*; 100 *mmol*) was dissolved in 150 *ml* deionized water and heated to about 80°C. Copper carbonate (16.6 *g*; 75 *mmol*) was added in portions over a period of 30 *min*. The reaction was stirred for an additional 30 *min*. The hot, deep-blue suspension was filtered through silica gel. The filter was washed with a small amount of water. On the following day, the lysine copper complex containing the combined filtrate was cooled in an ice bath, and 100 *ml* tetrahydrofuran was added. A solution of acryloyl chloride in methyl-*tert*-butylether (8.9 *ml*, 110 *mmol*) was added dropwise during a period of 1 *h*. The pH was initially maintained between 8 and 10 by parallel, dropwise addition of 10% sodium hydroxide solution. After half of the acryloyl chloride solution had been added, the product began to precipitate. When most of the acryloyl chloride had been added, addition of sodium hydroxide was

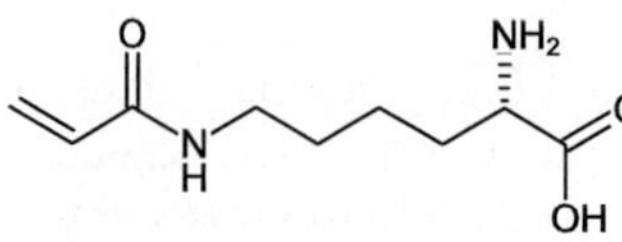

Acryloyl-*L*-lysine

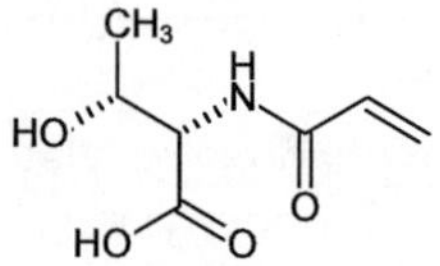

Acryloyl-*L*-threonine

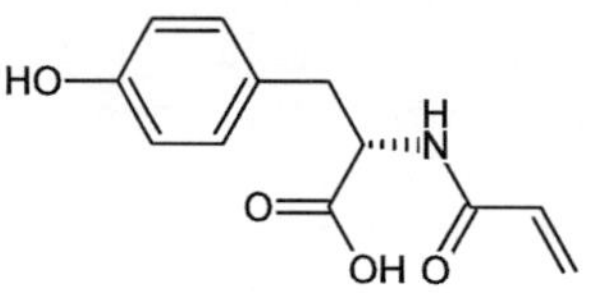

Acryloyl-*L*-tyrosine

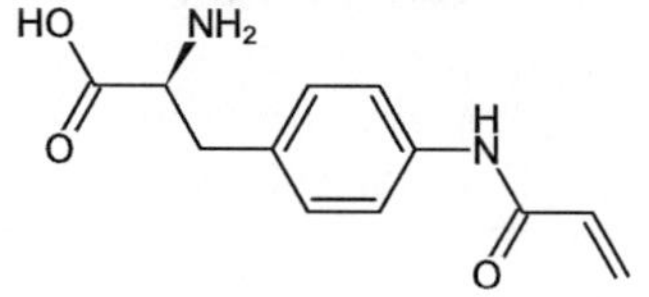

Acryloyl-*L*-amino-phenylalanine

Figure 1.1 Monomers for side-chain-linked amino acids.

slowed down to allow the pH to drop to about 6 and the temperature of the reaction mixture was allowed to reach room temperature. The blue suspension was stirred for an additional 2 *h* and was then filtered. The solid material retained on the filter was washed with water and acetone and then dried. A yield of 6.5 *g* of acryloyl-*L*-lysine copper complex was obtained. Acryloyl-*L*-lysine copper complex (29.5 *g*) was suspended in 300 *ml* deionized water and cooled in an ice bath. H_2S gas was bubbled into the suspension until copper sulfide precipitation was complete; then 3 *g* of active charcoal was added to the suspension. The suspension was heated briefly to 100°C. After cooling to room temperature, 500 *ml* acetone was added to the suspension which was then filtered on silica gel. The clear filtrate was put in a rotary evaporator. After evaporation of the solvent, the solid product was recrystallized from 200 *ml* of 50% aqueous acetone. A yield of 17.76 *g* (69.76%) of white powder was obtained. The structure of the compound was verified by nuclear magnetic resonance spectroscopy and LC-MS spectroscopy.

The preparation of a block copolymer containing a hydrophilic cellophil polymer and a lipid-like copolymer was done by raft polymerization as follows (18):

Preparation 1–2: Step A

In a 50 *ml* round-bottom flask, a solution of 2-(dodecylthiocarbonothioylthio)-2-methylpropionic acid (6.13 *mg*, 0.017 *mmol*), *N,N*-Dimethyl acrylamide (0.624 *ml*, 6.05 *mmol*), and *iso*-decyl acrylate (0.163 *ml*, 0.673 *mmol*) in 10 *ml* *N,N*-dimethylformamide was degassed using ultrasonic treatment. Subsequently, 2-benzyl-2-(dimethylamino)-4′-morpholinobutyrophenone (6.40 *mg*, 0.017 *mmol*) was added, and polymerization was induced by UV light. After 4 *h* of polymerization under stirring, the reaction mixture was purified by extensive dialysis against deionized water using a membrane with a 3.5 *kDa* MWCO. The mixture was subsequently lyophilized. The average molecular weight (12 *kDa*) and PDI (1.19) of the block copolymer was verified by GPC measurement.

Step B

The lyophilized macro-CTA prepared in step A (300 *mg*, 6.82 *μmol*) was mixed with acryloyl-*L*-lysine (100 *mg*, 0.499 *mmol*) in 10 *ml* deionized water. The mixture was degassed using ultrasonic treatment. 2,2′-Azobis(2-methylpropionamidine) dihydrochloride (4.62 *mg*, 0.017 *mmol*) was added to the mixture. The polymerization was induced by heating the mixture in a reaction vessel to 50°C. After 4 *h* of polymerization at 50°C, the resulting block copolymer was purified by extensive dialysis against deionized water using a membrane with a 3.5 *kDa* MWCO. The cellophil block copolymer was subsequently lyophilized. The average molecular weight (18 *kDa*) and PDI (1.25) of the block copolymer were verified by GPC measurement. Larger block copolymers (32 *kDa*, PDI 1.28; 58 *kDa*, PDI 1.24) were obtained by decreasing the ratio of CTA to monomers in step A from 1/100 to 1/200 (32 *kDa*) and 1/400 (58 *kDa*), respectively, whereas the molar ratios of *i*-decylacrylate (7.5 *mol* of 5), DMA (63.9 *mol* of 5) and AK (28.6 *mol* of 5) were kept constant.

Some of the compounds mentioned in Preparation 1–2 are shown in Figure 1.2.

1.3.2 *Silicone Acrylamides*

Examples of hydrophilic methacrylamide monomers are collected in Table 1.5. Some of these compounds are shown in Figure 1.3. Also, several other similar monomers have been detailed (22).

These alkyl and aryl groups can be straight or branched. Of these monomers, the *N*-(2-hydroxyethyl)methacrylamide monomer is preferable from a perspective of increasing the transparency of the so obtained polymer.

The monomer mixture for synthesizing the polymer additionally may contain between about 1% and about 30% of a hydrophilic

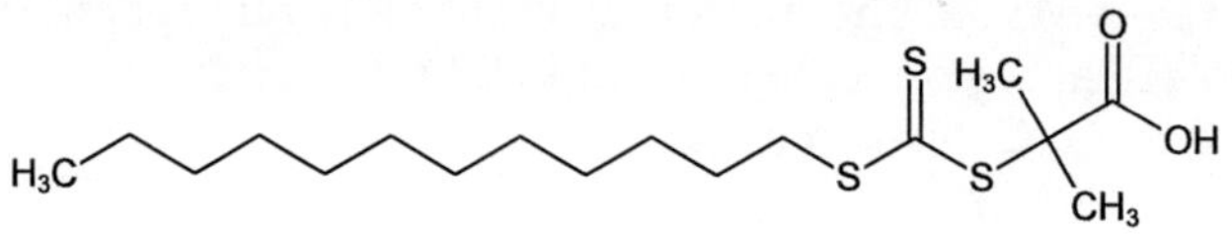

2-(Dodecylthiocarbonothioylthio)-2-methylpropionic acid

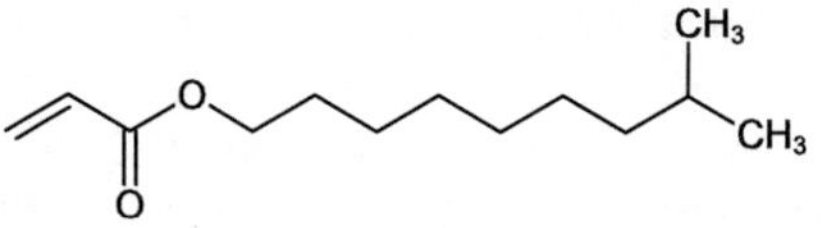

iso-Decyl acrylate

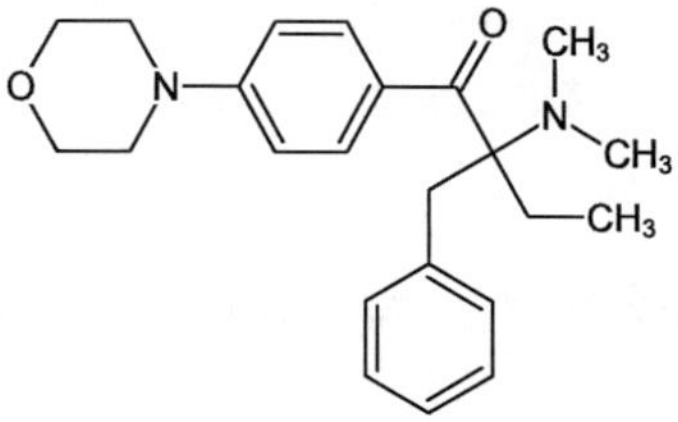

2-Benzyl-2-(dimethylamino)-
4′-morpholinobutyrophenone

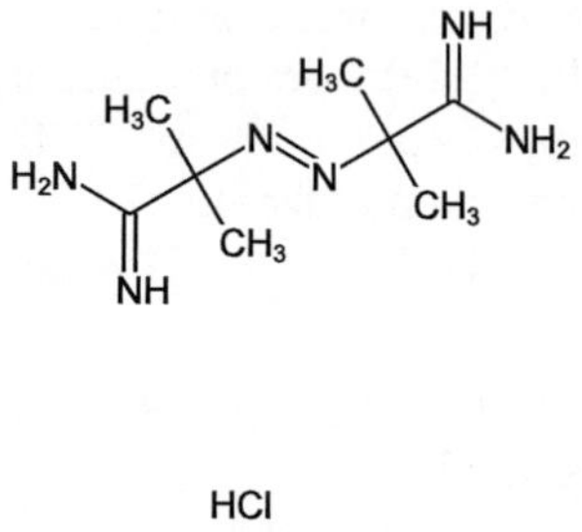

2,2′-Azobis(2-methylpropion-
amidine) dihydrochloride

Figure 1.2 Compounds for a block copolymer.

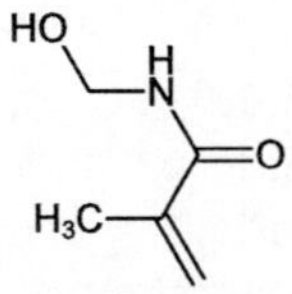

N-Hydroxymethyl methacrylamide

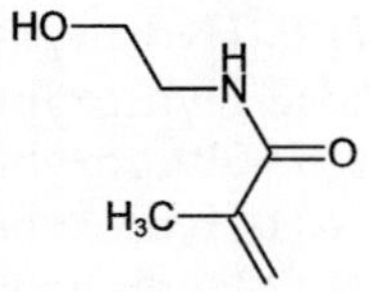

N-(2-Hydroxyethyl) methacrylamide

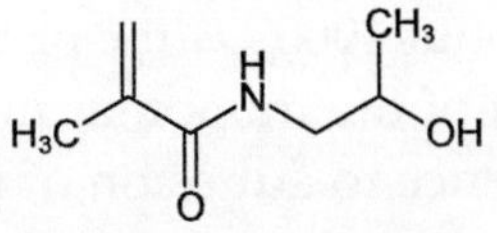

N-(2-Hydroxypropyl) methacrylamide

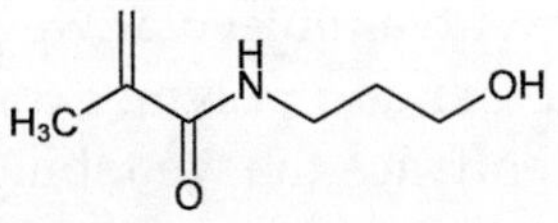

N-(3-Hydroxypropyl) methacrylamide

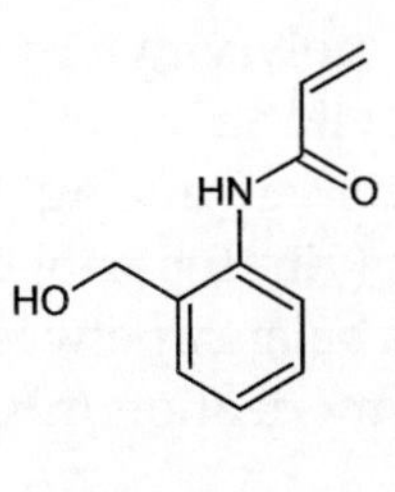

N-(2-Hydroxymethylphenyl) methacrylamide

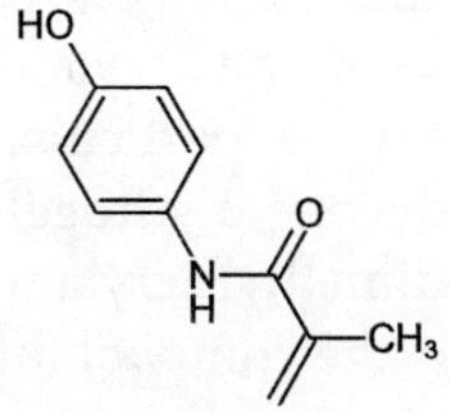

N-(4-Hydroxymethylphenyl) methacrylamide

Figure 1.3 Hydrophilic methacrylamide-based monomers.

Table 1.5 Hydrophilic methacrylamide-based monomers (23).

Compound
N-Hydroxymethyl methacrylamide
N-(2-Hydroxyethyl) methacrylamide
N-(2-Hydroxypropyl) methacrylamide
N-(3-Hydroxypropyl) methacrylamide
N-(2-Hydroxybutyl) methacrylamide
N-(3-Hydroxybutyl) methacrylamide
N-(4-Hydroxybutyl) methacrylamide
N-(2-Hydroxymethylphenyl) methacrylamide
N-(3-Hydroxymethylphenyl) methacrylamide
N-(4-Hydroxymethylphenyl) methacrylamide

polymer with a molecular weight of about 1000 *Dalton* or higher in the monomer and polymer component of the monomer mixture in order to enhance the wettability, resistance to adhesion of proteins, resistance to adhesion of lipids and combinations thereof.

Examples of hydrophilic polymers that can be used in the polymer are shown in Table 1.6. Some of the monomers of these compounds are shown in Figure 1.4.

Hydrophilic polymers selected from poly(vinyl pyrrolidone), poly(*N,N*-dimethyl acrylamide), poly(acrylic acid), and poly(vinyl alcohol) may be particularly effective for enhancing the wettability of silicone hydrogels (23). Poly(vinyl pyrrolidone) and poly(*N,N*-dimethyl acrylamide) provide a balance between the wettability and the compatibility of the polymerization mix in certain formulations.

The polymer can also include a monomer with two or more reactive groups as a copolymerization component. In this case, the polymer becomes solvent resistent.

Preferable monomers with two or more vinyl groups include bifunctional and polyfunctional acrylates. Examples are shown in Table 1.7. Some bisacrylamide monomers are shown in Figure 1.5. Polyfunctional methacrylate compounds are shown in Figure 1.6.

A polymerization initiator may be added to enhance the polymerization traction. Suitable initiators include thermal polymerization initiators, such as a peroxide compound or an azo compound, or

Table 1.6 Hydrophilic polymers (23).

Polymer compound
Poly(*N*-vinyl pyrrolidone)
Poly(*N*-vinyl-2-piperidone)
Poly(*N*-vinyl-2-caprolactam)
Poly(*N*-vinyl-3-methyl-2-caprolactam)
Poly(*N*-vinyl-3-methyl-2-piperidone)
Poly(*N*-vinyl-4-methyl-2-piperidone)
Poly(*N*-vinyl-4-methyl-2-caprolactam)
Poly(*N*-vinyl-3-ethyl-2-pyrrolidone)
Poly(*N*-vinyl-4,5-dimethyl-2-pyrrolidone)
Poly(2-vinylimidazole)
Poly(*N*-vinyl formamide)
Poly(*N*-vinyl acetamide)
Poly(*N*-methyl-*N*-vinyl acetamide)
Poly(*N*,*N*-dimethyl acrylamide)
Poly(*N*,*N*-diethyl acrylamide)
Poly(*N*-isopropyl acrylamide)
Poly(vinyl alcohol)
Poly(acrylate)
Poly(ethylene oxide)
Poly(2-ethyl oxazoline)
Heparine Polysaccharide
Poly(acryloyl morpholine)

Table 1.7 Multifunctional monomers (23).

Compound	Compound
Ethylene glycol acrylate	Ethylene glycol dimethacrylate
Diethylene glycol diacrylate	Diethylene glycol dimethacrylate
Triethylene glycol diacrylate	Triethylene glycol dimethacrylate
Neopentyl glycol diacrylate	Neopentyl glycol dimethacrylate
Tetraethylene glycol diacrylate	Tetraethylene glycol dimethacrylate
Glyceryl triacrylate	Glyceryl trimethacrylate
Pentaerythritol tetraacrylate	Pentaerythritol tetramethacrylate
Trimethylol propane triacrylate	Trimethylol propane trimethacrylate
N,*N*′-Methylene bisacrylamide	*N*,*N*′-Ethylene bisacrylamide
N,*N*′-Propylene bisacrylamide	

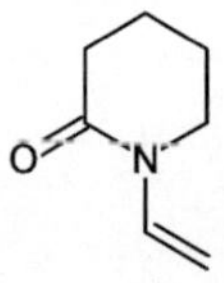 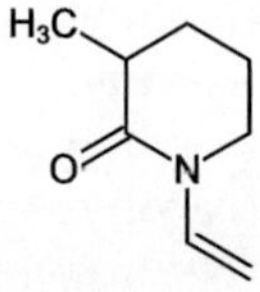

N-Vinyl-2-piperidone *N*-Vinyl-3-methyl-2-piperidone

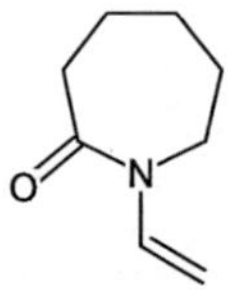 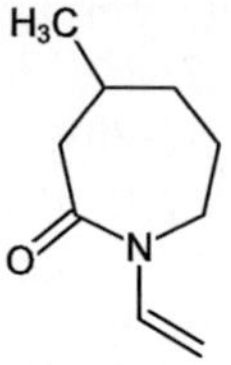

N-Vinyl-2-caprolactam *N*-Vinyl-4-methyl-2-caprolactam

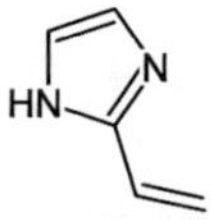 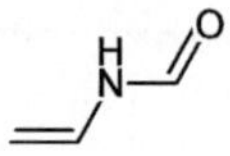

2-Vinylimidazole *N*-Vinyl formamide

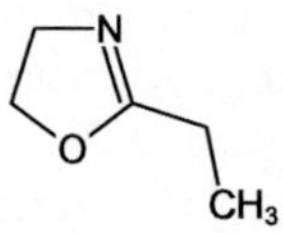 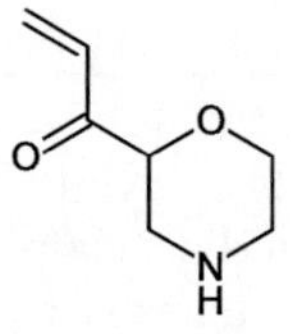

2-Ethyl oxazoline Acryloyl morpholine

Figure 1.4 Monomers for hydrophilic polymers.

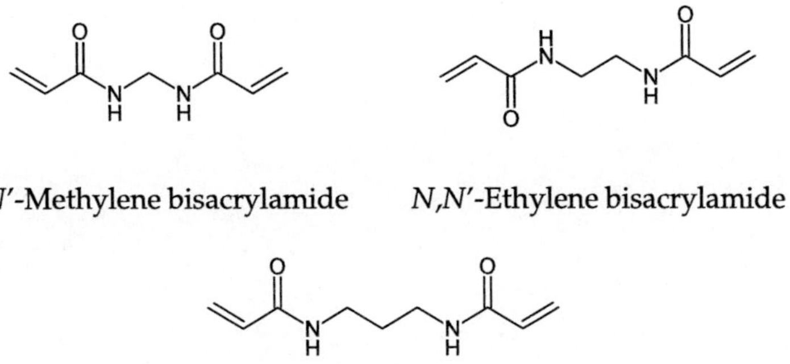

Figure 1.5 Bisacrylamide monomers.

photopolymerization initiators. Also, photoinitiators can be added in order to enhance the polymerization.

Several examples of the polymerization procedure have been detailed (23).

1.4 Soft Lenses

1.4.1 Hydrogels

Soft contact lens materials are made by polymerizing and crosslinking hydrophilic monomers such as 2-hydroxyethyl methyacrylate, *N*-vinyl-2-pyrrolidone, and combinations thereof (19).

The polymers produced by polymerizing these hydrophilic monomers exhibit significant hydrophilic character themselves, and are capable of absorbing a significant amount of water in their polymeric matrices. Due to their ability to absorb water, these polymers are often referred to as *hydrogels*.

These hydrogels are optically clear and, due to their high levels of water of hydration, are particularly useful materials for making soft contact lenses. However, the high levels of water of hydration of hydrogels contributes to their relative lack of physical strength, which results in hydrogel contact lenses being relatively easy to tear (19).

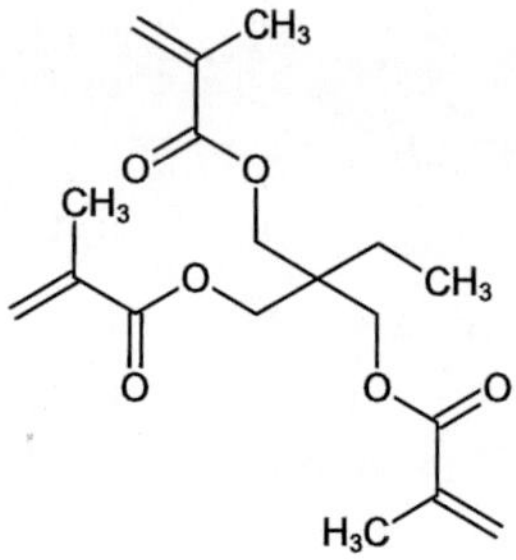

Trimethylol propane
trimethacrylate

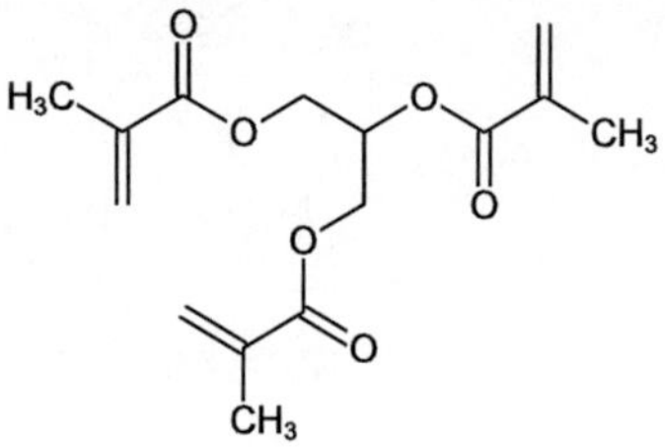

Glyceryl
trimethacrylate

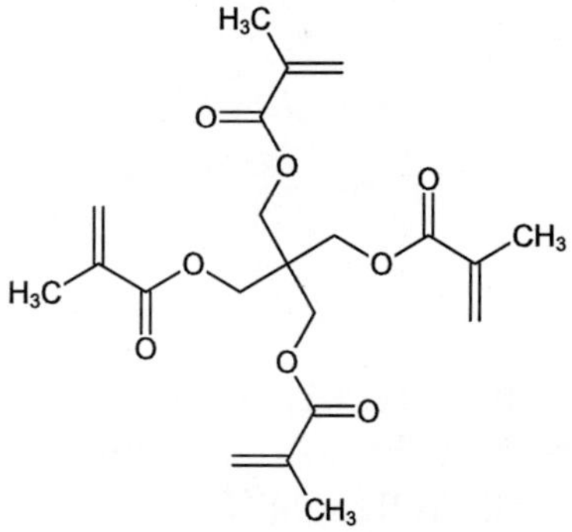

Pentaerythritol
tetramethacrylate

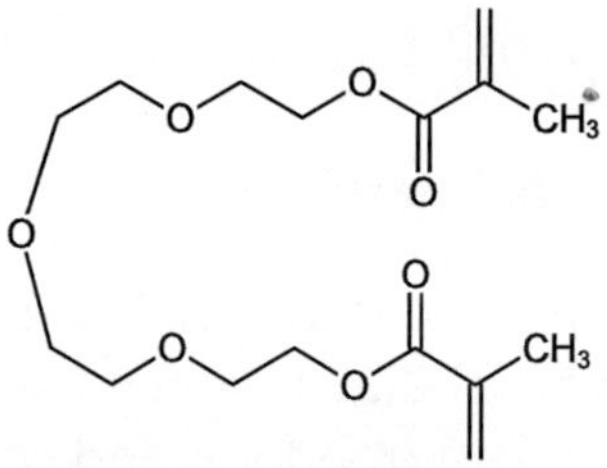

Tetraethylene glycol
dimethacrylate

Figure 1.6 Polyfunctional methacrylate compounds.

Various hydrophobic monomers have been copolymerized with these hydrophilic monomers in order to obtain polymers with an improved physical strength. Such hydrophobic monomers include styrene, and various acrylates and methacrylates such as methyl methacrylate, isobornyl methacrylate, and *tert*-butylcyclohexyl methacrylate. The last two compounds are shown in Figure 1.7.

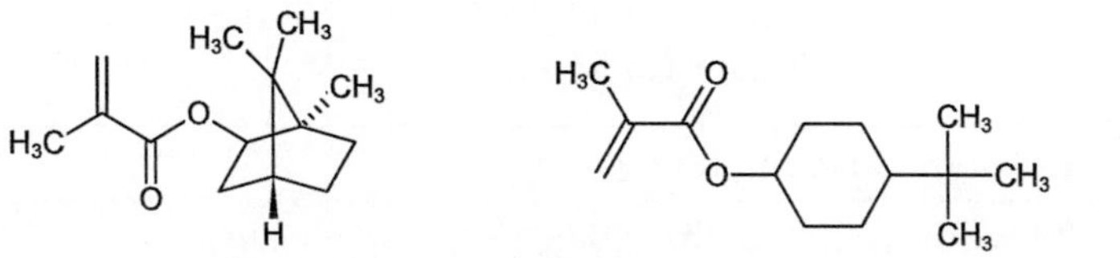

Figure 1.7 Hydrophobic monomers.

While these hydrophobic monomers do increase the physical strength of hydrogel polymers, they also produce polymers with lower levels of water of hydration than the unmodified hydrogels.

So, an attempt was made to provide polymeric materials with an increased physical strength and high levels of water of hydration (19).

It has been found that certain hydrophobic monomers act as strengthening agents when copolymerized with hydrophilic monomers and crosslinkers. Examples of these monomers are shown in Table 1.8 and in Figures 1.8, 1.9, and 1.10.

Most preferred contact lenses have an oxygen transport rate of at least about 2×10^{-6} $cm^3 sec^{-1} cm^{-2} atm^{-1}$, which makes them hydrolytically stable, biologically inert, transparent, and resilient. Furthermore, they should preferably have a softness of about 60 or below on the Shore hardness A scale when hydrated. The more preferred materials have a Shore hardness between 25 to 35 on the A scale.

The tensile modulus of elasticity of these hydrated polymers is at least about 50 $g\,mm^{-2}$, preferably from about 75 $g\,mm^{-2}$ to about 100 $g\,mm^{-2}$, and the tear strength is at least about 2.0 $g\,mm^{-1}$ thickness, preferably from about 2.0 $g\,mm^{-1}$ to about 250 $g\,mm^{-1}$ thickness.

Table 1.8 Monomers (19).

Hydrophilic monomers
2-Hydroxyethyl methacrylate
N-(2-Hydroxy ethyl)-methacrylamide
N-Vinyl-2-pyrrolidone
Glyceryl methacrylate
N-Methacryloyl glycine
2-Hydroxyl-3-methacryl(propyl)-4-methoxy phenyl ether
2-Hydroxy cyclohexyl methacrylate
Hydrophobic strengthening agent monomers
4-*tert*-Butyl-2-hydroxycyclohexyl methacrylate
4-*tert*-Butyl-2-hydroxycyclopentyl methacrylate
Methacryloylamino-4-*tert*-butyl-2-hydroxycyclohexane
6-Isopentyl-3-hydroxycyclohexyl methacrylate
Methacryloylamino-2-isohexyl-5-hydroxy cyclopentane
Crosslinking monomers
Allyl methacrylate
Ethylene glycol dimethacrylate
Divinyl ethylene urea
1,3-Bis(4-methacryloxybutyl) tetramethyl disiloxane

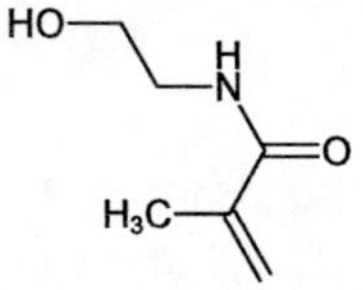

N-(2-Hydroxy ethyl)-methacrylamide

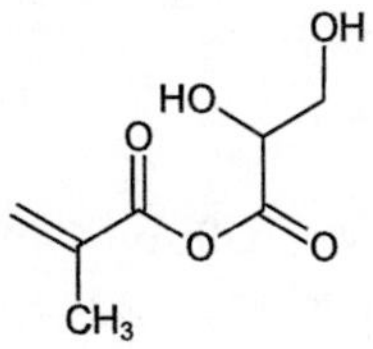

Glyceryl methacrylate

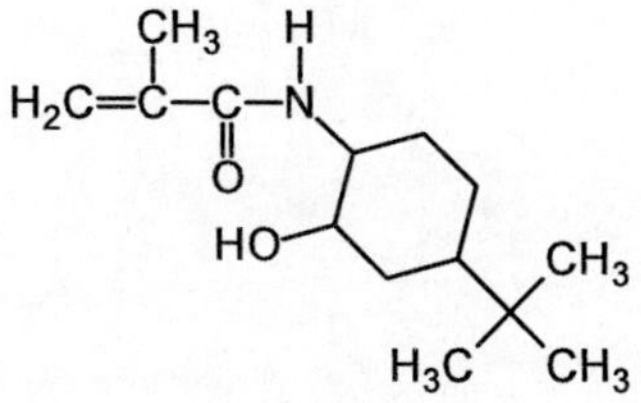

Methacryloylamino-4-*tert*-butyl-2-hydroxycyclohexane

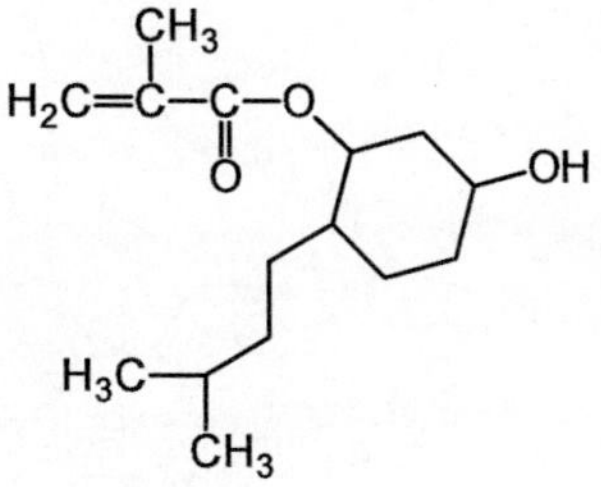

6-Isopentyl-3-hydroxy cyclohexyl methacrylate

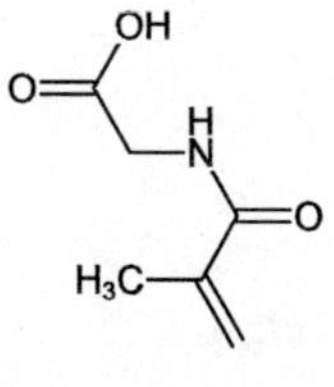

N-Methacryloyl glycine

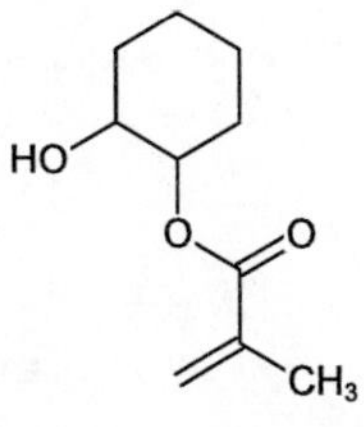

2-Hydroxy cyclohexyl methacrylate

Figure 1.8 Hydrophilic monomers.

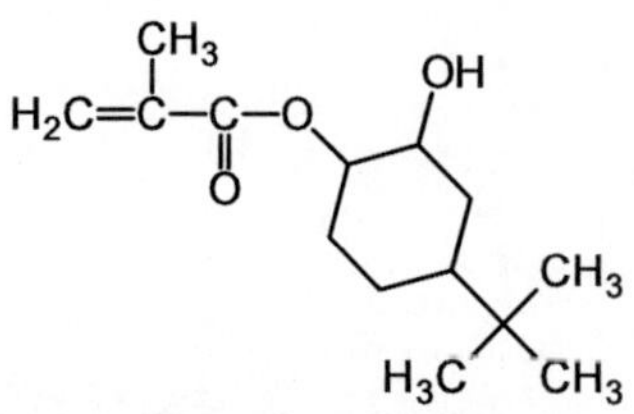

4-*tert*-Butyl-2-hydroxy-
cyclohexyl methacrylate

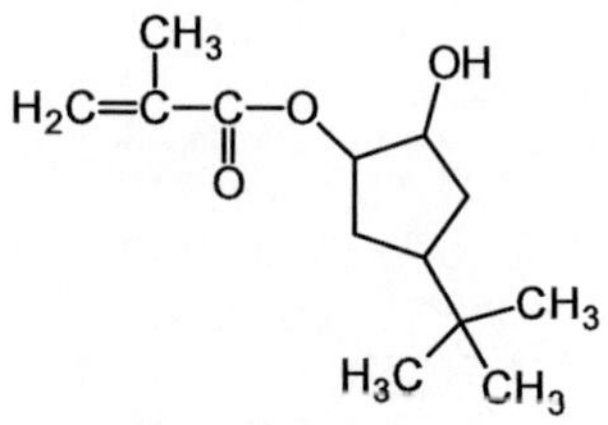

4-*tert*-Butyl-2-hydroxy-
cyclopentyl methacrylate

Figure 1.9 Hydrophobic strengthening monomers.

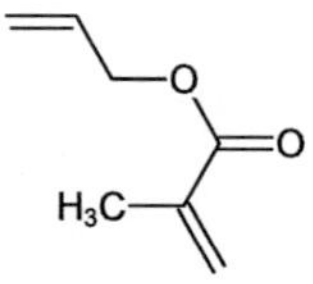

Allyl methacrylate

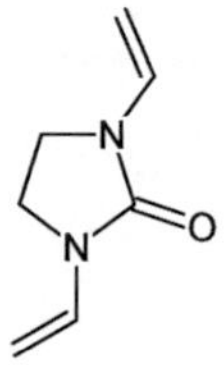

Divinyl ethylene urea

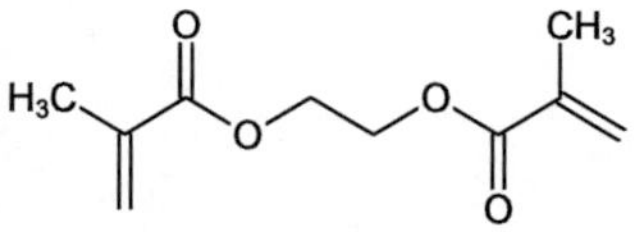

Ethylene glycol dimethacrylate

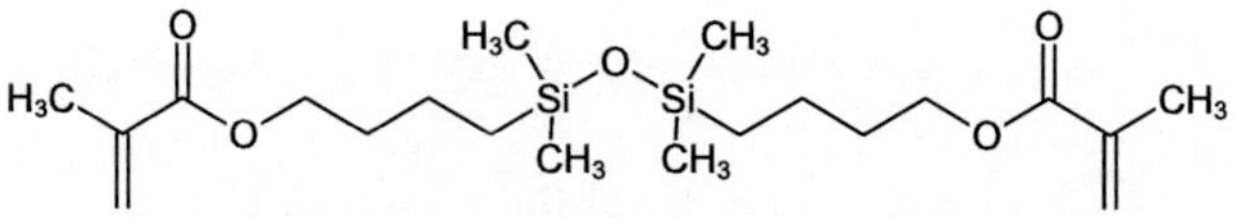

1,3-Bis(4-methacryloxybutyl) tetramethyl disiloxane

Figure 1.10 Crosslinking monomers.

High tensile modulus of elasticity is desirable for strength and durability. High tear strength is desirable in order to prevent damage to the contact lens due to tearing during patient use, i.e., the removing and placing of the lens on the eye, and to prevent damage to the lens during cleansing and disinfecting.

A soft contact lens formulation is illustrated in the following example (19):

Preparation 1–3: A mixture was made containing 77.0 *g* of glyceryl methacylate, 22.5 *g* of 4-*tert*-butyl-2-hydroxycyclohexyl methacrylate, and 0.5 *g* of ethylene glycol dimethacrylate. To this mixture was added 0.5 *g* of benzoin methyl ether, an ultraviolet-induced polymerization initiator. The solution was cast between glass plates separated by a Teflon perfluoro polymer gasket, 0.3 *mm* thick and cured. After curing, the film was released from the glass plates and hydrated and extracted in hot distilled water for 4 *h*.

Then, the film was placed in a borate buffered saline solution for testing. The resultant material was optically clear and had a water content of 53% and an oxygen permeability of 18×10^{-11} $cm^3 cmseccm^2 mmHg^{-1}$.

The mechanical properties were measured according to the following test methods and gave the results shown in Table 1.9.

Table 1.9 Mechanical properties (19).

Standard	Ref.	Name	Value
ASTM-D 1708	(24)	Young's modulus of elasticity	60 $g\,mm^{-2}$
ASTM-D 1708	(24)	Tensile strength	84 $g\,mm^{-2}$
ASTM-D 1708	(24)	% Elongation	164 %
ASTM-D 1938	(25)	Tear Initiation	3.8 $g\,mm^{-1}$

1.4.1.1 Polymerizable Contact Lens Formulations

Hydrogel contact lenses, polymerizable compositions useful for making such lenses, packaging systems for use with such lenses and methods of producing such lenses have been discovered (26). These contact lenses have a relatively low surface friction and are able to release hydrophilic polymers present in the contact lenses for prolonged periods of time.

The contact lenses have a lens body. The lens body is the reaction product of a polymerizable composition containing one or more monomers, and a crosslinker that crosslinks the monomers during a polymerization reaction to form a first polymer component. The polymerizable composition also contains a hydrophilic polymer component, which is substantially unreactive during the polymerization.

Thus, the resulting lens body includes a first polymer component formed from the one or more monomers present in the polymerizable composition, and the second polymer component, the hydrophilic polymer component that is physically entangled with the first polymer component in the lens body.

The hydrophilic polymer component is unreactive or substantially unreactive during the polymerization process. Thus, the resulting hydrogel lens body can be understood to be a network of a first polymeric component, formed from the monomers present in the polymerizable composition, and a second polymeric component, the hydrophilic polymer component, in which the hydrophilic polymer component is substantially physically entrapped by the first polymer component. Although there may be some small amounts of reactivity of the hydrophilic polymer component, the reactivity is not sufficient to prevent leaching or release of the hydrophilic polymer from the lens body. The present contact lenses can be understood to consist of an interpenetrating polymer network where the formation of the first polymer component occurs in the presence of the hydrophilic polymer component. However, as discussed herein, in the present contact lenses, it is possible for the hydrophilic polymer component to be released from the lens body even though it is entrapped by the first polymer component.

Examples of these monomers are shown in Table 1.10 and in Figure 1.11.

Polymerization initiators can be used in the polymerizable composition. Thermal initiators that may be used are azo or peroxide compounds, such as those having a half-life at the polymerization temperature of at least 20 *min*. Examples of initiators are shown in Table 1.11 and in Figure 1.12.

A tinting agent can be any agent that imparts a visibility to the otherwise clear hydrogel lens body. The tinting agent may be a water-soluble dye, or particles of pigment, or combinations thereof. Some examples of tinting agents include copper phthalocyanine

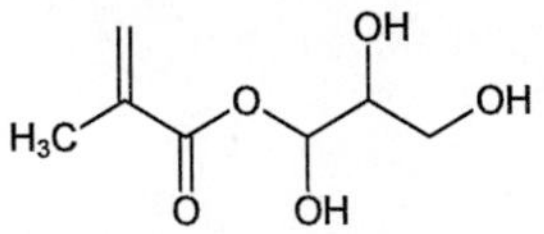

Glycerol mono methacrylate

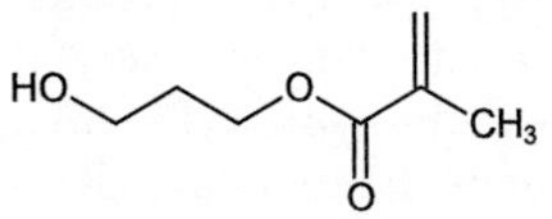

3-Hydroxypropyl methacrylate

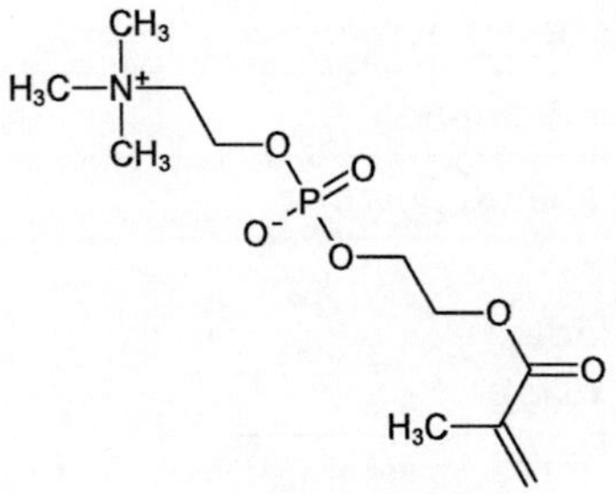

2-Methacryloyloxyethyl phosphorylcholine

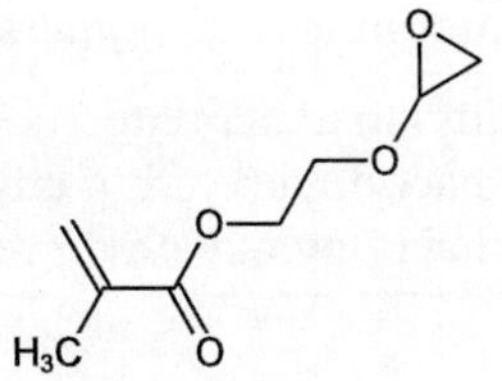

Methacryloyloxyethyl ethylene oxide

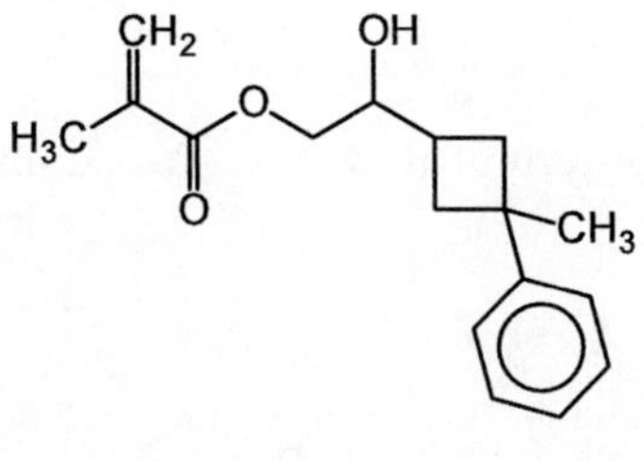

2-(3-Phenyl-3-methylcyclobutyl)-2-hydroxyethyl methacrylate

Figure 1.11 Monomers and comonomers.

Table 1.10 Monomers (26).

Monomers for the first polymer
2-Hydroxyethyl methacrylate 2-(3-Phenyl-3-methylcyclobutyl)-2-hydroxyethyl methacrylate 2-Hydroxyethyl acrylate 2-Hydroxypropyl methacrylate 2-Hydroxypropyl acrylate 3-Hydroxypropyl methacrylate Glycerol mono acrylate Glycerol mono methacrylate *n*-Vinyl pyrrolidone Acrylamide
Hydrophilic monomers for the second polymer
2-Methacryloyloxyethyl phosphorylcholine
Hydrophilic comonomers for the second polymer
n-Butyl methacrylate Methacryloyloxyethyl ethylene oxide Methacryloyloxyethyl propylene oxide

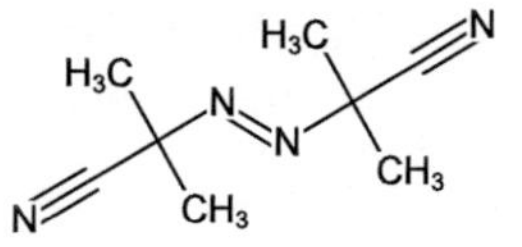

2,2′-Azo-bis-isobutyronitrile

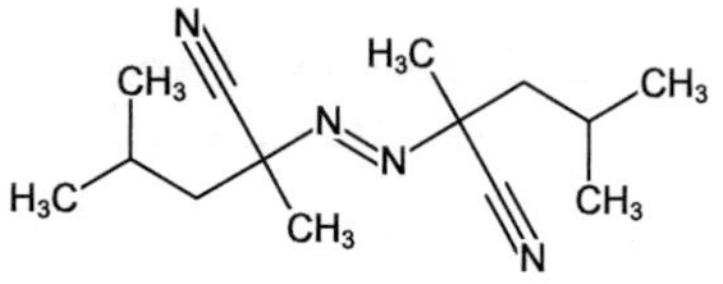

2,2′-Azo-bis(2,4-dimethyl-valeronitrile)

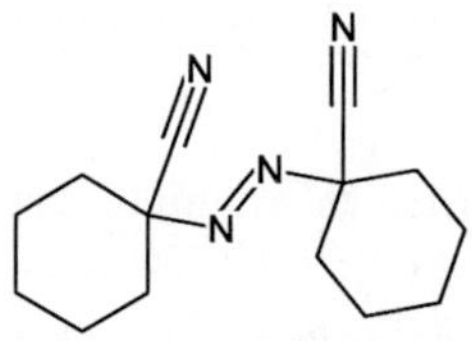

1,1′-Azo-bis(cyclohexane carbonitrile)

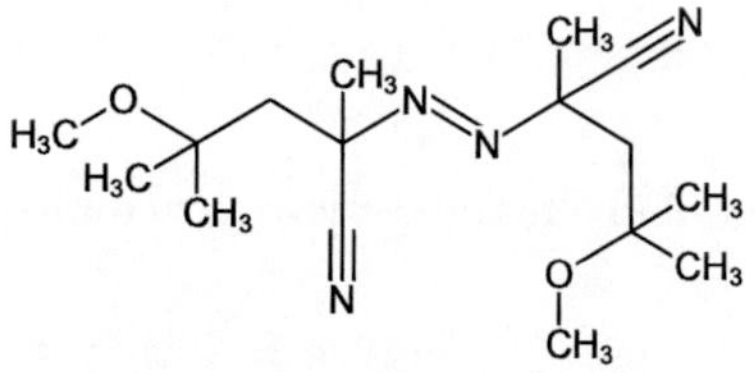

2,2′-Azo-bis(2,4-dimethyl-4-methoxy-valeronitrile

Figure 1.12 Azo initiators.

Table 1.11 Initiators (26).

Azo initiators
2,2′-Azo-bis-isobutyronitrile
2,2′-Azo-bis(2,4-dimethylvaleronitrile)
1,1′-Azo-bis(cyclohexane carbonitrile)
2,2′-Azo-bis(2,4-dimethyl-4-methoxyvaleronitrile)
Peroxy initiators
Isopropyl percarbonate
tert-Butyl peroctoate
Benzoyl peroxide
Lauroyl peroxide
Decanoyl peroxide
Acetyl peroxide
Succinic acid peroxide
Methyl ethyl ketone peroxide
tert-Butyl peroxyacetate
Propionyl peroxide
2,4-Dichlorobenzoyl peroxide
tert-Butyl peroxypivalate
Pelargonyl peroxide
2,5-Dimethyl-2,5-bis(2-ethylhexanoylperoxy)hexane
p-Chlorobenzoyl peroxide
tert-Butyl peroxybutyrate *tert*-Butyl peroxymaleic acid
tert-Butyl-peroxyisopropyl carbonate
Bis(1-hydroxycyclohexyl)peroxide
Photoinitiators (23, 26)
Diethoxyacetophenone
1-Hydroxycyclohexyl phenyl ketone
2,2-Dimethoxy-2-phenylacetophenone
Phenothiazine
Diisopropylxanthogen disulfide
Benzoin
Benzoin methyl ether
2-Hydroxy-2-methyl-1-phenyl-propan-1-one
Bis(2,6-dimethoxybenzoyl)-2,4-4-trimethylpentyl phosphine oxide
Bis(2,4,6-trimethylbenzoyl)-phenyl phosphine oxide
2,4,6-Trimethylbenzoyl diphenylphosphine oxide

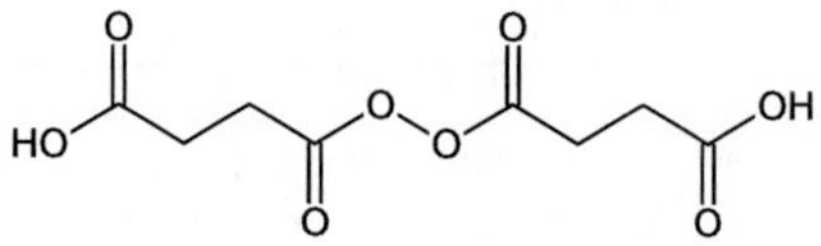

Succinic acid peroxide

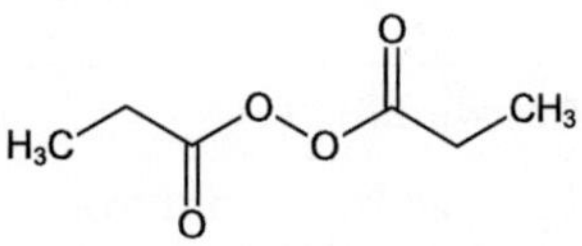

Propionyl peroxide

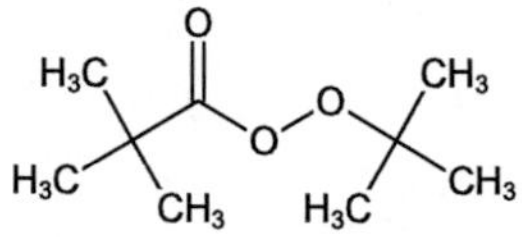

tert-Butyl peroxypivalate

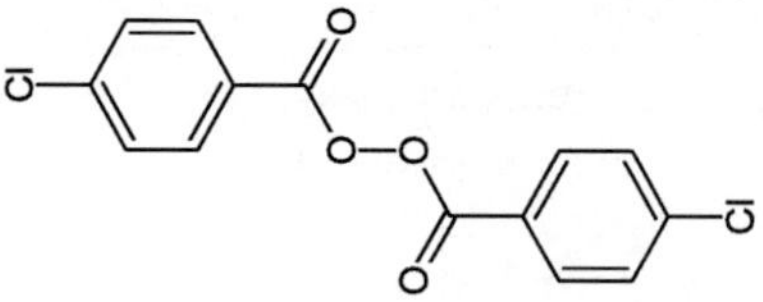

p-Chlorobenzoyl peroxide

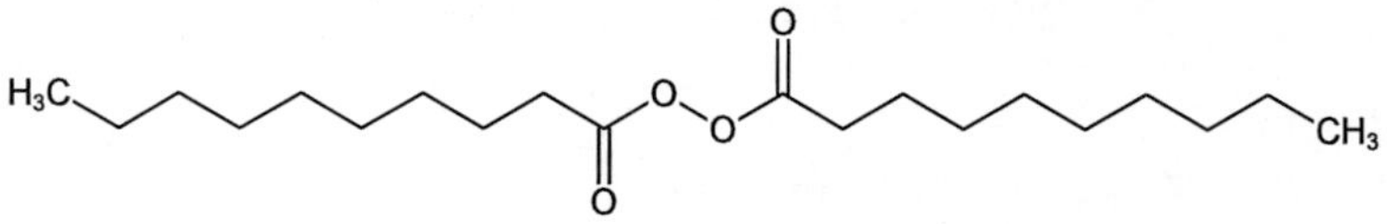

Decanoyl peroxide

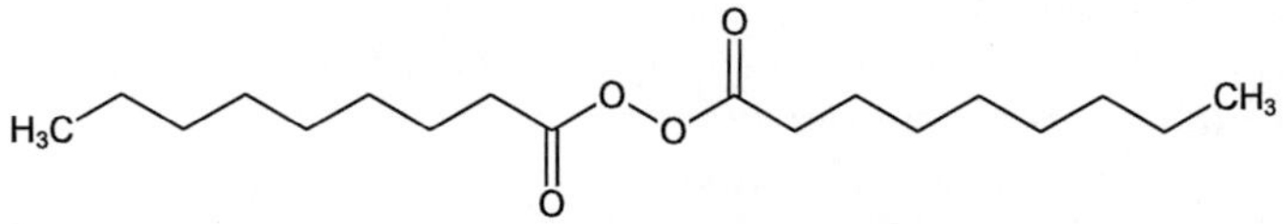

Pelargonyl peroxide

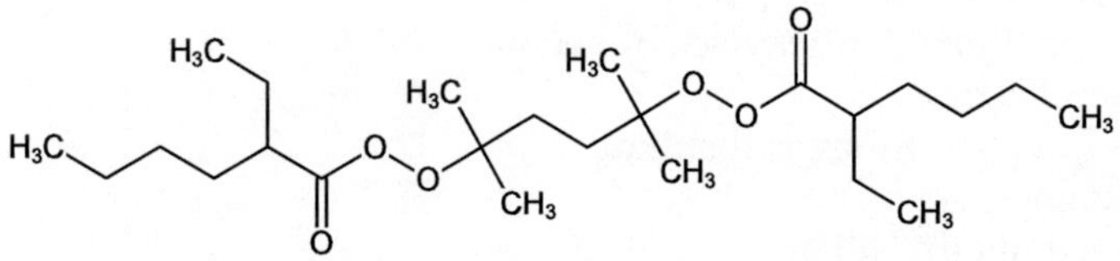

2,5-Dimethyl-2,5-bis(2-ethylhexanoylperoxy)hexane

Figure 1.12 (cont) Peroxy initiators.

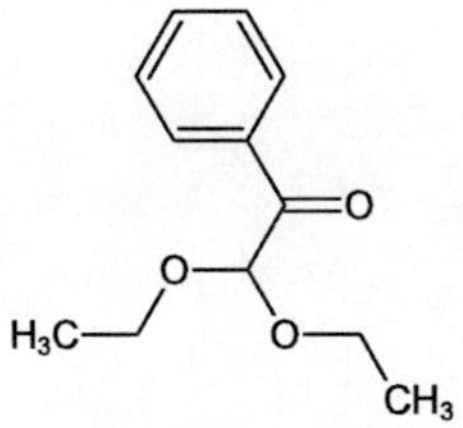

Diethoxyacetophenone

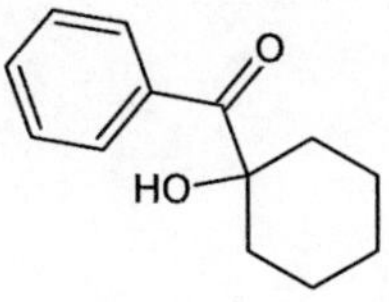

1-Hydroxycyclohexyl phenyl ketone

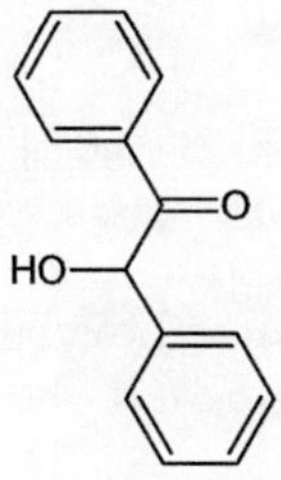

Benzoin

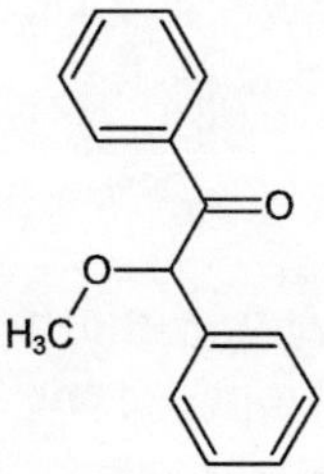

Benzoin methyl ether

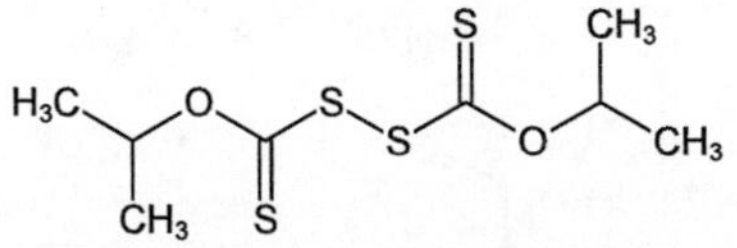

Diisopropylxanthogen disulfide

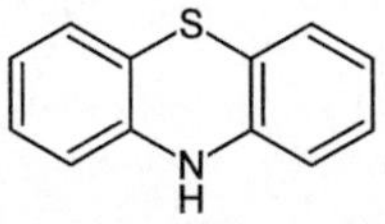

Phenothiazine

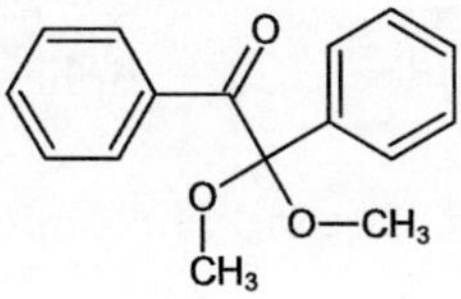

2,2-Dimethoxy-2-phenylacetophenone

Figure 1.12 (cont) Photoinitiators.

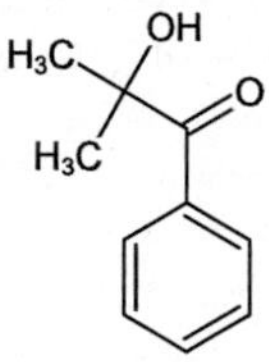

2-Hydroxy-2-methyl-1-phenyl-propan-1-one

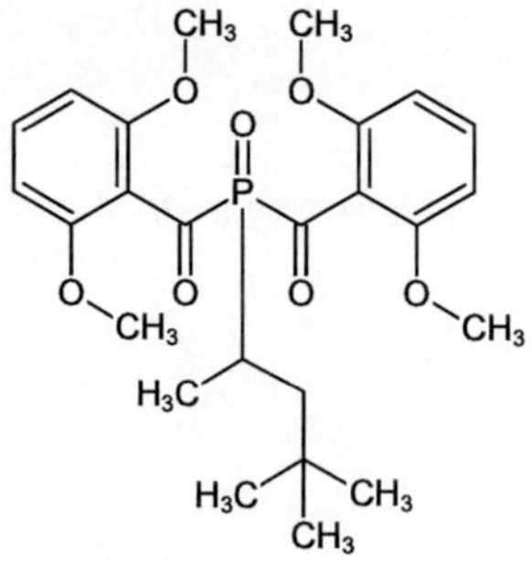

Bis(2,6-dimethoxybenzoyl)-2,4-4-trimethylpentyl phosphine oxide

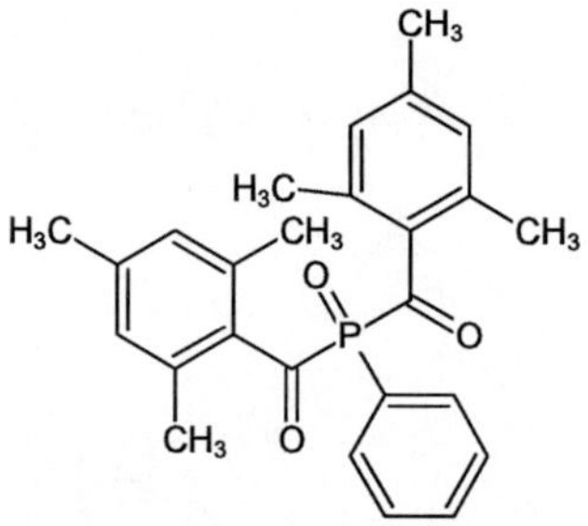

Bis(2,4,6-trimethylbenzoyl)-phenyl phosphine oxide

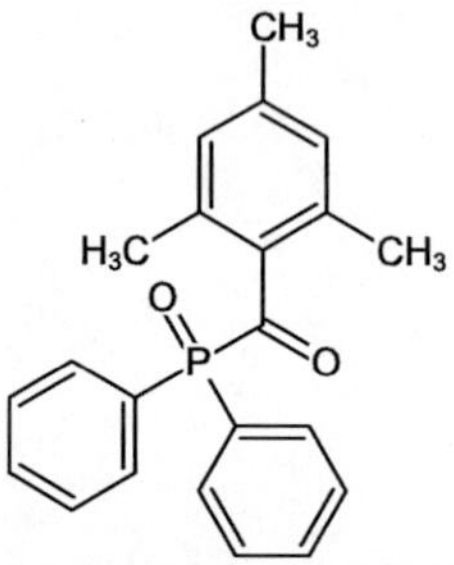

2,4,6-Trimethylbenzoyl diphenylphosphine oxide

Figure 1.12 (cont) Photoinitiators.

blue, Vat Blue 6, Reactive Blue 4, and Reactive Blue 19. These compounds are shown in Figure 1.13.

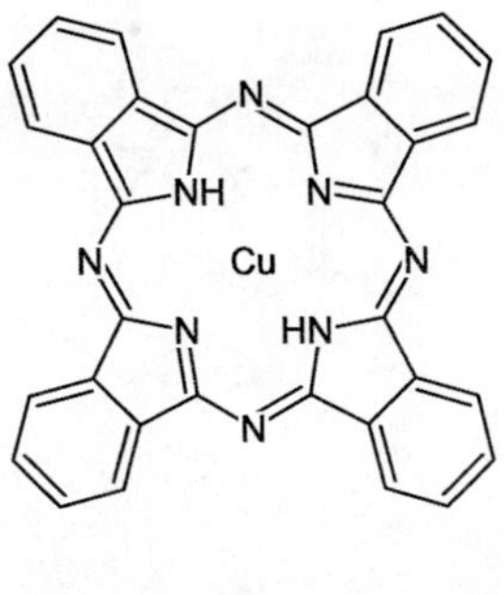

Copper phthalocyanine blue

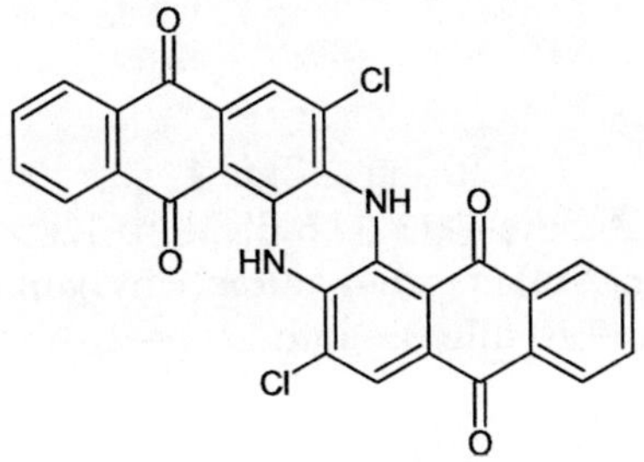

Vat Blue 6
7,16-Dichloro-6,15-dihydrodinaphtho[2,3-a:2′,3′-h]
phenazine-5,9,14,18-tetrone

Figure 1.13 Tinting agents.

An effective amount of the tinting agent used can vary depending on factors such as the type of tinting agent, the reactive monomer composition, or the non-reactive polymers present in the composition. In general, the amount of tinting agent used may be up to about 15% of the polymerizable composition (26).

1.4.1.2 Surface Treatment for Silicone Hydrogel Contact Lenses

The usage of transparent silicone rubber for corneal contact lenses was first described in 1966 (27).

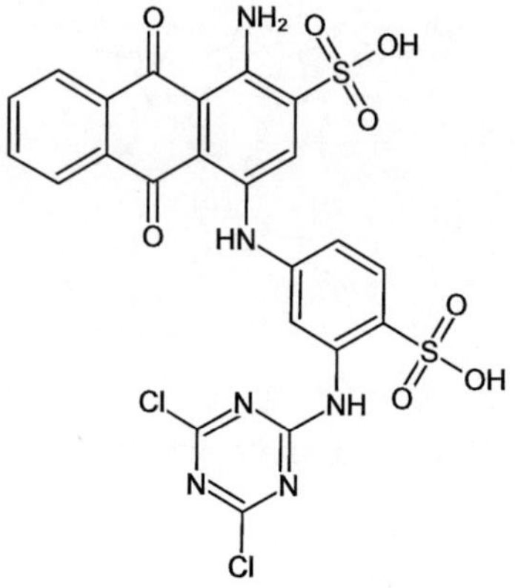

Reactive Blue 4
1-Amino-4-((3-((4,6-dichloro-1,3,5-triazin-2-yl)amino)-4-sulfophenyl)amino)-9,10-dioxo-9,10-dihydroanthracene-2-sulfonic acid

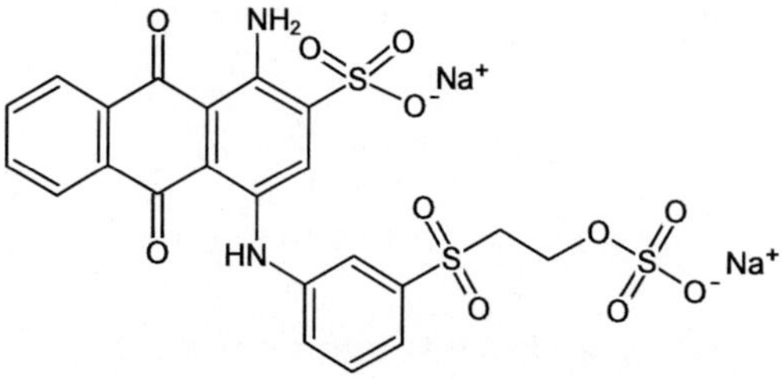

Reactive Blue 19
Disodium 1-amino-9,10-dioxo-4-[(3-{[2-(sulfonatooxy)ethyl]sulfonyl}phenyl)amino]-9,10-dihydroanthracene-2-sulfonate

Figure 1.13 (cont) Tinting agents.

Silicone lenses have been subjected to plasma surface treatment to improve their surface properties; for example, to make the surface more hydrophilic, deposit-resistant, or scratch-resistant (28).

A method of surface treatment has been described that consists of coating the device with a carbon layer, followed by the attachment of hydrophilic polymer chains to the surface of the carbon layer. Then, the carbon layer is plasma treated to form reactive functionalities containing oxygen, nitrogen, and/or sulfur. Complementary reactive functionalities in monomeric units along a hydrophilic reactive polymer are then reacted with the reactive functionalities on the carbon layer. Also, a contact lens surface can be pretreated with an oxidizing plasma prior to deposition of the carbon layer in order to improve adhesion of the carbon layer.

Silicone hydrogels generally have a water content of 10% to 80%. Such materials are usually prepared by polymerizing a mixture containing at least one silicone-containing monomer and at least one hydrophilic monomer. Either the silicone-containing monomer or the hydrophilic monomer may function as a crosslinking agent. Examples of silicon-containing monomeric units are bulky polysiloxanylalkyl(meth)acrylic monomers.

Plasma surface treatments involve passing an electrical discharge through a gas at low pressure (28). The electrical discharge may be at radio frequency (typically 13.56 *MHz*), although microwave and other frequencies can be used. Electrical discharges produce ultraviolet radiation, in addition to being absorbed by atoms and molecules in their gas state, resulting in energetic electrons and ions, atoms, molecules, and radicals. So, a plasma is a complex mixture of atoms and molecules in both ground and excited states, which reach a steady state after the discharge is begun. The circulating electrical field causes these excited atoms and molecules to collide with one another as well as the walls of the chamber and the surface of the material being treated.

The deposition of a coating from a plasma onto the surface of a material has been shown to be possible from high-energy plasmas without the assistance of sputtering. Monomers can be deposited from the gas phase and polymerized in a low pressure atmosphere, at preferably 0.001 *torr* to 1.0 *torr*, onto a substrate utilizing continuous or pulsed plasmas, suitably as high as about 1000 *W*. A modulated plasma may be applied 100 *ms* on then off. In addition, liquid nitrogen cooling has been utilized to condense vapors out of the gas phase onto a substrate and subsequently use the plasma to chemically react these materials with the substrate. However, plasmas do not require the use of external cooling or heating to cause the deposition. Low or high wattage (20 *W* to 500 *W*) plasmas can coat even the most chemical-resistant substrates, including silicones.

The method of fabrication can be done as follows (28):

1. Subjecting the surface of a lens substrate to a plasma polymerization deposition with a C_1 to C_{10} saturated or unsaturated hydrocarbon to form a polymeric carbonaceous layer (or *carbon layer*) on the lens surface,
2. Forming reactive functionalities on the surface of the carbon layer, and
3. Attaching hydrophilic polymer chains to the carbon layer by reacting the reactive functionalities on the carbon layer with complementary isocyanate or ring-opening reactive functionalities along a reactive hydrophilic polymer.

It has been found that in the case of silicone hydrogels, the use of diolefins, such as 1,3-butadiene or isoprene, are particularly preferred, resulting in coatings that are more flexible and expandable in water (28). More flexible coatings are especially preferred for high-water lenses that expand considerably upon hydration.

There are various ways to attach a polymer chain to a carbon layer, including plasma oxidation or other means to provide surface reactive functional groups that can react with the polymer. Preferably, a nitrogen-containing gas is used to form amine groups on the carbon layer. However, oxygen- or sulfur-containing gases may alternatively be used to form oxygen- or sulfur-containing groups, such as hydroxy or sulfide groups or radicals, on the carbon layer. Thus, the carbon layer is rendered reactive (functionalized) to promote the covalent attachment of the hydrophilic polymer to the surface.

To create a reactive functional group on the carbon layer, such an oxidation preferably utilizes a gas composition consisting of an oxidizing media such as ammonia, ethylene diamine, C_1 to C_8 alkyl amine, hydrazine, or other oxidizing compounds. Preferably, the oxidation of the hydrocarbon layer is performed for a period of about 1 *min* to 10 *min*, a discharge frequency of 13.56 *MHz* at about

20 *W* to 500 *W* and about 0.1 *torr* to 1.0 *torr*. The lens substrate may be treated on both sides at once or each side sequentially.

The hydrophilic reactive polymer may contain monomeric units derived from azlactone-functional, epoxy-functional and acid-anhydride-functional monomers. Azlactone monomers are listed in Table 1.12 and in Figure 1.14.

Table 1.12 Azlactone monomers (28).

2-Alkenyl azlactones
2-Ethenyl-1,3-oxazolin-5-one
2-Ethenyl-4-methyl-1,3-oxazolin-5-one
2-Isopropenyl-1,3-oxazolin-5-one
2-Isopropenyl-4-methyl-1,3-oxazolin-5-one
2-Ethenyl-4,4-dimethyl-1,3-oxazolin-5-one
2-Isopropenyl-4-dimethyl-1,3-oxazolin-5-one
2-Ethenyl-4-methyl-ethyl-1,3-oxazolin-5-one
2-Isopropenyl-4-methyl-4-butyl-1,3-oxazolin-5-one
2-Ethenyl-4,4-dibutyl-1,3-oxazolin-5-one
2-Isopropenyl-4-methyl-4-dodecyl-1,3-oxazolin-5-one
2-Isopropenyl-4,4-diphenyl-1,3-oxazolin-5-one
2-Isopropenyl-4,4-pentamethylene-1,3-oxazolin-5-one
2-Isopropenyl-4,4-tetramethylene-1,3-oxazolin-5-one
2-Ethenyl-4,4-diethyl-1,3-oxazolin-5-one
2-Ethenyl-4-methyl-4-nonyl-1,3-oxazolin-5-one
2-Isopropenyl-methyl-4-phenyl-1,3-oxazolin-5-one
2-Isopropenyl-4-methyl-4-benzyl-1,3-oxazolin-5-one
2-Ethenyl-4,4-pentamethylene-1,3-oxazolin-5-one
Cycloalkyl azlactones
2-Isopropenyl-4,4-dimethyl-2-oxazolin-5-one
2-Vinyl-4,4-dimethyl-2-oxazolin-5-one
Spiro-4′-(2′-isopropenyl-2′-oxazolin-5-one) cyclohexane
Cyclohexane-*spiro*-4′-(2′-vinyl-2′-oxazol-5′-one)
2-(1-Propenyl)-4,4-dimethyl-oxazol-5-one

The synthesis of such monomers has been described in detail (29). The synthesis of 2-isopropenyl-4,4-dimethyl-2-oxazolin-5-one can be done as follows (29):

Preparation 1–4: 1. Methacryloylation:

In a 500 *ml* 3-neck round-bottom flask equipped with a mechanical stirrer, thermometer and an addition funnel, 51.5 *g* (0.5 *mol*) of

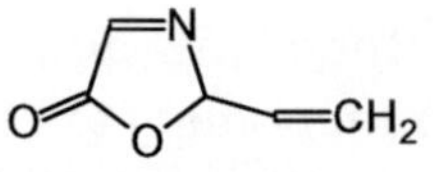

2-Ethenyl-
1,3-oxazolin-5-one

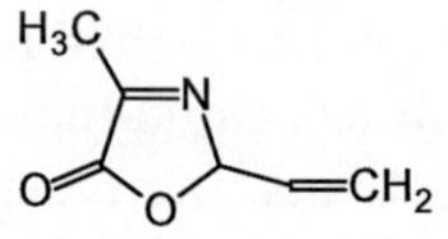

2-Ethenyl-4-methyl-
1,3-oxazolin-5-one

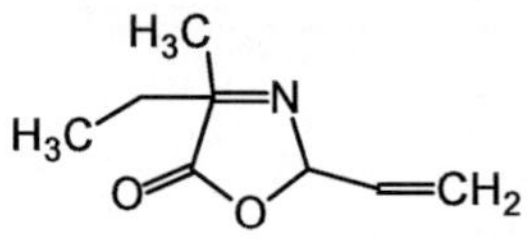

2-Ethenyl-4-methyl-ethyl-
1,3-oxazolin-5-one

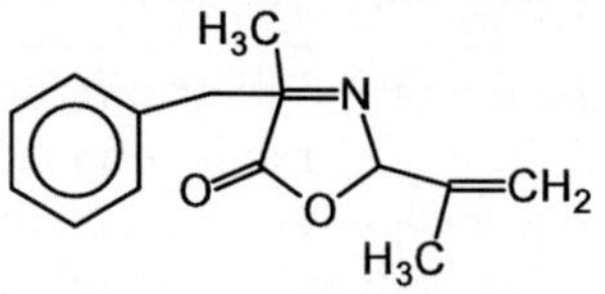

2-Isopropenyl-4-methyl-4-benzyl-
1,3-oxazolin-5-one

Figure 1.14 2-Alkenyl azlactones.

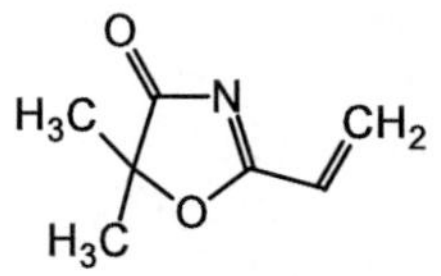

2-Vinyl-4,4-dimethyl-2-
oxazolin-5-one

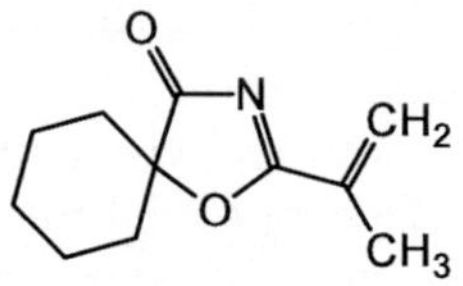

Spiro-4′-(2′-isopropenyl-2′-
oxazolin-5-one) cyclohexane

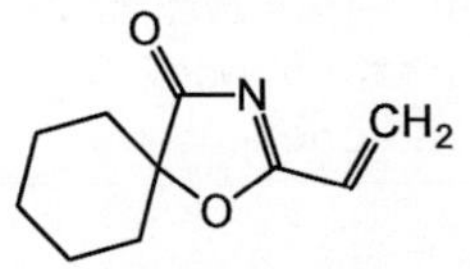

Cyclohexane-*spiro*-4′-(2′-vinyl-2′-
oxazol-5′-one)

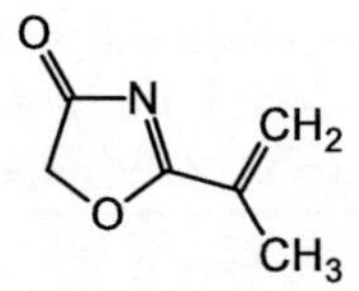

2-(1-Propenyl)-4,4-dimethyl-
oxazol-5-one

Figure 1.14 (cont) Cycloalkyl azlactones.

α-aminoisobutyric acid and 40 *g* (1 *mol*) of NaOH were dissolved in 150 *ml* of H_2O. The reaction flask was cooled to 0°C to 5°C in a CH_3OH ice bath and 0.5 *mol* of methacrylate chloride was added dropwise while the temperature of the reaction mixture was kept below 0°C. After stirring for an additional hour, the reaction mixture was acidified with concentrated HCl with a pH of 3 to precipitate out the intermediate, which was then filtered, washed with cold H_2O and air dried. Further drying was accomplished in a vacuum oven at 80°C overnight to obtain 44.9 *g* (0.26 *mol* 53%) *N*-methacryloyl-*α*-aminoisobutyric acid, which was suitable for the synthesis of 2-isopropenyl-4,4-dimethyl-2-oxazolin-5-one.

Cyclization, synthesis of 2-isopropenyl-4,4-dimethyl-2-oxazolin-5-one:

In a 500 *ml* dry 3-neck round-bottom flask, 0.26 *mol* of *n*-methacryloyl-*α*-aminoisobutyric acid was dispersed in 300 *ml* of dry hexane and allowed to react with mechanical stirring by dropwise addition of triethylamine (0.52 *mol*) while the temperature of the reaction mixture was maintained at 45°C to 0°C. During the addition, the copious evolution of carbon dioxide and the formation of white precipitate of TEA-HCl were observed. The reaction mixture was stirred for an additional 2 *h*. After cooling to room temperature, a white precipitate was filtered off and hexane evaporated off yielding an oil. Pure 2-isopropenyl-4,4-dimethyl-2-oxazolin-5-one was obtained after being recrystallized twice in hexane at dry ice/acetone temperature. The yield was 29 *g* (73%).

2-Isopropenyl-4,4-dimethyl-2-oxazolin-5-one is shown in Figure 1.15.

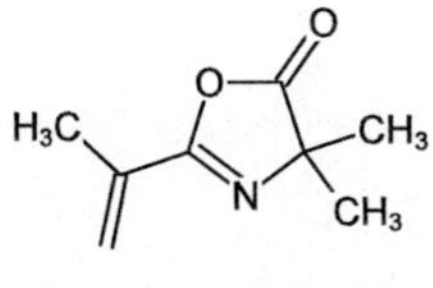

Figure 1.15 2-Isopropenyl-4,4-dimethyl-2-oxazolin-5-one.

Azlactone-functional monomers can be copolymerized with other monomers in various combinations of amounts (28). Using a monomer of similar reactivity ratio to that of an azlactone monomer will result in a random copolymer. Alternatively, use of a comonomer having a higher reactivity to that of an azlactone will tend to result in a block copolymer chain with a higher concentration of azlactone functionality near the terminus of the chain.

After producing a lens with the desired final shape, it is desirable to remove residual solvent from the lens before edge-finishing operations. This is because, typically, an organic diluent is included in the initial monomeric mixture in order to minimize phase separation of the polymerized products produced by polymerization of the monomeric mixture and to lower the glass transition temperature of the reacting polymeric mixture, which allows for a more efficient curing process and ultimately results in a more uniformly polymerized product. Sufficient uniformity of the initial monomeric mixture and the polymerized product are of particular concern for silicone hydrogels, primarily due to the inclusion of silicone-containing monomers which may tend to separate from the hydrophilic comonomer.

Suitable organic diluents include, for example, monohydric alcohols, such as *n*-hexanol and *n*-nonanol (cf. Figure 1.16), diols such as ethylene glycol, polyols such as glycerin, ethers such as diethylene glycol monoethyl ether (cf. Figure 1.17), ketones such as methyl ethyl ketone, esters such as methyl enanthate (cf. Figure 1.18), and hydrocarbons such as toluene.

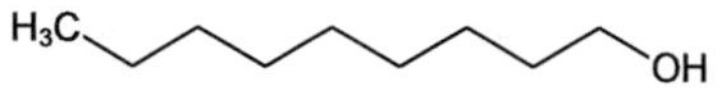

Figure 1.16 *n*-Nonanol.

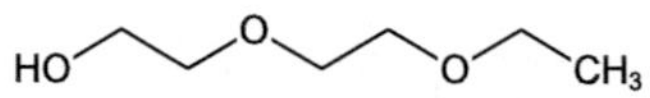

Figure 1.17 Diethylene glycol monoethyl ether.

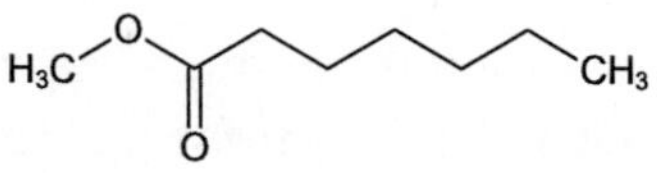

Figure 1.18 Methyl enanthate or Methyl heptanoate.

Preferably, the organic diluent is sufficiently volatile to facilitate its removal from a cured article by evaporation at or near ambient pressure. Generally, the diluent is included at 5% to 60% of the monomeric mixture, with 10% to 50% being especially preferred.

The cured lens is then subjected to solvent removal, which can be accomplished by evaporation at or near ambient pressure or under vacuum. An elevated temperature can be employed to shorten the time necessary to evaporate the diluent. The time, temperature and pressure conditions for the solvent removal step will vary depending on such factors as the volatility of the diluent and the specific monomeric components, as can be readily determined by one skilled in the art. According to a preferred embodiment, the temperature employed in the removal step is preferably at least 50°C. A series of heating cycles in a linear oven under inert gas or vacuum may be used to optimize the efficiency of the solvent removal. The cured article after the diluent removal step should preferably contain not more than 5%.

After solvent removal, the lens is next subjected to mold release and optional machining operations. The machining step includes, for example, buffing or polishing a lens edge and/or surface. Finally, the lens is subjected to a surface treatment (28).

1.4.1.3 Hydrophilicity Improvement

The hydrophilicity of the surface of a silicone hydrogel lens can be improved with a poly(oxy ethylene) derivative with a plurality of hydroxyl groups (30). The surface treatment can be done as follows (30):

Preparation 1–5: First, 60 parts by mass of 3-[tris(trimethylsiloxy)silyl] propyl methacryloyloxyethyl succinate, shown in Figure 1.19, 39 parts by mass of 2-hydroxyethyl methacrylate, 0.5 part by mass of ethylene glycol dimethacrylate, and 0.5 part by mass of azobisisobutyronitrile were mixed and dissolved. Then the solution was flowed into a cell sandwiched between a glass plate and a polypropylene plate through the use of a poly(ethylene terephthalate) sheet having a thickness of 0.1 *mm* as a spacer. After an oven had been purged with nitrogen, the solution was heated at 100°C for 2 *h* to be polymerized, followed by molding into a film shape. After polymerization, the cured film was removed from the cell, and was immersed in a mixed liquid containing ethyl alcohol and ion-exchanged water at a ratio of 3/1 for 12 *h*, and in ion-exchanged water for 12 *h* to produce a water-containing film. The produced water-containing film was placed in a discharging apparatus, and the pressure in a chamber was reduced to about 2.66 *Pa*. After that, a plasma discharge treatment was performed under an oxygen gas atmosphere at about 13.3 *Pa* for 10 *min* (frequency: 13.56 *MHz*, high-frequency output: 50 *W*). After that, a peroxide (peroxide group) was produced on the surface of the water-containing film by storing it under an oxygen gas atmosphere for a minimum of 10 *min*.

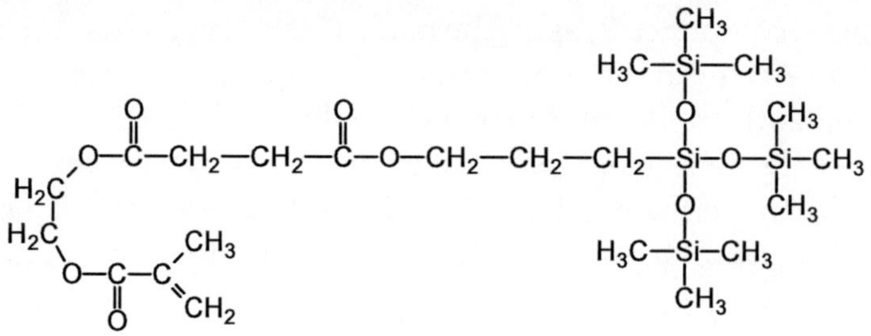

Figure 1.19 3-[Tris(trimethylsiloxy)silyl]propyl methacryloyloxyethyl succinate.

Examples of preferred monomers for use in the base material of a silicone hydrogel contact lens to control the water content include water-soluble monomers. These materials are collected in Table 1.13.

Table 1.13 Monomers for controlling water content (30).

Compound	Compound
(Meth)acrylic acid	Itaconic acid
Crotonic acid	Cinnamic acid
Vinylbenzoic acid	Glycerol (meth)acrylate
N-Vinylformamide	*N*-Vinylacetamide
2-Hydroxyethyl (meth)acrylate	2,3-Dihydroxypropyl (meth)acrylate
N-Methyl-*N*-vinylacetamide	*N*-Vinyl-2-pyrrolidone
2-(Meth)acryloyloxyethyl phosphorylcholine	
Polyalkylene glycol mono(meth)acrylate	
Polyalkylene glycol monoalkyl ether (meth)acrylate	

The usage amount of any monomer in Table 1.13 is typically from 10 parts by mass to 50 parts by mass, preferably from 20 parts by mass to 40 parts by mass with respect to 100 parts by mass of the monomer composition of the silicone hydrogel contact lens base material (30).

1.4.1.4 Interpenetrating Polymer Network Hydrogel Contact Lenses

Interpenetrating polymer network hydrogels have been described that have high oxygen permeability, strength, water content, and resistance to protein adsorption (20).

The hydrogels include two interpenetrating polymer networks. The first polymer network is based on a hydrophilic telechelic macromonomer. The second polymer network is based on a hydrophilic monomer. The hydrophilic monomer is polymerized and crosslinked to form the second polymer network in the presence of the first polymer network.

The telechelic macromonomer is preferably poly(ethylene) glycol diacrylate or poly(ethylene) glycol dimethacrylate. The hydrophilic monomer can be acrylic acid, acrylamide, *N*-hydroxyethyl acrylamide, *N*-isopropyl acrylamide, methacrylic acid (MA), 2-acrylamido-2-methylpropanesulfonic acid, 2-hydroxyethyl methacrylate, or 2-hydroxyethyl acrylate, cf. Figure 1.20.

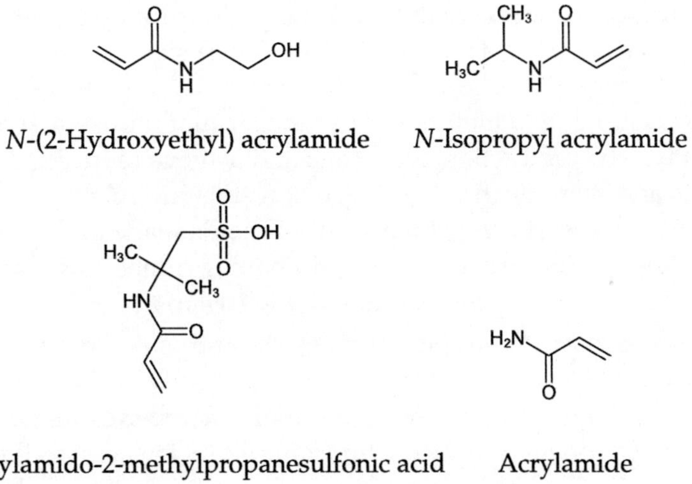

Figure 1.20 Monomers for telechelic macromonomers (20).

One surface of the interpenetrating polymer network hydrogel should be surface modified. Preferably, at least one surface is modified with a layer of poly(ethylene) glycol macromonomers, polymerized poly(ethylene) glycol diacrylate, or polymerized poly(ethylene) glycol dimethacrylate.

The steps required for synthesis of an interpenetrating polymer network hydrogel are as follows (20):

The starting material for the hydrogel is a solution of telechelic macromonomers with functional end groups. The telechelic macromonomers are polymerized to form a first polymer network. Next, hydrophilic monomers are added to the first polymer network. Hydrophilic monomers are then polymerized and crosslinked in the presence of the first polymer network to form a second polymer network.

1.4.1.5 *Poly(olefin) Contact Lenses*

New lens molds and methods useful in producing soft contact lenses have been discovered. Poly(propylene) (PP) contact lens molds and methods of making such soft contact lenses, such as hydrogel contact lenses, by using such molds have been described (31).

The present molds and methods provide contact lenses with consistent high optical quality; for example, producing lenses with fewer surface defects and with less severe surface defects or a reduced optical distortion caused by surface defects. Furthermore, the present molds and methods use reduced amounts of energy, shorten contact lens production cycle time and achieve reduced machinery wear and tear. Such advantageous results are relative to producing identical soft contact lenses from molds made of thermoplastic poly(olefin), in particular PP, resin having a melt flow rate of less than 10 $g\,(10min)^{-1}$, for example, 1.9 $g\,(10min)^{-1}$.

The term *melt flow rate* denotes the industry known standard ASTM D1238-13 (32). This parameter is usually available from suppliers of commercial resins. Such mold member or members may be conventionally produced, for example, by injection molding processing. Preferably, both mold members are injection molded from one or more of such resins.

These benefits of producing soft contact lenses can be obtained without requiring molds made from thermoplastic poly(olefin) resins having a melt flow rate of at least about $g\,(10min)^{-1}$, as described in a previous publication (33) for rigid gas-permeable contact lenses. Also, molds made out of Ziegler-Natta catalyst-based poly(olefin) resin are not required, as noted in a publication of Ansell and Yin (34).

Here, methods of producing soft contact lens products, e.g., soft hydrophilic or hydrogel contact lens products, are provided. These methods consist of placing a soft lens-forming composition in a cavity formed between a first mold member and a second mold member, subjecting the soft lens-forming composition in the cavity to conditions effective to form a contact lens product from the lens-forming composition, and repeating the placing and subjecting steps a plurality of times, for example, at least about 100 times or at least about 1000 times or at least about 10,000 times, thereby producing a plurality of soft contact lens products.

At least the first mold members, and advantageously all of the first and second mold members, consist of a nucleated thermoplastic poly(olefin) resin having a melt flow rate in a range of 10 $g\,(10min)^{-1}$ to about 40 $g\,(10min)^{-1}$ (31).

A nucleating agent is specifically utilized to increase the rate of crystallization of the poly(olefin) component as it cools from the melt as compared to the same or identical poly(olefin) component without the nucleating agent. Many nucleating agents are suitable for inclusion with the thermoplastic poly(olefin) resin formulations useful in the present invention.

Nucleating agents for PP have been described (35, 36). Examples of suitable nucleating agents are collected in Table 1.14 and shown in Figure 1.21.

The thermoplastic poly(olefin) resin acts to reduce the time required for crystallization of the poly(olefin) resin and/or to produce smaller crystals of the poly(olefin) resin relative to an identical thermoplastic poly(olefin) resin without the nucleating agent. Reducing poly(olefin) crystallization time is believed to allow for better and more precise control of poly(olefin) resin crystallization. Producing smaller poly(olefin) resin crystals is believed to allow the poly(olefin) resin (crystallized) to more closely conform to the desired shape of the mold member or members, in particular to the desired shape of the surface or surfaces of the mold member or

Table 1.14 Nucleating agents (31).

Compound
Sodium benzoate
Sodium sulfate
Sodium 2,2′-methylenebis(4,6-di-*tert*-butylphenyl) phosphate
Aluminum 2,2′-methylenebis(4,6-di-*tert*-butylphenyl) phosphate
Dibenzylidene sorbitol
Di(*p*-tolylidene) sorbitol
Di(*p*-ethylbenzylidene) sorbitol
Bis(3,4-dimethylbenzylidene) sorbitol
N′,N′-Dicyclohexyl-2,6-naphthalenedicarboxamide
Salts of disproportionated rosin esters

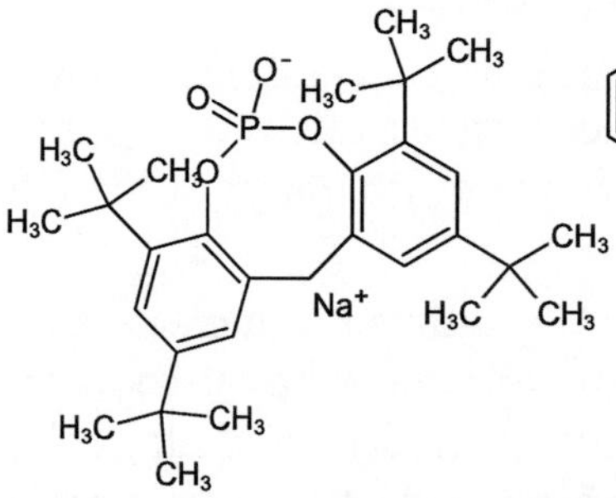

Sodium 2,2′-methylenebis(4,6-di-*tert*-butylphenyl) phosphate

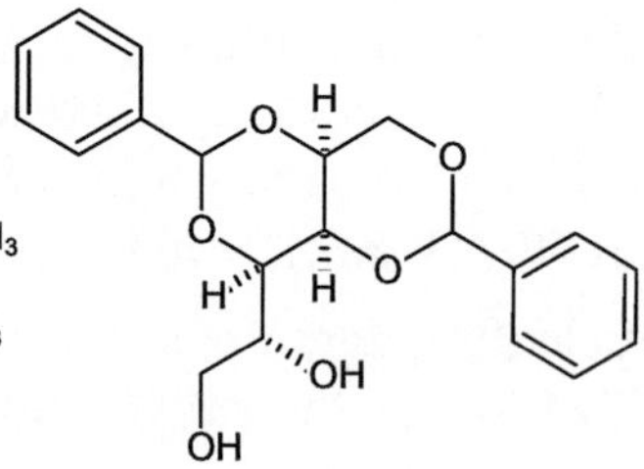

Dibenzylidene sorbitol

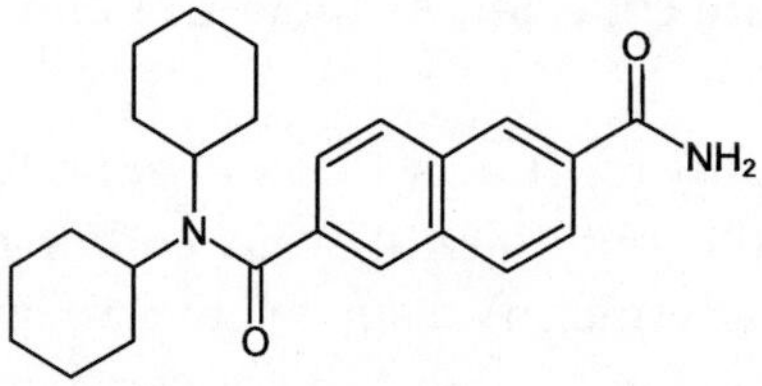

N′,N′-Dicyclohexyl-2,6-naphthalenedicarboxamide

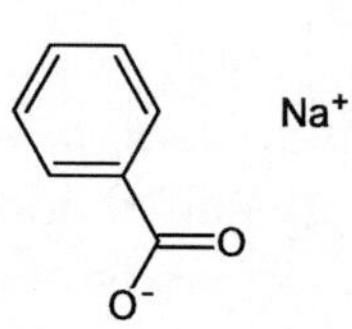

Sodium benzoate

Figure 1.21 Nucleating agents (31).

members which are shaped to produce the anterior and/or posterior surfaces of the contact lens product.

In addition, many other types of additives can be included in the thermoplastic poly(olefin) resin formulations. Such additives include lubricants, antistatic agents, slip agents, antiblocking agents, colorants, metal deactivators, mold release agents, fillers and reinforcements, fluorescent whitening agents, biostabilizers, and mixtures thereof.

These methods produce a plurality of soft contact lens products having fewer surface defects and/or less severe surface defects and/or reduced optical distortion caused by surface defects relative to an identical plurality of soft contact lens products produced in identical molds in which the first mold members comprise a thermoplastic poly(olefin) resin having a melt flow rate of less than 10 $g\,(10min)^{-1}$, for example, 1.9 $g\,(10min)^{-1}$.

Also, a method of producing soft hydrophilic cast-molded contact lenses having enhanced surface quality is assessed. Such a method consists of (31):

1. Providing first and second mold members structured to be assembled together to form a lens-shaped cavity therebetween, each of the first and second mold members comprises a nucleated, thermoplastic poly(olefin) resin having a melt flow rate in a range of about 10 $g\,(10min)^{-1}$ to about 40 $g\,(10min)^{-1}$,
2. Placing a soft hydrophilic contact lens-forming composition in the cavity,
3. Forming a soft hydrophilic contact lens product from the soft hydrophilic contact lens-forming composition in the cavity,
4. Removing the soft hydrophilic contact lens product from the first and second mold members; and repeating the above-noted providing, placing, forming and removing steps a plurality of times.

This method can produce a plurality of soft hydrophilic contact lens products having enhanced surface quality relative to an identically produced plurality of soft contact lens products made using first and second mold members consisting of thermoplastic olefin resin having a melt flow rate of 1.9 $g\,(10min)^{-1}$.

In an aspect, a method of producing soft hydrophilic contact lenses is provided which includes forming a plurality of soft hydrophilic contact lens products from a soft hydrophilic contact lens-forming composition in cavities formed by first and second mold members and removing the soft hydrophilic contact lens products from the first and second mold members. This method consists of using first and second molds consisting of a nucleated thermoplastic poly(olefin) resin having a melt flow rate in a range of about 10 $g\,(10min)^{-1}$ to about 40 $g\,(10min)^{-1}$, and producing a soft hydrophilic contact lens with enhanced surface quality (31).

A cross-sectional view of a contact lens mold assembly is shown in Figure 1.22.

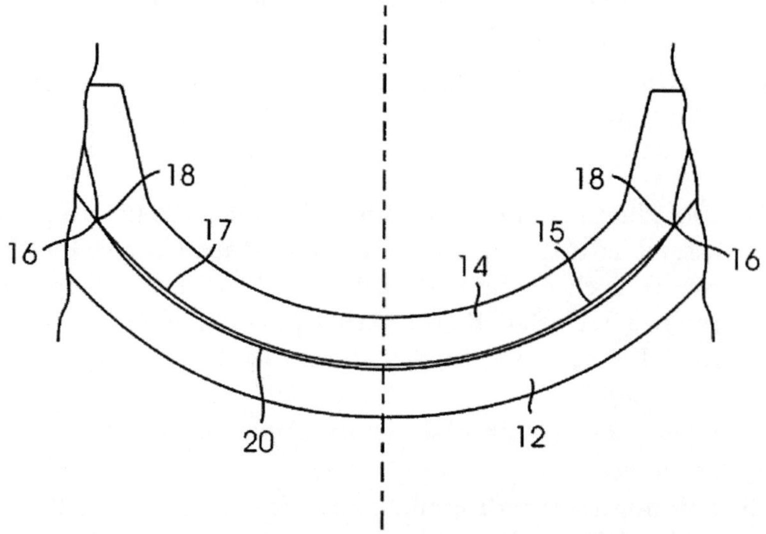

Figure 1.22 Cross-sectional view of a contact lens mold assembly (31).

The contact lens mold assembly, shown in Figure 1.22, includes a first or female mold member 12 coupled to a second or male mold member 14 to form a lens-shaped cavity 15 which has a circular periphery. In addition, the first and second mold members 12 and 14 can be structured to produce a contact lens having a rounded posterior lens edge surface. However, other embodiments of the mold members 12 and 14 may form non-rounded lens edge surfaces. As shown in Figure 1.22, lens-shaped cavity 15 contains a polymerizable contact lens precursor composition 17, which is discussed in detail elsewhere herein. The first and second mold members 12 and 14 are made of thermoplastic poly(olefin) resin and are interference fitted together. In particular, first and second mold members 12 and 14 are press fitted together at first peripheral region 16 (of first mold member 12) and second peripheral region 18 (of second mold member 14). Thus, first and second peripheral regions 16 and 18 are structured to be in direct, securing contact when the mold is assembled, as shown in Figure 1.22.

The first and second mold members 12 and 14 can be securely joined or coupled together simply by moving one or both of the mold members toward each other until the peripheral regions 16 and 18 come into direct, securing contact. When it is desired to separate the first and second mold members 12 and 14, the mold members can be pulled apart or a tool can be used to overcome the direct, securing contact at the peripheral regions 16 and 18, preferably without causing substantial damage to at least one of the first and second mold members and to the ophthalmic lens product formed in the lens-shaped cavity.

The contact lens precursor composition 17 within the lens-shaped cavity often includes one or more monomers, macromers, polymers, or other reactive agents, and combinations thereof, which are polymerized, such as by exposure to UV light and/or heat, to form a contact lens product. Other processing steps may include, without limitation, disassembling the mold assembly or demolding the mold assembly, removing the contact lens product from the first mold member or second mold member or delensing the contact lens product from a mold member, extracting extractable materials from the contact lens product, for example, extracting extractable materials from a silicone hydrogel contact lens product, hydrating the extracted contact lens product, inspecting the contact lens, packaging the contact lens, and sterilizing the contact lens. In certain lenses, a separate extraction step may not be necessary. The resulting contact lens is a cast-molded contact lens (31).

1.4.1.6 Carboxy Betaine Ester

A hydrogel contact lens has been described from a polymer composition that can be obtained by polymerizing a monomer mixture of a betaine ester (37). Betaine is also known as trimethylglycine or (trimethylammonio)acetate.

The synthesis of the carboxy betaine ester *N*-carbomethoxymethyl-*N*-methacryloylamidopropyl-*N*,*N*-dimethyl ammonium chloride is performed under a dry nitrogen atmosphere in dry acetone. Under these circumstances the carboxy betaine ester, which is a salt, precipitates from the solution. Being salts, the carboxy betaine esters are very hygroscopic since they absorb water rather quickly and thus must be stored under dry conditions to retain their quality.

In detail the synthesis runs as follows (37):

Preparation 1–6: First, 42.566 *g* (0.250 *mol*) *N*-[3-(dimethylamino)propyl]-methacrylamide in 100 *ml* of dry acetone was added to a three-necked flask and stirred. Then, 29.848 *g* (0.275 *mol*) methylchloro acetate in 30 *ml* dry acetone was added into a dropping funnel attached to the three-necked flask. The reaction commenced under a continuous slight dry nitrogen overpressure while the tip of the reaction flask touched the ice/water mixture, thus setting the initial temperature of the reaction solution at 15°C.

Now, methylchloro acetate was slowly added in about 30 *min*, while maintaining the reaction temperature just below 15°C by varying the immersion depth of the reaction flask in the ice/water mixture. During the addition of methylchloro acetate only a slight whitish haze developed in the reaction solution. After the addition of all methylchloro acetate, the reaction flask was lifted from the ice/water bath, and the reaction solution was allowed to warm to ambient temperature while still being stirred. Then the temperature slowly rose to about 30°C, slightly over ambient temperature, while more and more white crystals were formed. The temperature was controlled to avoid an increase above 30°C in order to prevent too much acetone being evaporated from the reaction solution. After one night of continuous stirring, a dense crust of white crystalline material had precipitated on the inside of the reaction flask, while a slurry of crystals had formed in the reaction solution. The crystals were isolated by filtration and washed with dry acetone under a flow of dry nitrogen gas to avoid water uptake. The crystals were dried in a vacuum oven at 50°C for one night. The yield was 60.215 *g* (79%).

The synthesis is also shown in Figure 1.23.

1.4.1.7 *Silver Nanoparticles*

The effect of the monomer composition on the binding capacity of hydrogels with silver nanoparticles was investigated and its antibacterial efficacy was evaluated (38).

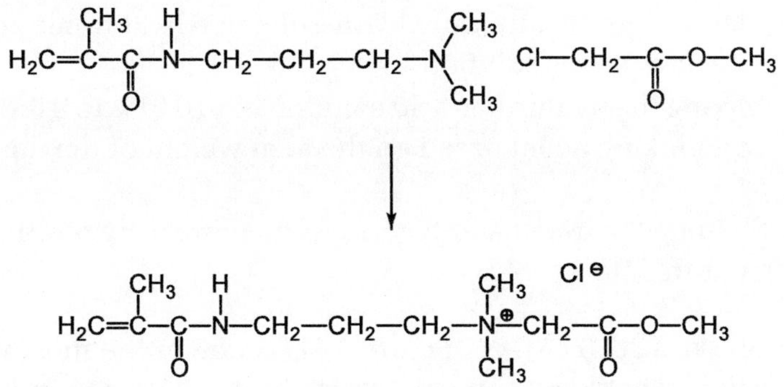

Figure 1.23 Synthesis of *N*-carbomethoxymethyl-*N*-methacryloylamido-propyl-*N*,*N*-dimethyl ammonium chloride.

Three series of poly(2-hydroxyethyl methacrylate) hydrogels were prepared using MA, methacrylamide, and 4-vinylpyridine as comonomers, and ethylene glycol dimethacrylate (EGDMA) as crosslinking agent (38).

The binding capacity of the hydrogels with the silver nanoparticles was evaluated in different concentrations of 2 *ppm*, 10 *ppm*, and 20 *ppm*. The *in-vitro* antibacterial activity of the silver nanoparticles-loaded hydrogels was studied against *Pseudomonas aeruginosa* (*P. aeruginosa*) isolated from the eyes of some patients. Then, the inhibitory effect of hydrogels in biofilm formation was evaluated in the presence of *Staphylococcus epidermidis* (*S. epidermidis*) (DSMZ 3270).

The obtained data indicated that poly(HEMA-*co*-MAA-*co*-EGDMA) showed a superior binding affinity for the silver nanoparticles in comparison to other hydrogels. All silver nanoparticle-loaded hydrogels showed excellent antimicrobial effects against *P. aeruginosa* and *S. epidermidis* after soaking in 10 *ppm* and 20 *ppm* silver nanoparticle suspensions (38).

1.4.1.8 Transparent Hydrogel Membrane

A method for preparing a transparent hydrogel membrane has been described. The method includes the following steps (39):

1. Preparing 6 to 10% of a hyaluronic acid solution based on a total weight of a mixture by dissolving a hyaluronic acid in a basic aqueous solution,
2. Mixing the hyaluronic acid solution with 0.01% to 0.05% of a crosslinking agent based on the total weight of the mixture, and
3. Shaping the transparent hydrogel membrane by pouring the mixture into a mold.

Hyaluronic acid (HA), cf. Figure 4.41, is one of the most widely used biocompatible polymers for medical use. It is a polymer consisting of two sugars, glucuronic acid and *N*-acetylglucosamine. These sugars are shown in Figure 1.24.

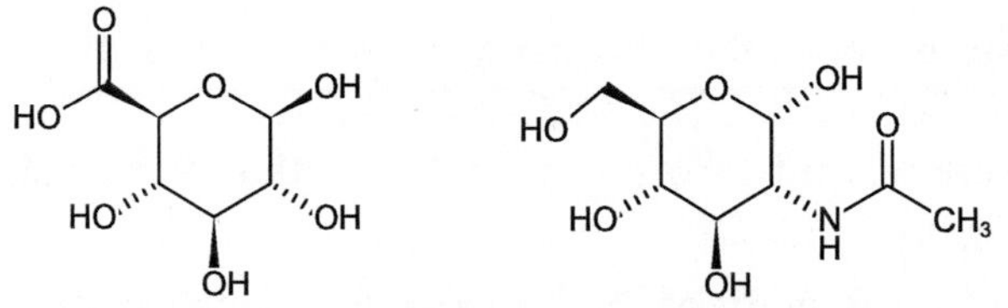

Glucuronic acid   *N*-Acetylglucosamine

Figure 1.24 Sugars in hyaluronic acid.

Hyaluronic acid is a natural mucopolysaccharide that is widely distributed in the interstices of tissues, is present in a large amount in the synovial fluid, cartilage, skin, eyeballs, and the like of a human, serves as a three-dimensional crosslinker of intercellular molecules, and protects cartilages between the cartilages due to its high viscosity. Furthermore, hyaluronic acid contains a large amount of carboxyl groups, which is a hydrophilic group, and thus has a feature by which its mechanical strength is reduced when it comes into contact with moisture.

The crosslinking agent serves to link and copolymerize hyaluronic acid monomers, and an internal structure of the transparent hydrogel membrane may form a network structure by the copolymerization. Suitable crosslinking agents are listed in Table 1.15 and shown in Figure 1.25.

Table 1.15 Crosslinking agents (39).

Compound
1,4-Butanediol diglycidyl ether
1-Ethyl-3-(3-dimethylaminopropyl)carbodiimide
Diepoxyoctane
1,2-Bis-(2,3-epoxypropyl)-2,3-ethylene

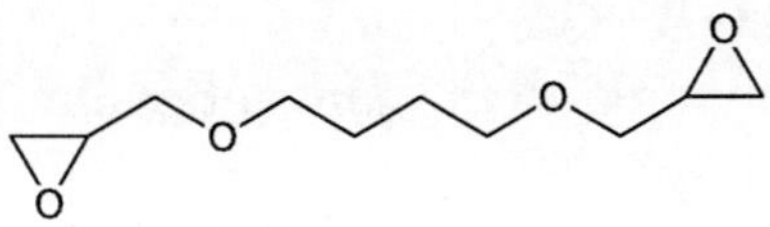

1,4-Butanediol diglycidyl ether

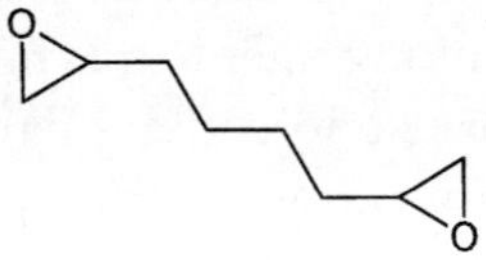

Diepoxyoctane

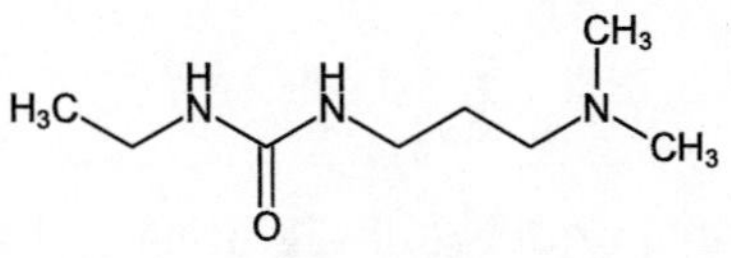

1-Ethyl-3-(3-dimethylaminopropyl) carbodiimide

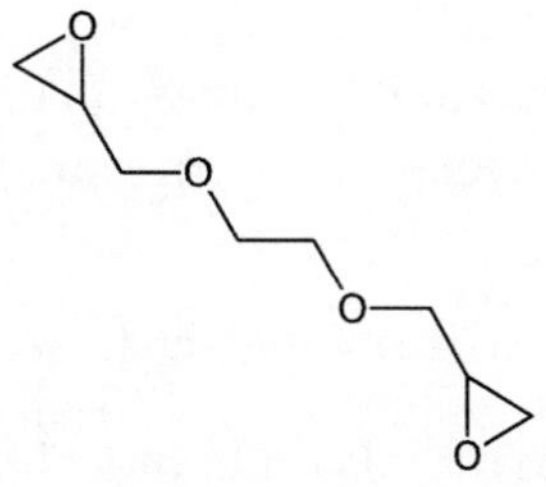

1,2-Bis-(2,3-epoxypropyl)-2,3-ethane

Figure 1.25 Crosslinking agents.

The preparation of a hyaluronic acid contact lens can be done as follows (39):

Preparation 1–7: A uniform hyaluronic acid mixture was prepared by dissolving a non-crosslinked hyaluronic acid in an amount of 8% in an aqueous sodium hydroxide solution with a pH of 8 and adding 0.01% of 1,4-butanediol diglycidyl ether thereto. The hyaluronic acid mixture was poured into a poly(carbonate) mold and dried in an oven at 40°C for 30 *h*. The hyaluronic acid contact lenses of a predetermined size prepared by drying the hyaluronic acid mixture were washed three times in total with distilled water every 24 *h*, and after a washing process of 72 *h* was performed, a hyaluronic acid hydrogel film was obtained. The hyaluronic acid hydrogel membrane had a diameter of 9 *mm* and a thickness of 20 μm.

1.4.2 *PVA Hydrogel*

A highly transparent poly(vinyl alcohol) (PVA) hydrogel can be obtained by freeze-thawing aqueous PVA solutions repeatedly at a relatively higher temperature. There is no need to use a chemical crosslinking agent. It is believed that these materials could be superior for use in contact lenses compared to the conventionally used 2-hydroxyethyl methacrylate (HEMA) (40).

Aqueous solutions of PVA are obtained by dissolving PVA in water at 80°C. The concentration of the polymers is around 5–20%. The solutions are then stored at room temperature for two weeks. Repeated freeze-thawing cycles are then performed. This procedure consists of 8 *h* freezing at 0°C. The thawing lasts 16 *h* at 37°C. A total of 15 cycles is appropriate (41).

1.4.3 *Clear Contact Lenses*

The materials for contact lenses have undergone significant changes over the past 20 years, in particular due to the introduction of silicone hydrogel materials (42).

The wettability of contact lenses is still an important part of biocompatibility. Contact lenses can be made more wettable by incorporation of surfactants into blister packs, internal wetting agents, surface treatments or care solutions (42). However, there is no clear association between contact lens wettability and comfort. This makes it challenging to predict these properties.

Most contact lenses are used on a daily wear, reusable basis, which requires them to be disinfected when not worn. The ideal disinfecting solution would also improve comfort during wear. However, balancing these requirements with other factors, including biocompatibility, remains a challenge.

Contact lens materials can sorb components of the tear film. These interactions are complex and may change the biochemistry of the tear film, which in turn may affect their comfort.

So, the interaction between lens materials, tear film and disinfection solution plays an important role in the biocompatibility of lenses.

The best available evidence to examine such complex relationships and the opportunities for practitioners to enhance the in-eye comfort of lenses have been reported (42).

1.5 Water Absorbable Formulations

It has been discovered that when a soft contact lens absorbs water and is hydrophilic, the lens will move on the eye sufficiently so that no physical damage will occur to the cornea and sufficient tear exchange will occur so that corneal metabolism will proceed normally.

It was found that poly(siloxane) soft contact showed some adhering to the eye. This problem has been a major obstacle in preventing the use of poly(siloxane)s as a soft contact lens material.

This major obstacle has now been overcome. Most unexpectedly, the instant poly(siloxane) copolymers are not only hydrophilic but are also water-absorbing. Therefore, the instant copolymers make excellent material for manufacturing contact lenses which not only do not stick to the eye but move sufficiently during normal wear so that corneal metabolism will proceed normally.

The contact lenses are made from a copolymer containing poly(siloxane) monomers copolymerized with acrylic acid.

The monomers that may be used are collected in Table 1.16. Some of these monomers are shown in Figure 1.26.

The monomers shown in Table 1.16 may be copolymerized in solution. A particularly preferred solvent is *p*-xylene. Poly(siloxane) monomers are collected in Table 1.17 and shown in Figure 1.27.

Table 1.16 Monomers (43).

Compound	
Cyclohexyl acrylate	Cinnamyl methacrylate
Cinnamyl acrylate	Cyclohexyl methacrylate
Phenoxyethyl methacrylate	Phenoxyethyl acrylate
tert-butyl-styrene	Vinyl toluene
Methacrylic acid	Acrylonitrile
Allyl methacrylate	Allyl acrylate
N-Vinyl pyrrolidone	Isopropyl acrylate
Isoamyl acrylate	2-Chloroethyl methacrylate
Cyclopentyl acrylate	*n*-Decyl acrylate
Phenyl acrylate	Tetrahydrofurfuryl acrylate
Benzyl acrylate	Hexafluoroisopropyl acrylate
Naphthyl acrylate	

Table 1.17 Poly(siloxane) monomers (43).

Compound
1,1,3,3-Tetramethyl-1,3-disila-2-oxacyclohexane
Octamethylcyclotetrasiloxane
1,3-Bis(4-methacryloxybutyl) tetramethyl disiloxane

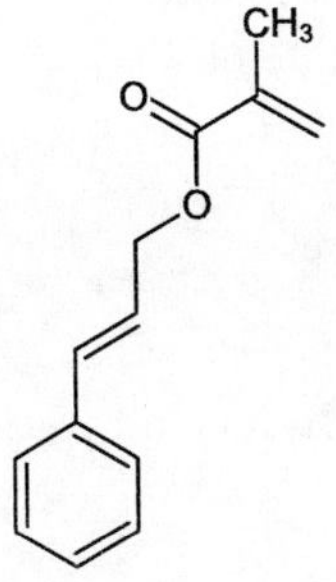

Cinnamyl methacrylate

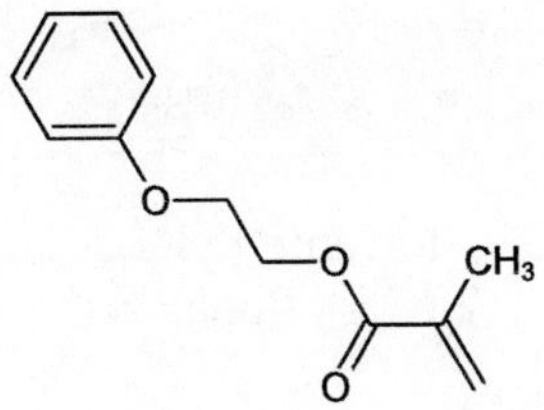

Phenoxyethyl methacrylate

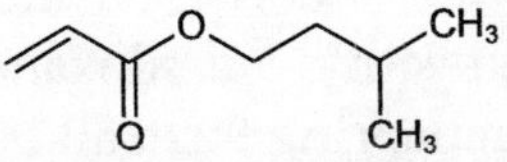

Isoamyl acrylate

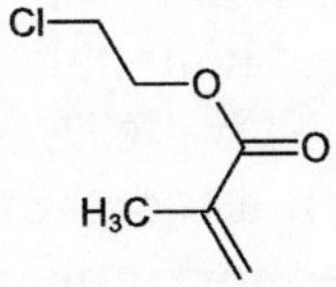

2-Chloroethyl methacrylate

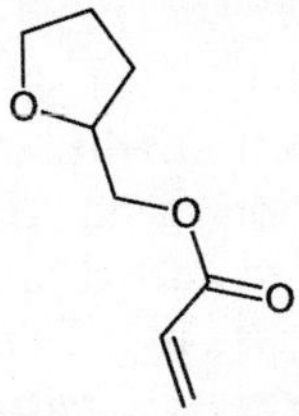

Tetrahydrofurfuryl acrylate

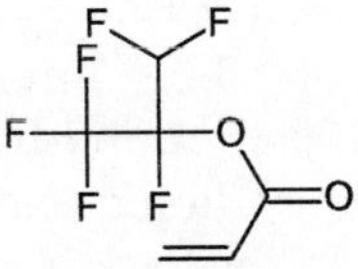

Hexafluoroisopropyl acrylate

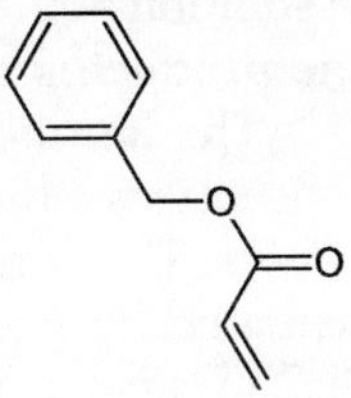

Benzyl acrylate

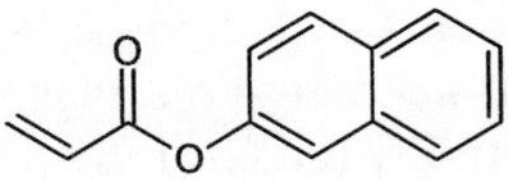

Naphthyl acrylate

Figure 1.26 Monomers.

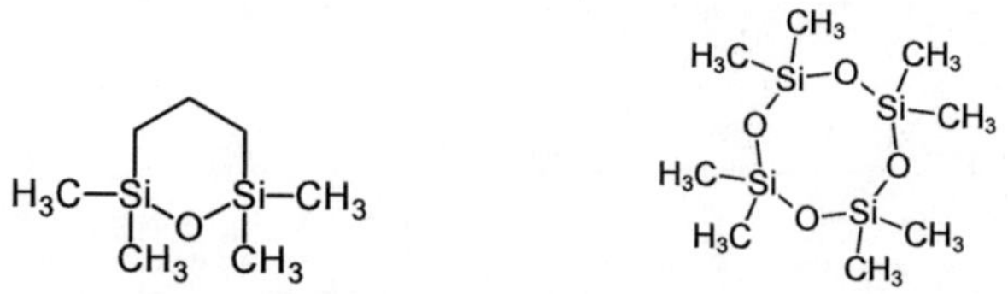

1,1,3,3,-Tetramethyl-1,3-disila-2-oxacyclohexane   Octamethylcyclotetrasiloxane

Figure 1.27 Poly(siloxane) monomers.

The copolymerization of cyclic siloxanes was first presented in 1960 (44). These materials are copolymerized with silethylene siloxane, $-Si - O - Si - CH_2 - CH_2 - O - Si-$, and then the rates of polymerization are determined. The silethylene siloxane is used because it does not equilibrate between the ring form and the linear form. Once the ring form is broken the ring stays open, i.e., the reaction is kept going in one direction. The preparation of the materials can be done as follows (43):

Preparation 1–8: First, 96.9 *g* 1,1,3,3-tetramethyl-1,3-disila-2-oxacyclohexane and 3.1 *g* of 1,3-bis(4-methacryloxybutyl) tetramethyl disiloxane are charged in a 200 *ml* round-bottom polymerization flask. Then, 1.3 *ml* of trifluoromethanesulfonic acid, cf. Figure 1.28, are added to the polymerization flask and the flask is stoppered. An increase in the viscosity of the flask's contents and the evolution of heat are observed 2 *min* to 3 *min* after the addition of the acid to the flask. The contents of the flask are agitated on a shaker overnight.

Then, the polymerization is quenched by the addition of 10 *g* Na_2CO_3. Hexane is added to the viscous product and the solution filtered to remove the insoluble salts. The hexane solution of the product is then washed three times with water and dried over $MgSO_4$. The hexane is removed from the product at a reduced pressure. The viscosity of the product as measured with Gardner viscosity tubes is 910 *Stokes*. The number average and weight average molecular weights as measured by gel permeation chromatography (GPC) are 12.3 *k Dalton* and 31.7 *k Dalton* respectively.

Also, several other examples of preparation have been reported (43).

The oxygen transportability of poly(siloxane)s is substantially greater in comparison to the conventional contact lens polymers

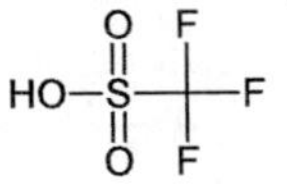

Figure 1.28 Trifluoromethanesulfonic acid.

such as PMMA or poly(2-hydroxyethyl methacrylate). The oxygen transportability of these materials can be varied by altering the percentage of siloxane units in the poly(siloxane) monomer. A high percentage of siloxane units results in a product that is more capable of transporting oxygen as compared with a lower percentage of siloxane units which results in a material with less ability to transport oxygen (43).

1.6 Bandage Contact Lenses

A bandage contact lens is used to protect an injured or diseased cornea from the mechanical rubbing of the blinking eyelids, therefore allowing it to heal (45). The bandage lens often makes the eye feel more comfortable, but has no focusing power. Usually a bandage contact lens is made from a soft lens material.

The materials employed as bandage contact lenses are basically those designed for use in the uncompromised eye for refractive contact lens purposes (46). Thus, there is an unmet challenge for therapeutic bandage lenses that are specifically designed for the injured (accident or surgery) or diseased cornea to aid healing.

1.6.1 Antimicrobial Bandage Contact Lens

Microbial adhesion to contact lenses is governed by many factors, including surface wettability, surface roughness and surface adhesion energy (47), and these factors differ substantially between silicone hydrogel contact lenses and conventional hydrogel contact lenses (48–50).

An antimicrobial bandage contact lens has been described wherein the antimicrobial bandage contact lens shields the eye from the environment while providing continuous long-term treatment (51).

The antimicrobial bandage contact lens can act as a prophylactic device that prevents microbial infections in an eye using inherently antimicrobial biomaterials with nanotopography. Furthermore, the antimicrobial bandage contact lens treats existing infection by dispensing antimicrobial medication at controlled rates over a period of up to 10 *d*. The antimicrobial bandage contact lens diminishes the risk of infection while simultaneously allowing damaged tissues to heal. The device allows the user to maintain vision to the extent allowed by the nature of the injury (51).

The antibacterial and antifungal surface is designed to be placed over the ocular lens to prevent ocular microbial infections while simultaneously delivering a drug at a controlled release rate that aids in healing of an injured or infected eye.

A transparent, therapeutic bandage material was designed that harnesses advanced nanotechnology to combine inherently antimicrobial biomaterials, antimicrobial nanoarchitectures, and an innovative biocomposite modality for antimicrobial drug delivery (51). The architecture of the antifungal bandage device contains three layers: A drug-eluting hydrogel-composite core layer sandwiched between two surface layers of lubricating hydrogel with antimicrobial nanopillars. The functions of the three layers are: The central layer of hydrogel-chitin composite provides structural and shape stability and strength, and acts as a reservoir for the long-term release of the antifungal and antibacterial drugs, and the outer layers provide wearability and antimicrobial shielding.

The ophthalmologic bandage must deliver antimicrobial drugs to the injured cornea. The current treatment for fungal keratitis involves hourly applications of topical agents such as natamycin that penetrate the posterior stroma to kill the hyphae. A mixture of drugs can also be coformulated for simultaneous delivery with natamycin, such as Voriconazole (2-(2,4-difluorophenyl)-3-(5-fluoro-4-pyrimidinyl)-1-(1H-1,2,4-triazol-1-yl)-2-butanol) or erythromycin (51). These compounds are shown in Figure 1.29.

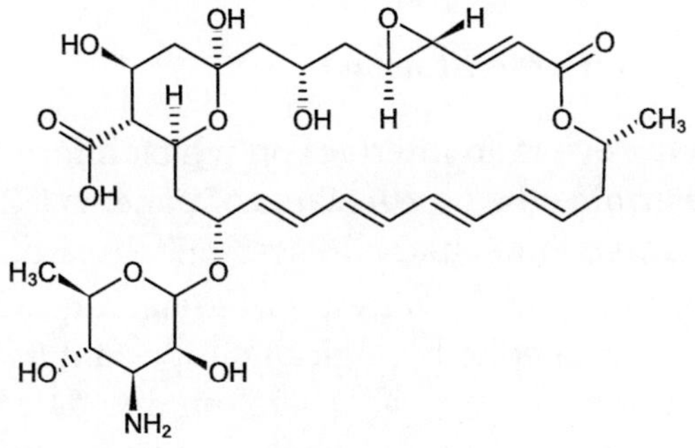

Natamycin

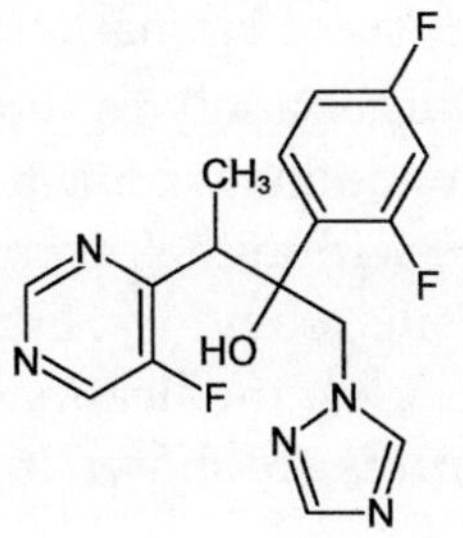

Voriconazole

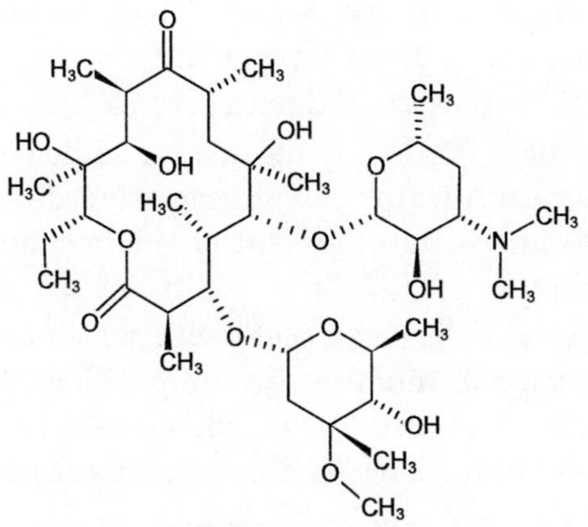

Erythromycin

Figure 1.29 Drugs.

1.7 Functional Contact Lenses

1.7.1 *Remote Health Monitoring*

The surface of the eye is an interface on which information may be gathered to determine the health status of patients (52). Tears are a source of biomarkers for ocular and systemic diseases (53–55).

The tear fluid contains a variety of biomarkers whose concentrations can be correlated to biologically important health markers, such as blood composition (52). Therefore, the detection of these biomarkers may provide a route towards noninvasive analysis of human health, with the help of a functional contact lens. Functional contact lenses are an emerging technology which provide a platform for the detection and analysis of biomarkers in the human tear (52).

Target biomarkers or target analytes that may be sensed by the biosensors used in the functional contact lenses described herein may be molecules that are within the precorneal tear, such as acids, ions, carbohydrates, proteins, enzymes, lipids, antigens, hormones, nucleic acids, small molecules, medications, or recreational drugs. Examples of such compounds are shown in Table 1.18 and in Figure 1.30.

In the functional contact lens at least one sensing element is disposed on the substrate for sensing a target analyte and undergoing a physical change representing a sensed signal. An antenna coupled to the sensing element is disposed on the substrate for transmitting the sensed signal to an external device (52).

The opportunities afforded by using a functional contact lens for remote wireless health status monitoring were discussed and the progress to date in the development of this technology platform was detailed (56).

A functional contact lens complete with sensors and embedded circuitry can be used to monitor the composition of the tear fluid and, by extension, a number of health-status-related parameters in the body in a noninvasive and continuous fashion. The data collected by a disposable contact lens may be sent wirelessly to a mobile phone that, in turn, can relay the information to a medical practitioner via the cellular phone network.

If successfully developed and deployed, such a system can be used for monitoring a variety of health indicators over a large geo-

Table 1.18 Target biomarkers (52).

Compound	Compound
Ascorbic acid	Lactic acid
Pyruvic acid	Fructose
Glucose	Sucrose
Galactose	Maltose
Lactose	Lysozyme
Lipocalin	Cytokine
Albumin	Interleukins
Glycoproteins	Orosomucoid
Transferrin	Lactoferrin
Ceruloplasmin	Ferritin
Procalcitonin	Hexokinase
Aldolase	Triose phosphate isomerase
Phosphoglucose isomerase	Pyruvate kinase
Enolase	Lactic dehydrogenase
Citrate synthase	Aconitase
Phosphofructokinase	Phosphoglyceratemutase
Pyruvate dehydrogenase	Isocitric dehydrogenase
Succinate dehydrogenase	Fumarase
Matalate dehydrogenase	Peroxidase
Wax esters	Cholesterol
Cortisol	Catecholamines
Endorphins	Insulin
Ibuprofen	Acetaminophen
Alrex	Betaxon
Besivance	Cosopt
Lucentis	Metformin
Adriamycin	Adrucil
Cytoxan	Ethyol
Psychedelics	Barbiturates
Benzodiazepines	Amphetamines

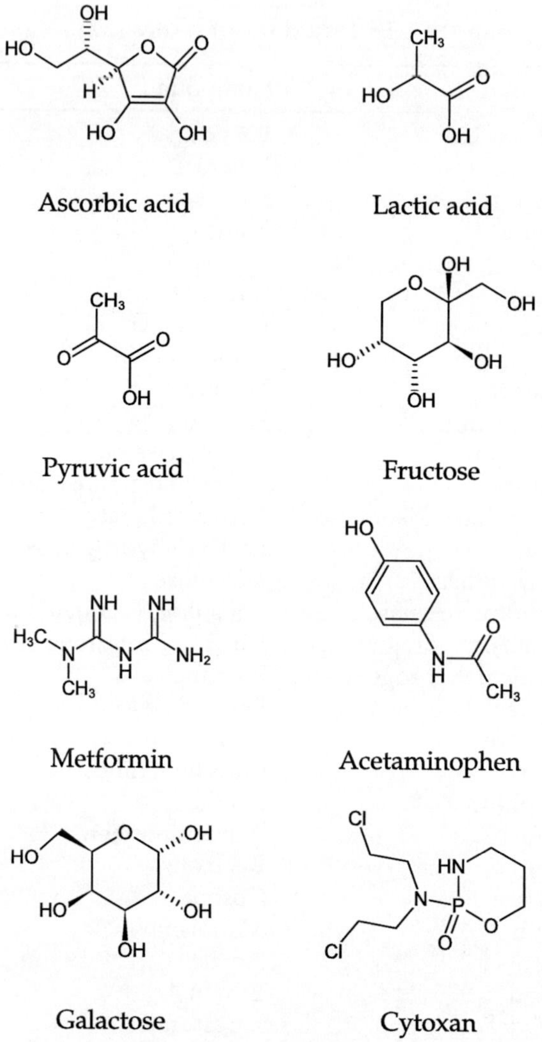

Figure 1.30 Target biomarkers.

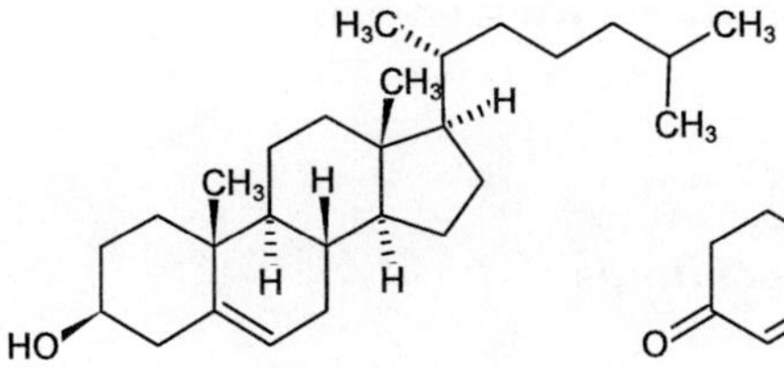

Cholesterol

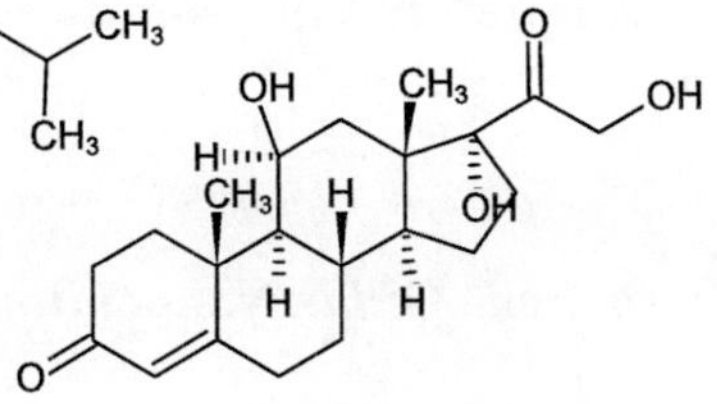

Cortisol

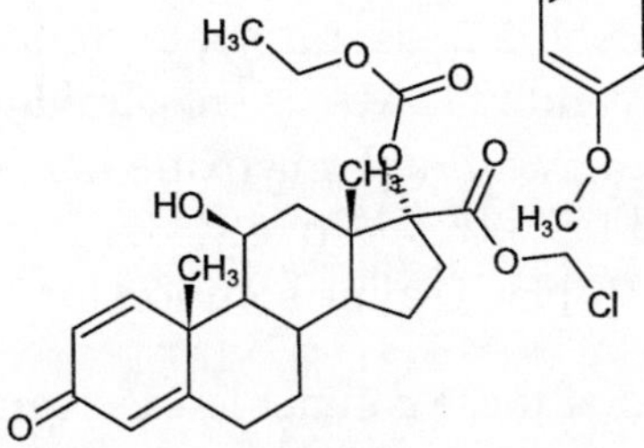

Alrex

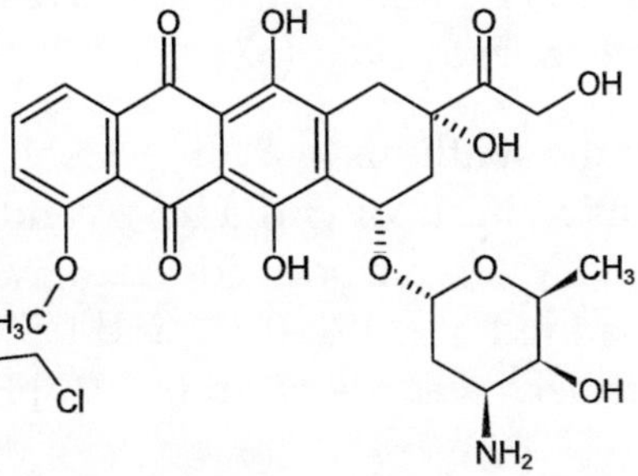

Adriamycin

HCl

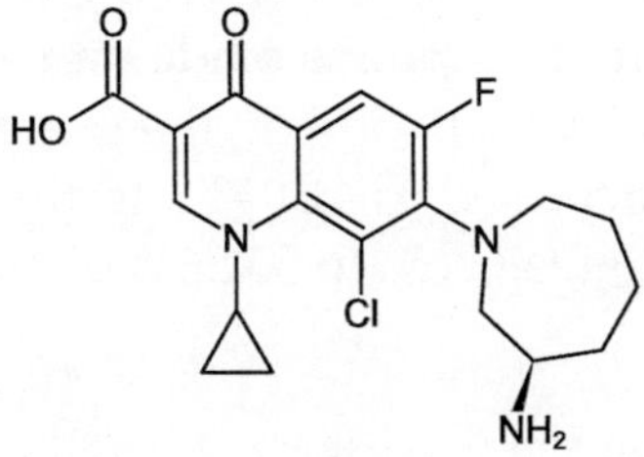

Besivance

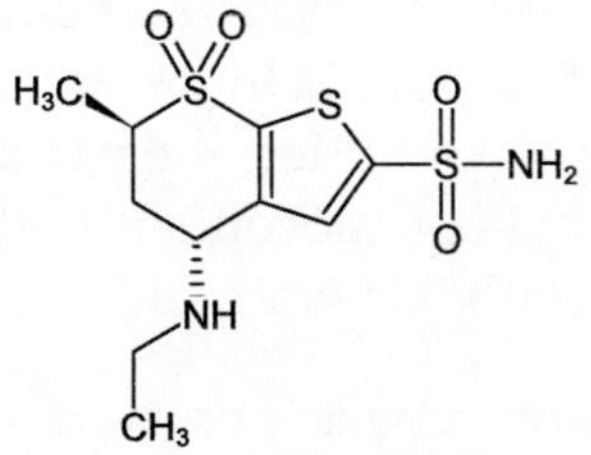

Cosopt

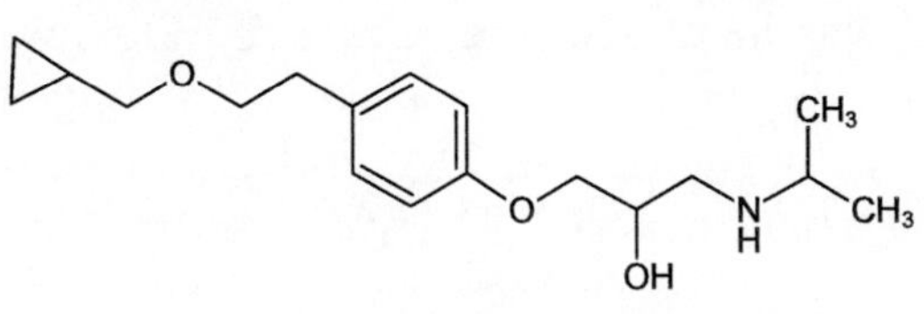

Betaxon

Figure 1.30 (cont) Target biomarkers.

graphic area and population distribution with a minimal need for the physical presence of healthcare providers (56).

1.7.2 *Graphene Oxide Nanocolloids*

The physical properties of contact lenses made by adding hydrophilic HA and MA as additives, and graphene oxide nanocolloids were evaluated (57).

For the synthesis of a contact lens, 2,2´-azobisisobutyronitrile was used as an initiator with HEMA and EGDMA as crosslinking agent. HA and MA were both added at 5%. Graphene oxide nanocolloids were added at 0.1%, 0.3% and 0.5%, respectively. Each prepared contact lens was hydrated in 99% NaCl saline solution for 24 *h* (57).

The basic physical properties of these contact lenses were evaluated and compared. The refractive index of the sample with HA and MA added was 1.4390, which was not significantly different from that of the basic combination contact lens sample. When graphene oxide nanocolloids, a nanomaterial, were added, the refractive index decreased with increasing amount of graphene oxide nanocolloids from 1.4209 to 13959. In the case of water content, the sample with 5% HA and MA added slightly increased to 41.01%. In the case of graphene oxide nanocolloids added, 48.76% to 53.56% of graphene oxide nanocolloids were added.

Especially, it was observed that the water content increased sharply in the 0.1% sample of graphene oxide nanocolloids. When the amount of graphene oxide nanocolloids added to the contact lens material was increased, the refractive index, which is a basic physical property, gradually decreased as the contact lens material was added together with HA, MA, and graphene oxide nanocolloids added as a nanomaterial. The water content tended to increase gradually.

Therefore, the combination of graphene oxide and hydrophilic materials shows a synergistic effect of physical properties, which is considered to be suitable as a material for contact lenses (57).

1.7.3 *Diabetic Diagnosis*

1.7.3.1 *Tear Glucose Analysis*

A contact lens is an ideal vehicle for continuous tear glucose monitoring of glucose concentration in the tear film (58).

An approach for noninvasive monitoring of the concentration of blood glucose is to monitor the glucose concentrations in the human tear fluid. The understanding of the physiology of glucose transport in tears has been assessed, in addition to the regulation of the aqueous tear fraction (53).

The various tear collection methods employed greatly influence the measured tear glucose concentrations. Studies that involve mechanical irritation of the conjunctiva during sampling measure the highest tear glucose concentrations, while studies that avoid tear stimulation measure the lowest concentrations.

Attempts to monitor tear glucose concentration *in situ* by using contact lens-based sensing devices were discussed. These studies indicate the importance of the sampling method in determining tear glucose concentrations (53).

A methodology has been reported for possible tear glucose monitoring using glucose-sensitive silicone hydrogel contact lenses. An interpenetrating polymer network was assessed, with nearly pure silicone and water regions existing in the silicone hydrogels, using the polarity-sensitive probe Prodan, cf. Figure 1.31.

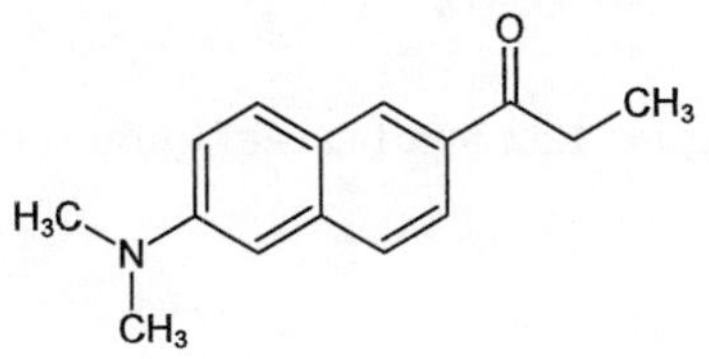

Figure 1.31 Prodan (1-(6-(Dimethylamino)naphthalen-2-yl)propan-1-one).

Then, a glucose-sensitive fluorophore Quin-C18 was synthesized with a hydrophobic side chain for localization of probe at the interfacial region. The synthesis of Quin-C18 is shown in Figure 1.32.

Here, glucose is bound to the boric acid moieties of Quin-C18.

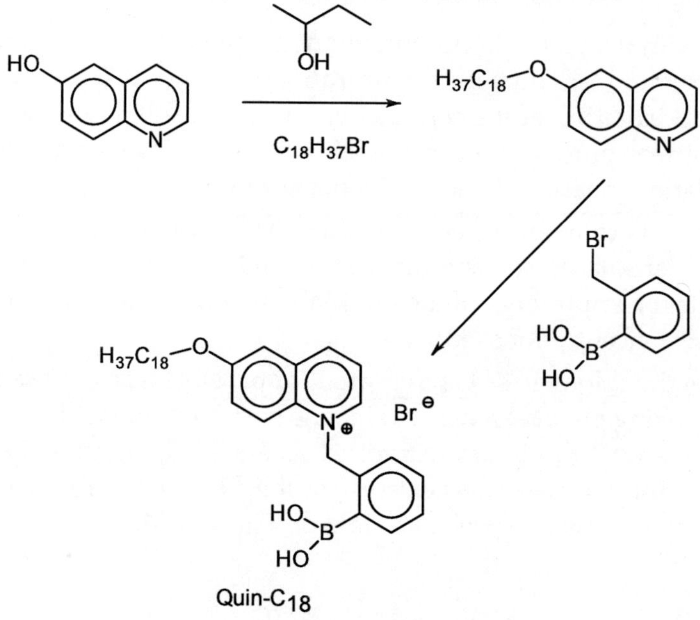

Figure 1.32 Synthesis of Quin-C18.

Using the glucose-sensing contact lens, it was possible to measure varying concentrations of glucose in an *in-vitro* system. The Quin-C18 strongly bound to the lenses with insignificant leaching even after multiple rinses. The lenses displayed a similar response to glucose after three months of storage in water. So the study demonstrated that it may be possible to develop a contact lens for continuous glucose monitoring in the near term, using the concept of fluorophore binding at the silicone-water interface.

1.7.3.2 Wireless Smart Contact Lenses

A smart contact lens can be used as an excellent interface between the human body and an electronic device for wearable healthcare applications (59). Despite wide investigations of smart contact lenses for diagnostic applications, hitherto there has been no report on electrically controlled drug delivery in combination with real-time biometric analysis.

Smart contact lenses were developed for both continuous glucose monitoring and the treatment of diabetic retinopathy. The smart contact lens device, built on a biocompatible polymer, contains ultrathin, flexible electrical circuits and a microcontroller chip for real-time electrochemical biosensing, on-demand controlled drug delivery, wireless power management, and data communication.

In diabetic rabbit models, tear glucose levels could be measured and compared by the conventional invasive blood glucose tests. So the feasibility of smart contact lenses for noninvasive and continuous diabetic diagnosis and diabetic retinopathy therapy was confirmed (59).

1.7.3.3 Capacitive Sensing

Certain medical conditions or states can be characterized by slow changes of a physiological property, e.g., a blood glucose concentration, over long periods of time by infrequent, short time scale events (60). Such physiological properties can be measured periodically.

An implanted or wearable device can be employed to provide a continuous or near-continuous measurement of such physiological properties. Such implantable or wearable devices can be battery powered or powered by radio frequency energy or other wireless energy sources. Furthermore, such devices can be configured to indicate measured physiological properties wirelessly, e.g., by using an RFID antenna and transmitter or a Bluetooth antenna and transmitter (60).

An eye-mountable device has been described (60). The eye-mountable device includes a substrate, a capacitance sensor disposed proximate to the substrate, and a controller disposed proximate to the substrate. The substrate is at least partially embedded within a shaped polymeric material.

The capacitance sensor includes at least two sensor electrodes. At least one sensor electrode of the two sensor electrodes is operable to carry out an additional function. The controller is communicatively coupled to at least two of the sensor electrodes. The controller is configured to receive data indicative of a change in mutual capacitance between the two sensor electrodes. The controller is further configured to detect an eye-related movement based on the change in mutual capacitance being greater than a threshold capacitance. The controller is also configured to produce a signal in response to detecting the eye-related movement.

The method of measuring includes receiving data indicative of a change in mutual capacitance between at least two sensor electrodes of a capacitance sensor (60). At least one sensor electrode of these two sensor electrodes is operable to carry out an additional function. The capacitance sensor is disposed proximate to a substrate. The substrate is at least partially embedded within a shaped polymeric material. The shaped polymeric material is configured to be mounted proximate to an eye.

Such a sensor may be operable to measure a level of glucose in the tear fluid.

The method also includes detecting an eye-related movement based on the change in mutual capacitance being greater than a threshold capacitance. The method further includes producing a signal in response to detecting the eye-related movement.

The detection of the eye-related movement may be useful to trigger an electrochemical sensor reading of a glucose level or another type of sensor reading or action. For example, a detected eye-related movement may cause a display to indicate a measured value, which may relate to a value of the analyte measured by the electrochemical sensor. Alternatively, the detection of an eye-related movement may trigger a communication signal to other components of the eye-mountable device or another device.

A block diagram of such a sensor is shown in Figure 1.33.

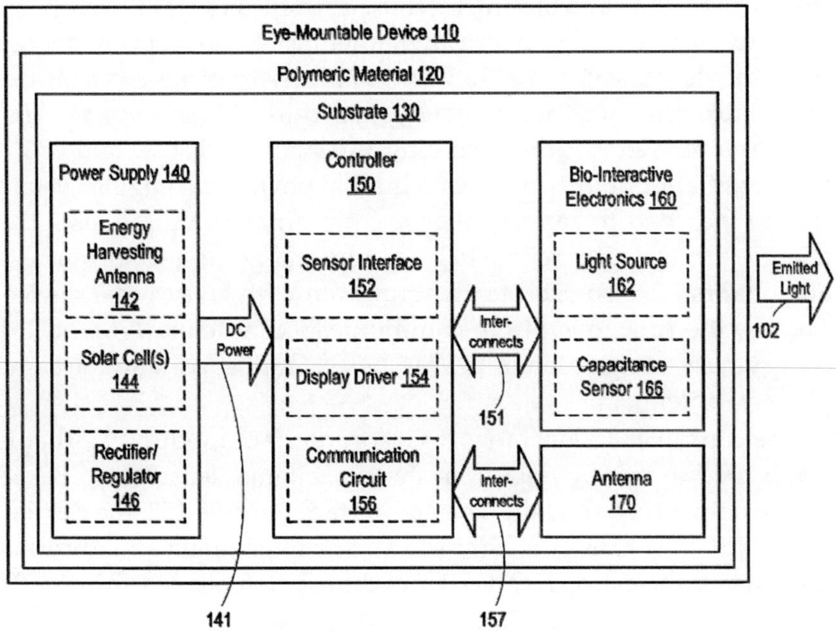

Figure 1.33 Block diagram of sensor (60).

The exposed regions of the eye-mountable device 110 are made of a polymeric material 120 formed to be contact-mounted to a corneal surface of an eye. A substrate 130 is embedded in the polymeric material 120 to provide a mounting surface for a power supply 140, a controller 150, bio-interactive electronics 160, and an antenna 170. The bio-interactive electronics 160 are operated by the controller 150. The power supply 140 supplies operating voltages to the controller 150 and/or the bio-interactive electronics 160. The antenna 170 is operated by the controller 150 to communicate information to and/or from the eye-mountable device 110, e.g., to communicate with an external device. The antenna 170, the controller 150, the power supply 140, and the bio-interactive electronics 160 can all be situated on the embedded substrate 130. Alternatively, one or more of the elements of the eye-mountable device 110 may be situated on a plurality of substrates 130 embedded within the polymeric material 120. Because the eye-mountable device 110 includes electronics and is configured to be contact-mounted to an eye, it is also referred to herein as an ophthalmic electronics platform.

The power supply 140 is configured to harvest energy to power the controller 150 and bio-interactive electronics 160. For example, a radio frequency energy harvesting antenna 142 can capture energy from incident radio radiation, for example, from an external device. Additionally or alternatively, solar cells 144 (*photovoltaic cells*) can capture energy from incoming ultraviolet, visible, and/or infrared radiation. Furthermore, an inertial power scavenging system can be included to capture energy from ambient vibrations. The energy-harvesting antenna 142 can optionally be a dual-purpose antenna that is also used to communicate with an external device. That is, the functions of the communication antenna 170 and the energy-harvesting antenna 142 can be accomplished with the same physical antenna.

The controller 150 includes a sensor interface module 152 that is configured to receive data from the capacitance sensor 166. Based on the data received by the sensor interface module 152, the display driver 154 may cause the light source 162 to generate an indication related to information received from the capacitance sensor 166 (60).

1.7.4 *Target Analyte Sensing*

Functional contact lenses for detecting at least one target analyte contain a substrate for supporting electronic components and provide a structural support for the functional contact lens (61). At least one sensing element is disposed on the substrate for sensing at least one target analyte and undergoes a physical change representing a sensed signal. Furthermore, an antenna is disposed on the substrate for transmitting the sensed signal to an external device, the antenna being coupled to the sensing element.

Target biomarkers or target analytes that may be sensed by the biosensors used in the functional contact lenses may be molecules that are within the precorneal tear, such as acids, ions, carbohydrates, proteins, enzymes, lipids, antigens, hormones, nucleic acids, small molecules, medications, and recreational drugs.

Specific compounds are collected in Table 1.19 and some hormones are shown in Figure 1.34.

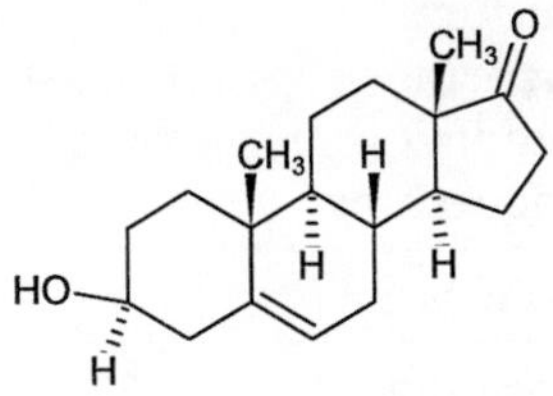

Dehydroepiandrosterone

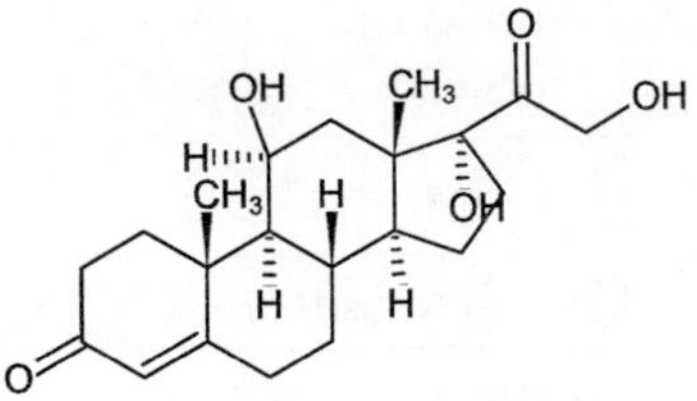

Cortisol

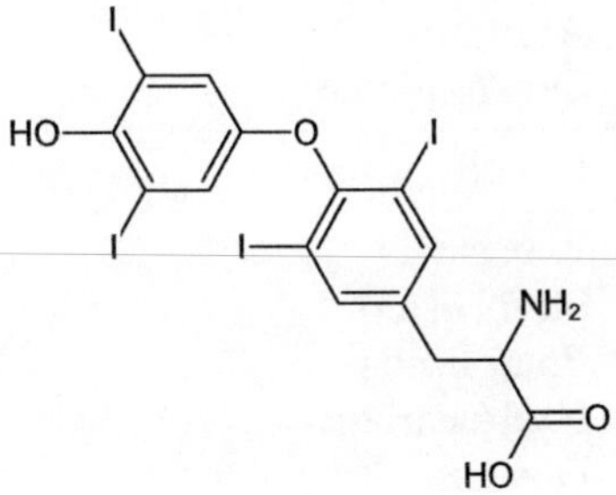

Thyroxine

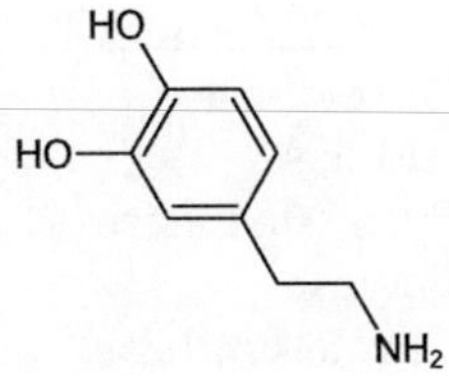

Dopamine

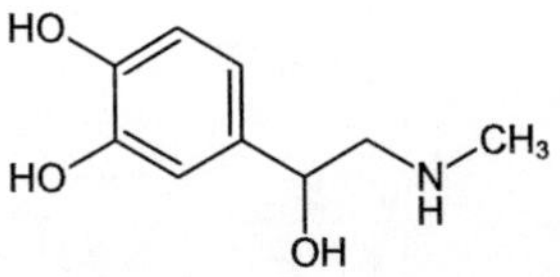

Epinephrine

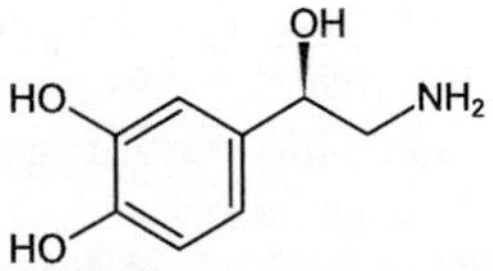

Norepinephrine

Figure 1.34 Hormones.

A schematic view of a chipless functional contact lens is shown in Figure 1.35.

Here, the functional contact lens does not have any integrated circuits or devices for processing, sensing, communication, or power. Instead, the sensing element is coupled with the antenna. The sensing element is a one-electrode system that uses a working electrode. The antenna may have one or more loops. When the antenna is

Table 1.19 Examples of target analytes (61).

Acids	Ions
Ascorbic acid Lactic acid Pyruvic acid Uric acid	Calcium Potassium Sodium Magnesium
Carbohydrates	**Proteins**
Fructose Glucose Sucrose Galactose Maltose Lactose	Lysozyme Lipocalin Cytokine Lipocalin Albumin Orosomucoid
Enzymes	**Lipids**
Hexokinase Aldolase Pyruvate kinase Enolase Citrate synthase Aconitase Phosphofructokinase Phosphoglyceratemutase Pyruvate dehydrogenase Isocitric dehydrogenase Succinate dehydrogenase Fumarase Matalate dehydrogenase Transketolase Transaldolase	Wax esters Sterol esters Polar lipids Hydrocarbons Diesters Triglycerides Free sterols Free fatty acids
Antigens	**Hormones**
Adenoviruses Staphylococcus bacteria Streptococcus bacteria Hemophilus influenza bacteria Chlamydia Gonorrhea	Cortisol Catecholamines Endorphins Insulin Dehydroepiandrosterone Thyroxine Epinephrine Dopamine

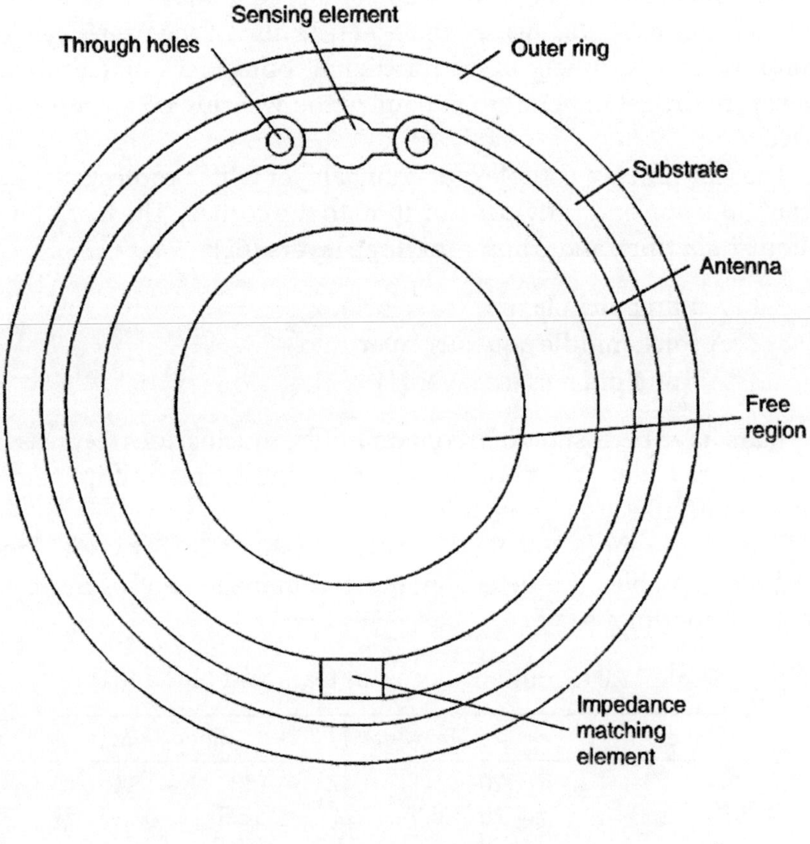

Figure 1.35 Chipless functional contact lens (61).

multilayered, then vias or through-holes may be used to vertically physically couple portions of the antenna that are on different layers of the substrate.

The sensing structure may be a biosensor, which may be an artificial enzymatic biosensor or an artificial non-enzymatic biosensor. Other types of sensors that may be used include label-free electrochemical immunoassay.

The thickness of the functional contact lens may be about 300 μm in order to reside inside the basal tear film of the user's eye for comfort. The periphery of the functional contact lens may be made of soft hydrogel material to maximize the wearing comfort for the user.

The tear film is a complex functional layer which protects the eye from infection and provides nutrition to the cornea. The tear film is about 7 μm thick and consists of three layers (62):

1. A thin mucin layer,
2. A thick middle aqueous layer, and
3. A thin lipid surface layer [1].

Tears have been shown to contain lipids, mucins, ions, proteases, immunoglobulins, catecholamines, endorphins, and multiple other small molecules (62).

The close compositional similarity, cf. Table 1.20, between blood and tears enables the detection and the management of multiple medical conditions.

Table 1.20 Common species in tears and blood (61).

Marker	Tear/[mM]			Blood/[mM]		
Na^+	120	–	165	130	–	145
K^+	20	–	42	3.5	–	-5
Ca^{2+}	0.4	–	1.1	2.0	–	2.6
Mg^{2+}	0.5	–	0.9	0.7	–	1.1
Cl^-	118	–	135	95	–	125
HCO^{3-}	20	–	26	24	–	30
Glucose	0.1	–	0.6	4	–	6
Urea	3.0	–	6.0	3.3	–	6.5
Lactate	2	–	5	0.5	–	0.8
Pyruvate	0.05	–	0.35	0.1	–	0.2
Ascorbate	0.008	–	0.04	0.04	–	0.06

A cortisol sensor has been formed using a graphene field-effect transistor that can measure cortisol concentration with a detection limit of 10 $pg\,ml^{-1}$, which is low enough to detect the cortisol concentration in human tears (63).

This soft contact lens only requires the integration of the cortisol sensor with transparent antennas and wireless communication circuits to make a smartphone the only device needed to operate the lens remotely without obstructing the wearer's view. *In-vivo* tests using live rabbits and the human pilot experiment confirmed the good biocompatibility and reliability of this lens as a noninvasive, mobile healthcare solution (63).

1.7.5 Adaptive Tuning

An augmented reality system including a source and a contact lens display can be used to project information from the contact lens display onto the retina of the wearer's eye (64). The source provides energy to the contact lens display and operates at a source frequency.

The source includes a source circuit including a conductive coil. The contact lens display includes a resonant circuit including another conductive coil and a capacitive circuit. The resonant circuit receives energy from the conductive coil of the source via a magnetic field, inductively coupling the conductive coils. The contact lens display additionally includes a feedback circuit to adjust the capacitance of the capacitive circuit to control a resonant frequency of the resonant circuit. The feedback circuit can control the capacitive circuit to maintain the resonant frequency of the resonant circuit near the source frequency as the wearer's eye blinks. The contact lens contains (64):

1. A resonant circuit including:
   (a) A first conductive coil to receive energy from an external source via inductive coupling, and
   (b) A capacitive circuit coupled parallel with the first conductive coil, the capacitive circuit having a capacitance that is adjustable to control a resonant frequency of the resonant circuit of the contact lens.
2. A contact lens display, and
3. A load coupled parallel with the first conductive coil and the capacitive circuit, the load consisting of:

(a) A projector to project images from the contact lens display towards a human retina based on data received wirelessly by the contact lens display, and
(b) An energy recovery circuit to recover energy from the resonant circuit and provide power for the projector.

A time-varying magnetic field is generated from a necklace, i.e., a source, worn about the neck of the wearer of the augmented reality system (64). The necklace includes a conductive coil and a time-varying current source, which generates a time-varying magnetic field.

The source provides energy to the contact lens display via the time-varying magnetic field, thereby resulting in wireless power transfer between the source and the contact lens displays. The contact lens display includes a resonant circuit with a conductive coil inductively coupled to the conductive coil of the necklace via the time-varying magnetic field.

The inductive coupling between the source and the resonant circuit allows energy generated by the source to be transferred to the contact lens display. The contact lens display recovers energy from the inductively coupled source and resonant circuit.

However, as the environment of the eye changes, e.g., the wearer's eye blinks, the eyeball rotates, the temperature changes, or the eyeball generates tears, the efficiency of the power transfer between the source and the resonant circuit fluctuates. Accordingly, the resonant circuit of the augmented reality system can include a tunable capacitance that can be adjusted to increase the efficiency of the power transfer.

Generally, constantly tuning the resonant circuit works to maximize the voltage across the resonant circuit and increase the efficiency of power transfer between the source and the resonant circuit. However, at times, the efficiency of power transfer is not maintained at maximum levels for any number of reasons, i.e., misalignment between the source and the contact lens display (64).

1.7.6 *Wireless Communication*

Developments in mobile communications combined with the increasing computing power have enabled significant processing and rich real-time feedback to be employed within wearable device systems (65). Advances in miniaturization have further enhanced wearables by allowing electronic devices and sensors to be located on a human in a continually shrinking footprint. For example, a wearable miniaturized device may be implemented within a contact lens to provide a variety of functions, including the ability to communicate with other peripheral accessory devices proximate to the contact lens.

A device for communicating data with a contact lens through a communication interface has been presented (65). Here, an accessory device identifies one or more wireless channels to communicate with a contact lens. The scheduling of this wireless communication is performed such that a preferred channel is selected based on noise and/or interference. A centralized scheduler, such as a Wi-Fi access point, can be used to reserve the preferred channel within the associated wireless network so that clients within the network do not use this channel.

A general illustration of a secure electronic contact lens system is shown in Figure 1.36.

The electronic contact lens contains a contact lens material, a projector and one or more electronic modules (65). The contact lens material may be made from relatively rigid material that provides sufficient structural support for mounting the electronic modules on the contact lens. The projector may be a femtoprojector, which is a miniaturized video or image projector, and may couple with the modules that are electronic circuits and devices, such as a transceiver circuit, sensors, and data processing devices. The modules may perform a variety of functions, some or all of which may require the wireless communication of data between an accessory device and the contact lens.

A schematic diagram of an accessory device is shown in Figure 1.37.

The accessory device may remain in a sleep mode to reduce the energy consumption and wake up to start communication with the contact lens via a communication interface. When the accessory device wakes up, the interference determination unit may scan the communication environment to map the noise and interference within its environment.

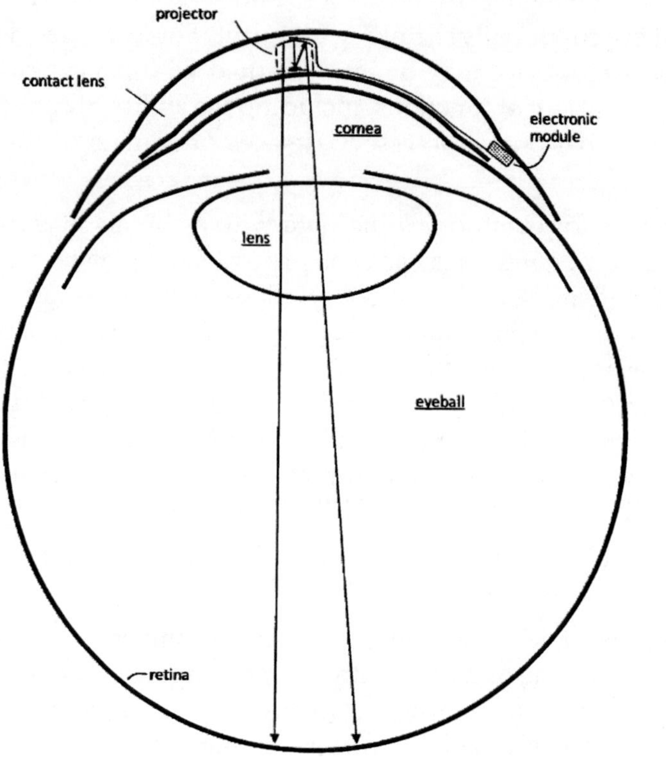

Figure 1.36 Electronic contact lens system (65).

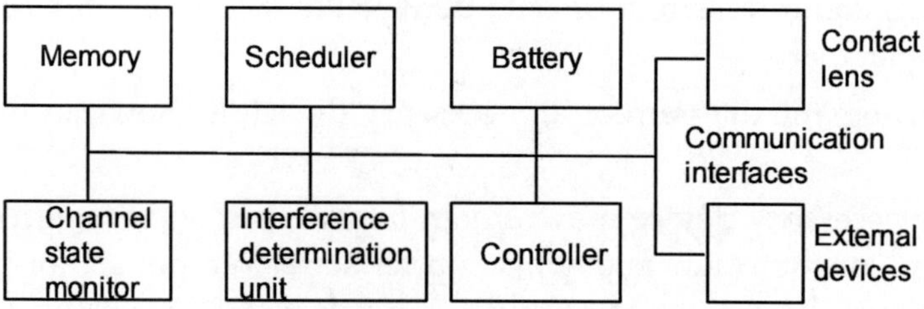

Figure 1.37 Accessory device (65).

Also, the interference determination unit may check for each Wi-Fi channel, whether the channel is not being used using signals received through a communication interface, and, if the channel is used, the interference determination unit may determine the level of interference in the channel.

The scheduler within the accessory device schedules the transmission of data on both the uplink and downlink of the wireless channel. This scheduling will depend on various factors, including the interference pattern within the channel and the sensitivity of the data to be transmitted. In performing this scheduling operation, a coordinator may communicate with other external device(s) that are also transmitting wireless signals within the area (65).

The accessory device may have multiple antennas to do the signal transmission.

The scheduler may select a channel and send the data to the contact lens in two steps:

1. The Wi-Fi manager 320 may send a control signal through the control channel, where the control data may notify the contact lens of the time slot during which the contact lens can anticipate data from the accessory device, and
2. The Wi-Fi manager may transmit data to the contact lens through the data channel during the notified time slot. In embodiments, the control channel may be the same as the data channel.

Figure 1.38 shows a schematic diagram of a beam pattern generated by an accessory device.

The accessory device may have multiple transmission antennas and use the antennas in such a way that the transmission signals from the antennas experience constructive interference at particular angles.

The left lobe shows the power distribution of the left downlink signal over an azimuthal angle, where the lobe is directed toward the left contact lens. Using the beamforming technique, the accessory device may use less power to deliver the signal compared to a omnidirectional transmission. The same is true for the right eye. Alternatively, the accessory device may generate one lobe for each contact lens at a point in time if both contact lenses cannot be cov-

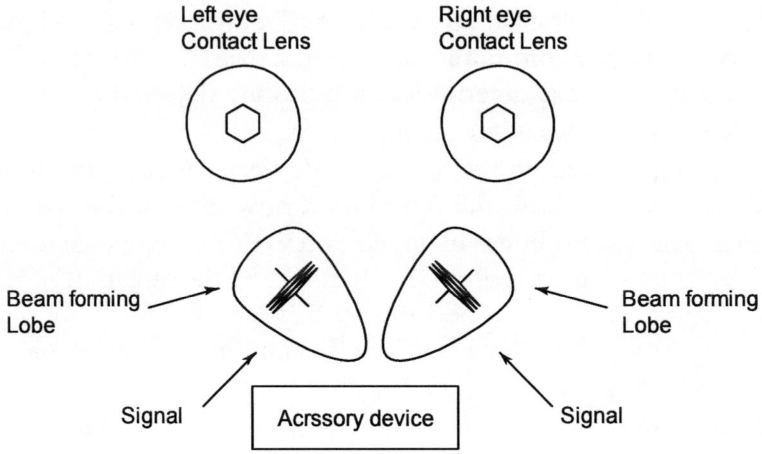

Figure 1.38 Beam pattern generated by an accessory device (65).

ered by one lobe. Otherwise, the accessory device may generate a single lobe to transmit a signal to both contact lenses (65).

1.7.7 Glucose Biosensors

Glucose detection using a biosensor can be categorized into either optical or electrochemical methods (66). Examples are shown in Table 1.21.

Table 1.21 Glucose biosensors developed for contact lenses (66).

Mode of detection	Glucose sensor	Reader	Reference
Fluorescence	Boronic acid, Concanavalin A	External detector	(67)
Colorimetric	Boronic acid	Color chart	(68)
Fluorescence	Boronic acid	Photodetector	(69)
Fluorescence, colorimetric	Boronic acid, Concanavalin A	External detector	(70)
Fluorescence, colorimetric	Boronic acid, Concanavalin A	Photodetector	(71)
Fluorescence	Boronic acid, Concanavalin A	External detector	(72)
Light emitted	Boronic acid	Photodetector	(73)
Electrochemical	Boronic acid	Electrode	(74)
Fluorescence, luminescence	Boronic acid	External reader	(75)
Light emitted	Boronic acid	Smartphone	(76)
Optical	Boronic acid	External reader	(77)
Absorbance	Concanavalin A	Spectrophotomer	(78)
Fluorescence	Concanavalin A	Handheld photofluorometer	(79)
Fluorescence	Concanavalin A	Handheld photofluorometer	(80)
Electrochemical	Glucose oxidase	Electrode	(81)
Electrochemical	Glucose oxidase	Handheld reader or smartphone	(82)
Electrochemical	Glucose oxidase	External receiver	(83)
Electrochemical	Glucose oxidase	On lens display	(84)
Electrochemical	Metal oxides	External receiver	(61)

Boronic acids are reversibly binding to carbohydrates. They show unique optical properties when bound to glucose, resulting in a colorimetric change or a change of fluorescence.

Concanavalin A is a lectin or carbohydrate binding protein. It is originally extracted from the jack bean (*Canavalia ensiformis*). In the absence of glucose, concanavalin is bound to a ligand, such as fluorescein-labeled dextran, and so shows a minimal fluorescence. In the presence of glucose, the ligand is displaced and instead glucose binds to concanavalin, resulting in an increase of the fluorescence.

1.7.8 Cancer Detection

It was found that the tear film is well suited to the detection of cancer biomarkers since it is less biologically complex than blood (85, 86). In addition, tear sampling is a relatively noninvasive method in comparison to the collection of blood samples (66).

In the early work in the detection of cancer in a tear film, the presence of a tear film protein called lacryglobin was detected (87).

Lacryglobin has similarities to mammaglobins upregulated in breast cancer (88). Lacryglobin is present in the tear film of patients with colon, lung, breast and prostate cancer, as well as patients with a family history of cancer (89).

Time-of-flight mass spectroscopy was used to compare the tear film of cancer patients and healthy controls, identifying differences in 20 tear film biomarkers (90–92).

1.8 Scleral Contact Lenses

Modern scleral lenses are a potentially life-changing technology (93). The growth in the scleral lens market and in the number of speciality contact lens practitioners in recent years (94) demonstrates their utility in the therapeutic treatment of ocular surface disease, the visual restoration of the irregular cornea, and the correction of simple refractive errors in patients who have normal corneas.

A theoretical model based on the Harvitt-Bonanno criteria was first developed in 2012 (95) and was soon followed by another model using a mathematical approach (96).

Both models suggested that scleral lenses may generate hypoxia-related stress in the central cornea if the lens material has limited oxygen permeability and if the lens is designed such that it has increased thickness and results in increased tear fluid reservoir thickness. Consequently, both authors recommended that scleral lenses should be manufactured in high oxygen permeable materials (D_k greater than 150), with a maximum thickness of 250 μm and fitted with a central tear reservoir of 200 μm or less.

For these models some questions were raised about their clinical significance (97), in particular in light of the favorable outcomes regularly encountered in clinical practice under adverse conditions (98, 99).

It was also suggested that in the absence of obvious clinical signs, any hypoxia-related ocular sequelae would be minimal. However, clinical studies were needed to determine a correct approach (93). Hypoxia is a condition in which the body or a region of the body is deprived of adequate oxygen supply at the tissue level (100).

Any scleral lens can and should be fitted to minimize a hypoxia-related stress. This means limiting lens thickness, increasing material oxygen permeability, limiting the tear reservoir depth, and, for certain patients, limiting the wearing time (93).

It was suggested that the lens thickness, and not the tear reservoir depth, was the significant factor leading to hypoxia-related stress (101).

However, this is contrary to current theoretical modeling derived from the understanding of the permeability of fluids and solutions (102). However, if true, it is imperative to collaborate with manufacturers to produce thinner lens designs (93).

1.8.1 *Fabrication of Scleral Lenses*

Soft contact lenses have been limited in their ability to correct irregular refractive errors because the soft lens material is deforming and takes the irregular shape of the underlying eye (103).

Furthermore, rigid contact lenses have been limited in their use due to the complexity of fitting the lenses, the difficulty in reducing or eliminating the pressure of the rigid lens material on the underlying eye, and the problems relating to stagnation of the post-lens tear environment.

Hybrid bimodulus contact lenses with a rigid gas-permeable material surrounded by a soft flexible material have solved some of the problems associated with rigid and soft contact lenses. However, lens flexure and the need to fit the lenses with a curvature that is substantially shorter in radius of curvature than the underlying eye are challenges to hybrid lens success. Furthermore, in some cases the soft peripheral skirt of hybrid lenses fails to elevate the rigid central zone above the cornea and the resultant bearing of the rigid gas-permeable material on the cornea is reported to cause discomfort and lens intolerance.

Because of the uncurving nature of the sclera near the limbus, often neither a concave downward curve nor an uncurved landing zone can contact the sclera at just inside the lens edge to accomplish appropriate edge lift without impinging on the more peripheral sclera to the point of penetration. Such landing zone curves may cause the entire lens to be supported further above the cornea and contact the sclera with a very narrow support zone.

To solve the abovementioned problems, scleral lenses have been designed. These lenses have a central zone and at least one peripheral zone defined by an angle (103).

Here, a peripheral zone is curved in either a concave or convex direction or is uncurved. In an exemplary embodiment, the angle for a plurality of semi-meridians or transverse sections can be varied to create a transverse undulation of a peripheral zone. These scleral lenses do not demonstrate excessive pressure on the sclera and allow for post-lens tear exchange.

The lens can be made from fluorosilicon acrylate, silicon acrylate, polymethylmethacrylate, a silicon hydrogel, or other suitable materials. In general, any gas-permeable, biocompatible material is suitable for use herein (103).

An illustration of a lens manufacturing system is shown in Figure 1.39.

The lens manufacturing system includes a controller, a lathe, and a scleral lens (103). The controller is a computer system, such as a data processing system. The controller causes the lathe to apply a modification to the scleral lens.

The tool is an object that removes material from the scleral lens when the lathe is rotating the scleral lens and the tool is in contact with the posterior surface of the scleral lens. The controller also causes the tool to move in some directions according to instructions

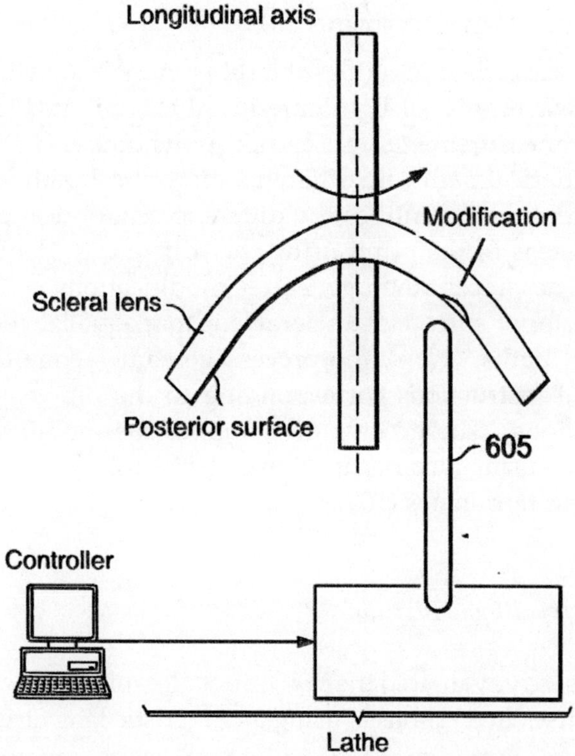

Figure 1.39 Lens manufacturing system (103).

received by the controller. For example, the controller may receive a plurality of computer numeric control codes.

The process of fabrication starts by generating an optical coherence tomography scan of an eye to identify the shape of the eye. The process then generates dimensions for the scleral portion of the scleral lens that correspond to the shape of the eye. Then the process performs wavefront aberrometry on the eye to identify alterations to wavefronts of light traveling through the areas of the pupil of the eye to generate measurements (103).

The process then identifies the differences in optical paths traveled by wavefronts of light entering the pupil at different points using the measurements and Zernike polynomials (104). The differences in optical paths are differences in optical path lengths (103). The process then identifies the differences in optical paths for additional areas of the pupil using the differences identified for the points. The process then generates modifications to the thickness of the posterior surface of a scleral lens that equalize the differences in optical paths. Next, the process generates computer numeric controlled instructions corresponding to the dimensions and the modifications. The process then applies the modifications to the scleral lens using a computer numeric controlled lathe. Thereafter, the process terminates (103).

1.8.2 Scleral Lens Fitting

A recent study evaluated the practitioner learning curve when fitting scleral lenses in 85 subjects using a diagnostic lens fitting (105).

Here, scleral lenses were fit by a single licensed optometrist who did not have a history of clinical experience fitting scleral lenses. In this study, the initial trial lens was selected based on the manufacturer's guidelines, severity of the corneal condition and clinical evaluation of the ocular surface.

Corneal topography, simulated keratometry measurements and corneal asphericity of the flat and steep corneal meridians were analyzed for each group. Objective measurements, such as scleral topography and ocular coherence tomography, were not utilized (106).

1.8.3 *Ocular Drug Delivery Systems*

Eyedrops are the standard method for delivering medications to the front of the eye. Eyedrops for long-term use have the same risk of any chronic patient-administered medication, requiring treatment adherence (107).

Scleral lenses provide a protected environment in which the corneal surface is continuously bathed in preservative-free fluid. These lenses are inherently stable to provide lasting ocular penetration of a drug. The main detriments of scleral lenses include handling and cost, along with a variety of other complications (108).

Various publications have reported the use of scleral lenses as ocular drug delivery systems. Treatment of corneal infiltrates with topical fortified non-preserved antibiotics in the bowl of the lens has been described (109).

Also, preservative-free antibiotics in the bowl of the scleral lens worn continuously to treat persistent epithelial defects has been reported (110).

Anti-VEGF agents have been used in the bowl of a scleral lens to treat corneal neovascularization (111, 112). The use of stem cells on a scleral lens carrier for management of a chemical burn in an animal model has also been described (113).

1.9 Multifocal Contact Lenses

The state of scientific publications concerning the multifocal contact lenses field was analyzed with a bibliometric study (114). A total of 346 articles were published between 1960 and 2019. The growth in the number of publications matches the exponential adjustment slightly better. The duplication time was found to be 13.2 years.

So, the research on multifocal contact lenses is seeing exponential growth, without evidence of having reached a saturation point. The main countries for scientific production in this field are the United States and Australia (114).

1.9.1 *Bifocal Contact Lenses*

Bifocal lenses contain two or more areas or zones, with different optical powers, typically including a far-power optic zone for distance vision, and a near-power optic zone for near or close-up vision (115). The two zones may be subdivided into additional power zones, in which case a lens may be called a multifocal lens. Previously known multifocal lenses have been limited by known manufacturing apparatus, such as, for example, cast-molding, standard lathing or tooling technology, and injection molding technology.

The retinal image and the visual percept that results from it are dependent upon the light that enters an eye through the entrance pupil. In order for a bifocal contact lens to function properly, the entrance pupil must be covered at least partly or, more effectively, completely by the distance-power zone of a lens when an eye observes a distant object, and covered at least partly or, more effectively, completely by a near-power zone of a lens when an eye observes a near object. This function may be accomplished by the principle of alternating vision in which a shifting action or translation of a contact lens is made to occur in order to place one or the other zones in front of the entrance pupil as an eye alternates between viewing distant and near objects (115).

Alternatively, a principle known as simultaneous vision may be utilized whereby a lens is designed and fitted in such a way as to position part or all of both the far- and near-power zones in front of the entrance pupil at the same time so that each contributes to the retinal image simultaneously. There is little or no translation required with this type of lens; however, as a consequence two images are seen simultaneously, compromising vision.

Generally, the two types of conventional bifocal contact lenses are segmented and concentric. Segmented bifocal contact lenses or translating contact lenses, generally have two or more divided optical power zones. A far-power zone is usually the upper zone and a near-power zone is usually the lower zone. With such a translating lens, a far-power zone of a lens is in front of the entrance pupil of an eye in straight-ahead gaze, while in downward gaze, the add power or near-power zone of a lens is over the entrance pupil. Concentric bifocal contact lenses generally have a central power zone and one or more annular power zones that function usually, but not always, by the simultaneous vision principle. It is recognized that these lenses do not provide good vision for both distance and near viewing, and are only worn successfully by those who are willing to accept less than optimal vision (115).

The effective use of a bifocal contact lens requires the translation of an ocular system between vision surfaces when an eye changes from gazing at an object at a distance to gazing at a nearby object. Alternatively, there may be a desire to have a translating multi-focal contact lens that may have one or more intermediate-power zones in addition to far-power and near-power optic zones. Such a translating contact lens may have to have an ability to control and optimize the amount of movement of a lens when the pupil translates from distance vision, to intermediate vision, to near vision, or any combination thereof (115).

1.9.2 Silicone Hydrogels

A contact lens product has been described that includes a multifocal contact lens and a buffer solution (21). The multifocal contact lens is immersed in the buffer solution. The buffer solution is a cycloplegic agent. The cycloplegic agent is favorable to relax the ciliary muscle and reduce the probability of drug side effects.

The multifocal contact lens includes a central region and at least one annular region. The annular region concentrically surrounds the central region, wherein a diopter of the annular region is different from a diopter of the central region.

Also, the multifocal contact lens can include a blue-light blocking agent. Therefore, the multifocal contact lens can block high--energy blue lights, and the probability that the retina hurt by the blue lights can be reduced. The blue-light blocking agent can be 4-(phenyldiazenyl) phenyl methacrylate. 4-(Phenyldiazenyl) phenyl methacrylate is shown in Figure 1.40.

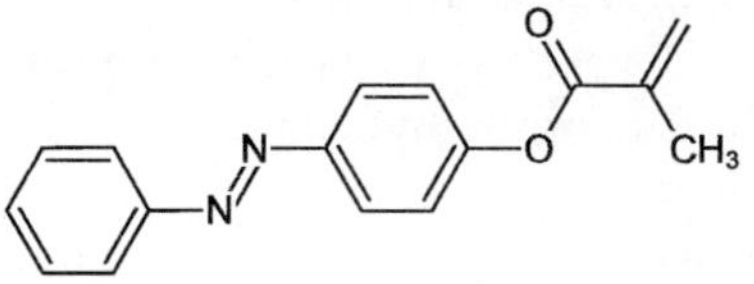

Figure 1.40 4-(Phenyldiazenyl) phenyl methacrylate.

However, the composition may contain a UV-blocking agent. Therefore, the multifocal contact lens can block high-energy UV lights, and the probability that the retina hurt by the UV lights can be reduced. UV-blocking agents are collected in Table 1.22 and shown in Figure 1.41.

Table 1.22 UV-blocking agents (21).

Compound
4-Methacryloxy-2-hydroxybenzophenone
2-Phenylethyl acrylate
2-Phenylethyl methacrylate
2-(2′-Hydroxy-5′-methacryloxyethylphenyl)-2*H*-benzotriazole
2-(4-Benzoyl-3-hydroxyphenoxy)ethyl acrylate

The multifocal contact lens is made from a silicone hydrogel or hydrogel. The silicone hydrogel can be a contact lens material, classified as Group V by the U.S. Food and Drug Administration (116, 117), such as Balafilcon A, Comfilcon A, Efrofilcon A, Enfilcon A, Galyfilcon A, Lotrafilcon A, Lotrafilcon B, Narafilcon A, Narafilcon B, Senofilcon A, Delefilcon A and Somofilcon A.

The monomers for a composition for manufacturing the silicone hydrogel are shown in Table 1.23 and in Figure 1.42.

Table 1.23 Silicone monomers (21).

Compound
2-Hydroxyethyl methacrylate
3-Methacryloxypropyltris(trimethylsiloxy) silane
2-Hydroxy-2-methyl-propiophenone *N*-Vinyl-2-pyrrolidinone
N,N-Dimethyl acrylamide
Ethylene glycol dimethacrylate
3-(3-Methacryloxy-2-hydroxypropoxy)propyl-bis(trimethylsiloxy)methylsilane
Isopropyl alcohol
Methacrylic acid

A composition for manufacturing a hydrogel is listed in Table 1.24.

So, the multifocal contact lens can block UV lights by adding 2-(2′-hydroxy-5′-methacryloxyethylphenyl)-2*H*-benzotriazole.

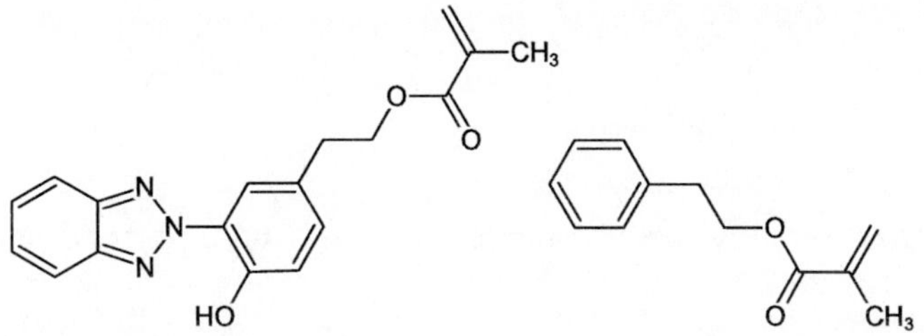

2-(2′-Hydroxy-5′-methacryloxy ethylphenyl)-2*H*-benzotriazole

2-Phenylethyl methacrylate

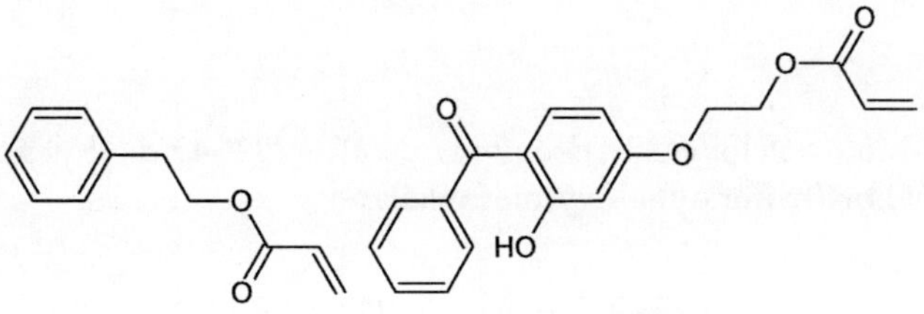

2-Phenylethyl acrylate

2-(4-Benzoyl-3-hydroxyphenoxy) ethyl acrylate

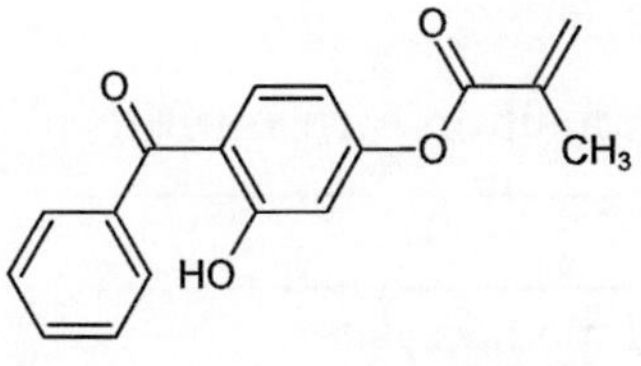

4-Methacryloxy-2-hydroxybenzophenone

Figure 1.41 UV-blocking agents.

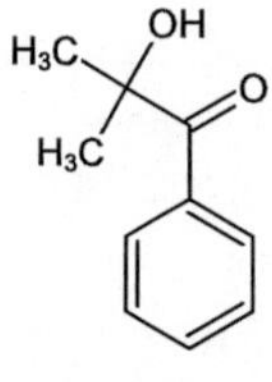

2-Hydroxy-2-methyl-propiophenone

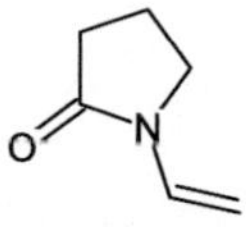

N-Vinyl-2-pyrrolidinone

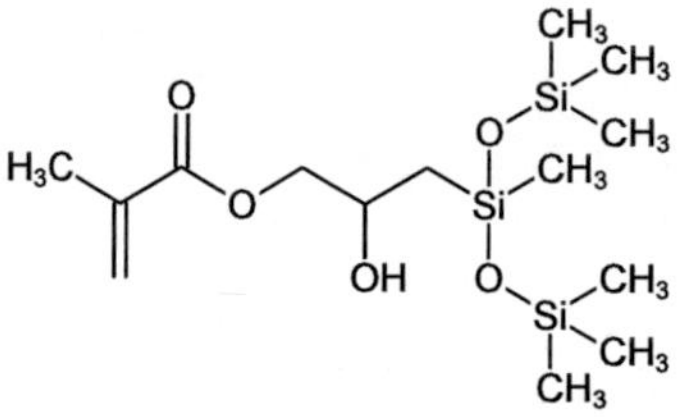

3-(3-Methacryloxy-2-hydroxypropoxy) propyl bis(trimethylsiloxy)methylsilane

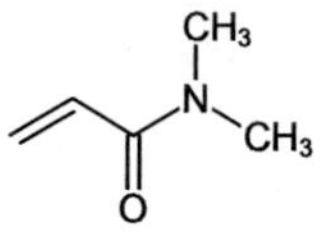

N,N-Dimethyl acrylamide

Figure 1.42 Silicone monomers.

Table 1.24 Composition for a multifocal contact lens (21).

Ingredient	Content/[%]
2-Hydroxyethyl methacrylate	82.0
2-(2′-Hydroxy-5′-methacryloxyethylphenyl)-2H-benzo triazole	1.2
Ethylene glycol dimethacrylate	0.4
2-Hydroxy-2-methyl-propiophenone	0.5
Glycerol	13.5
Trimethylol propane trimethacrylate	0.2
Methacrylic acid	2.2

1.9.3 *Non-Silicone Hydrogels*

Non-silicon-containing hydrogel compositions contain monomers or monomer mixtures which are polymerized to form non-silicon-containing soft or hydrogel contact lens products in the mold assembly comprised of the two mold members or halves (31). Monomers for these types are collected in Table 1.25. Some of these compounds are also shown in Figure 1.43.

Table 1.25 Monomers for non-silicone hydrogels (31).

Monomer	Monomer
Methyl acrylate	2-Hydroxyethyl methacrylate
Methyl methacrylate	2-Hydroxyethyl acrylate
N-Vinyl pyrrolidone	*N*-vinyl acrylamide
2-Hydroxypropyl methacrylate	Isobutyl methacrylate
Styrene	Ethoxyethyl methacrylate
Dimethylamino ethyl acrylate	Glycidyl methacrylate
Diacetone acrylamide	Vinyl acetate
Acrylamide	Hydroxytrimethylene acrylate
Methoxyethyl methacrylate	Acrylic acid
Methacrylic acid	Glycerol methacrylate
Methoxy triethylene glycol methacrylate	

The non-silicon-containing precursor compositions preferably contain a small amount of a crosslinking agent, usually from 0.05% to 2% and most frequently from 0.05 to 1.0%, of a diester or triester. Examples of representative crosslinking agents are collected in Table 1.26 and shown in Figure 1.44.

Typical crosslinking agents may have at least two ethylenically unsaturated double bonds.

The non-silicon-containing precursor compositions generally also include a catalyst, usually from about 0.05% to 1% of a free radical catalyst. Typical examples of such catalysts are shown in Table 1.27 and in Figure 1.45.

The polymerization of the monomer or monomer mixture in the mold assembly is preferably carried out by exposing the composition to polymerization-initiating conditions (31). The preferred technique is to include initiators in the composition which work upon exposure to thermal radiation, and exposing the composition to thermal radiation of an intensity and duration effective to initiate

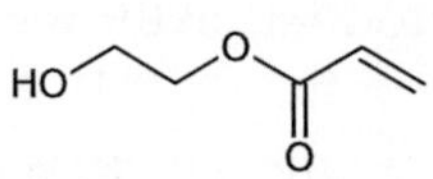

2-Hydroxyethyl acrylate

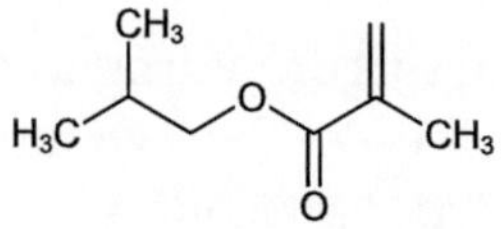

Isobutyl methacrylate

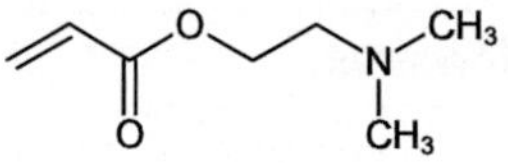

Dimethylamino ethyl acrylate

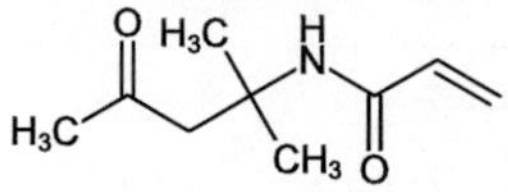

Diacetone acrylamide

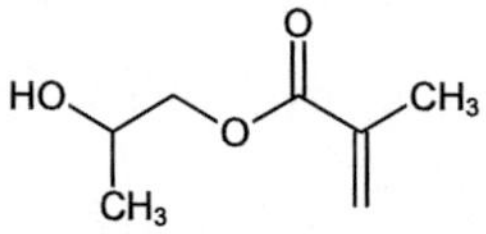

2-Hydroxypropyl methacrylate

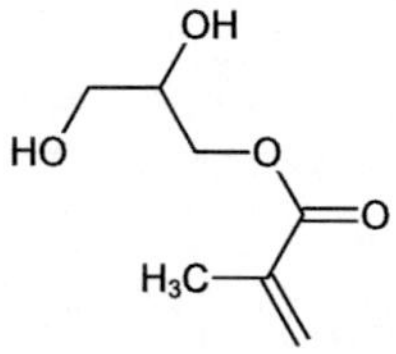

Glycerol methacrylate

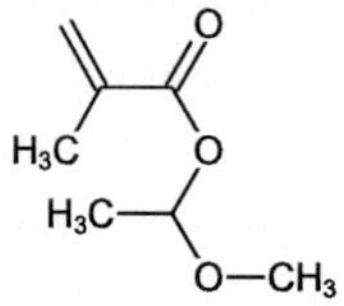

Methoxyethyl methacrylate

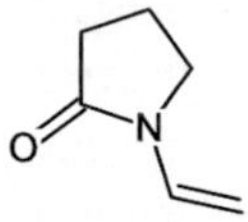

N-Vinyl pyrrolidone

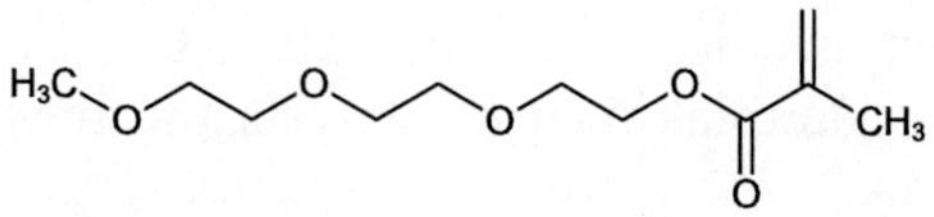

Methoxy triethylene glycol methacrylate

Figure 1.43 Monomers for non-silicone hydrogels.

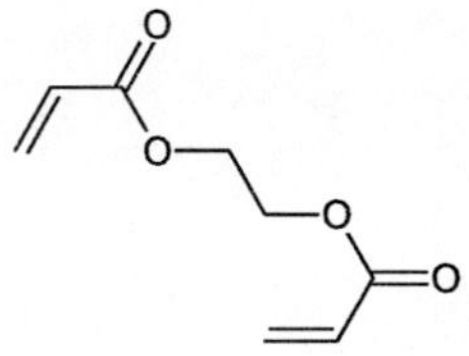

Ethylene glycol diacrylate

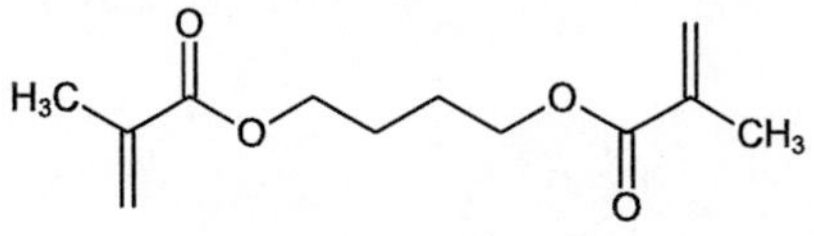

1,4-Butylene dimethacrylate

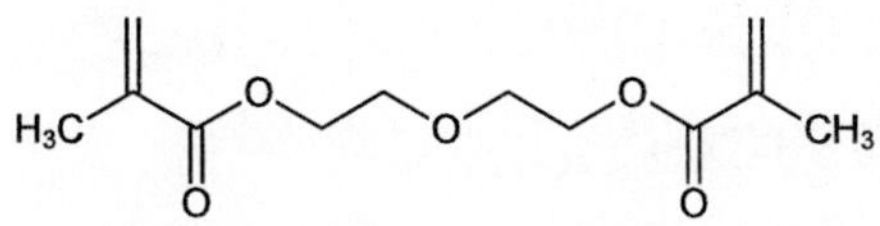

Diethylene glycol dimethacrylate

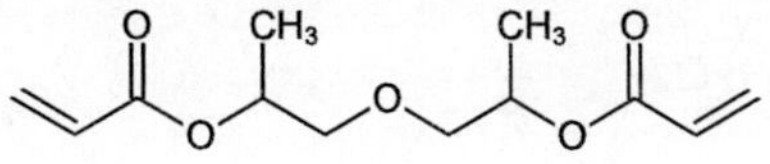

Dipropylene glycol diacrylate

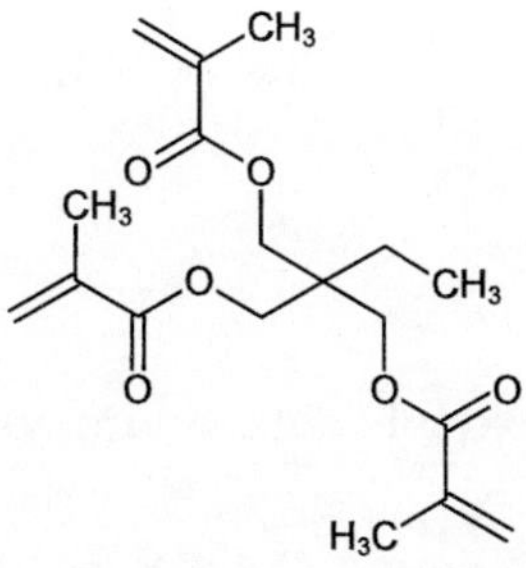

Trimethylol propane trimethacrylate

Figure 1.44 Crosslinking agents.

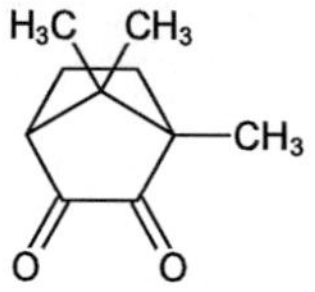

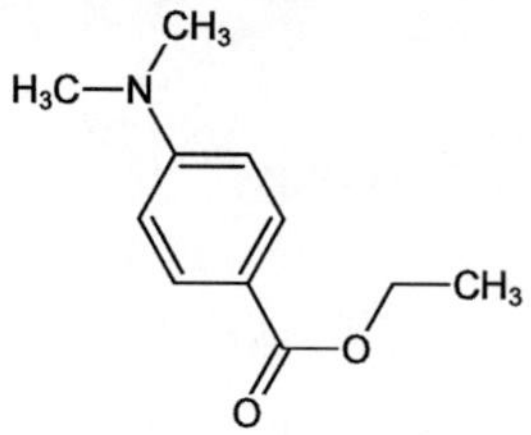

Camphorquinone Ethyl-4-(*N*,*N*-dimethyl-amino)benzoate

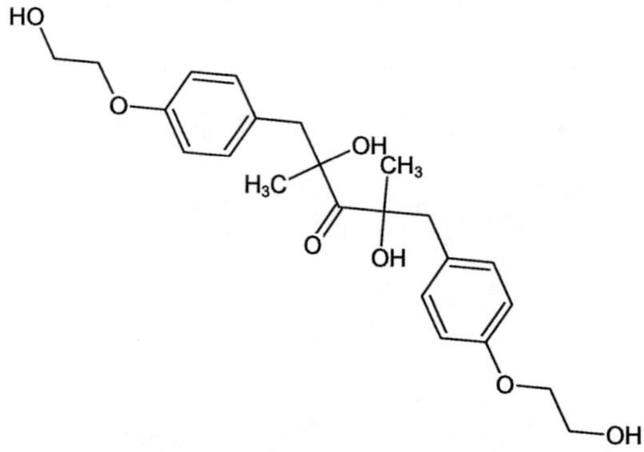

4-(2-Hydroxyethoxy)phenyl-2-hydroxy-2-propyl-ketone

Figure 1.45 Catalysts.

Table 1.26 Crosslinking agents for non-silicone hydrogels (31).

Monomer	
Ethylene glycol diacrylate	1,2-Butylene dimethacrylate
1,3-Butylene dimethacrylate	1,4-Butylene dimethacrylate
Propylene glycol diacrylate	Propylene glycol dimethacrylate
Diethylene glycol dimethacrylate	Dipropylene glycol dimethacrylate
Diethylene glycol diacrylate	Dipropylene glycol diacrylate
Glycerine trimethacrylate	Trimethylol propane triacrylate
Ethylene glycol dimethacrylate	
Trimethylol propane trimethacrylate	

Table 1.27 Free radical catalysts and initiators (31).

Initiators	Catalysts
Lauroyl peroxide	Ethyl-4-(*N*,*N*-dimethyl-amino)benzoate
Isopropyl percarbonate	Camphorquinone
Benzoyl peroxide	4-(2-Hydroxyethoxy)phenyl-2-hydroxyl-2-propyl ketone

polymerization and to allow the polymerization of the composition to proceed to form a polymerized contact lens product.

After polymerization of the lens precursor composition, the mold assembly can be demolded, the polymerized contact lens product can be delensed from one of the mold members, either the female or male mold member, the delensed contact lens product can then be inspected and packaged in a packaging solution and sterilized. In certain embodiments, such as silicone-containing hydrogel contact lenses, the delensed contact lens product can be extracted and hydrated prior to packaging the lenses in a packaging solution (31).

1.9.4 Tilted-Wear Type Contact Lenses

For the purpose of correcting presbyopia, it is widely known to prescribe multifocal contact lenses, such as bifocal lenses having multiple diopter power regions, and specifically a distance region provided as a first diopter power regions and a near region provided as a second diopter power region having more positive additional diopter power than that of the distance region. A multifocal contact lens has been described having a plurality of diopter power regions (118).

The tilted-wear type contact lens contains an optical zone situated in a lens center section, with a first diopter power region and a second diopter power region having a lens diopter power that is more positive than that of the first diopter power region (118).

Here, the contact lens has a lens profile that is axisymmetric with respect to a symmetrical meridian defined by one diametrical line of the optical zone; a superficial center of at least one of the first diopter power regions and the second diopter power region is decentered on the symmetrical meridian against a geometric center of the optical zone; a circumferential positioning member is provided to afford stable positions in a lens circumferential direction when worn in an eye, an orthogonal meridian that is orthogonal to the symmetrical meridian is tilted by a prescribed angle with respect to the vertical line of the eye. The circumferential positioning member is adapted to give rise to a first stable state in which, with the lens placed in a right eye, the orthogonal meridian is tilted by a first tilt angle in the circumferential direction relative to the vertical line of the eye, and to a second stable state in which, with the lens placed in a left eye with an orientation thereof flipped vertically from that when worn in the right eye, the orthogonal meridian is tilted relative to the vertical line of the eye by a second tilt angle to an opposite side in the circumferential direction from the first tilt angle; and a visible indicator mark is provided for identifying normal position and flipped position in relation to the orientation in a lens vertical direction (118).

1.9.5 *Neutral Density Filters*

The effect of wearing neutral density filters with different transmittance levels over multifocal contact lenses on pupil size, visual functions and the dynamic accommodative response under daylight conditions in early presbyopes was investigated (119).

There was no effect of the optical conditions on the accommodative response. However, there was a significant effect on the fixation distance.

So, the results of the study demonstrated that wearing neutral density filters over multifocal contact lenses was enough to induce a pupil size variation. However, pupil size changes induced by tinted lenses may not improve distance vision while wearing multifocal contact lenses under brightly illuminated conditions.

In addition, neutral density filters with less than 50% of visible light transmittance have a negative effect on distance visual acuity. Anecdotal suggestions to improve distance by enlarging the pupil when wearing a center-near design of a multifocal contact lens were not supported by the findings of this study. Therefore, adjustment of the prescription should be considered first for improving near or distance visual acuity with multifocal contact lens wear (119).

1.10 Augmented Reality Contact Lens Systems

General information about augmented reality technology has been provided which acts as a resource for special education researchers and teachers who are interested in using augmented reality as a learning/teaching material (120). In addition, the research that used augmented reality as a learning material in the education of individuals with special needs was examined and the obtained results revealed. In the education of individuals with special needs, 19 articles published between 2013 and 2019, addressing the use of augmented reality as learning material and meeting the inclusion criteria, were analyzed using descriptive content analysis in terms of general characteristics.

Also, the properties of augmented reality contents and development environments were examined in detail. The findings of the research indicate that the use of augmented reality as a learning material gives positive results in the education of individuals with special needs (120). Augmented reality contents are mostly used to support effective teaching strategies.

Augmented reality adds computer-generated information to a person's view of the world around them (121, 122). When the augmented reality system is displaying images, reacting to speech or receiving messages, it provides functions like that of a smartphone but in a more natural way.

1.10.1 *Electronic Contact Lenses*

An augmented reality system has been described that includes an electronic contact lens and a plurality of conductive coils to be worn, e.g., around a neck, around an arm, or on the chest of a user (121).

The conductive coils can inductively couple to the electronic contact lens by producing magnetic fields that the electronic contact lens can convert into power. A direction of the resulting magnetic field at the electronic contact lens can rotate over time, enabling the electronic contact lens to periodically form a strong inductive coupling with the plurality of conductive coils despite the orientation of the electronic contact lens.

The electronic contact lens can also output a feedback signal representative of the power produced at the electronic contact lens or an orientation signal representative of the orientation of the eye, and the magnetic fields produced by the conductive coils can be altered based on the feedback signal or orientation signal (121).

1.10.2 *Smart Contact Lenses*

In another study, methods of manufacturing smart contact lenses were detailed (122). A method of manufacturing such a smart contact lens consists of the following steps:

1. Forming a display unit. This step uses:
    (a) Forming a transparent substrate layer on a curved surface of a mold layer,
    (b) Transferring a switch array layer to the transparent substrate layer,
    (c) Transferring a light emission layer to the switch array layer, and
    (d) Forming wires to connect the devices of the switch array layer with devices of the light emission layer.
2. Mounting the display unit in a center region of a first contact lens, the mounting includes forming a groove in the center region of the first contact lens, and disposing the display unit in the groove, a size of the groove corresponding to a size of the display unit,
3. Forming a peripheral device on the first contact lens around the display unit and in connection with the display unit,

forming the peripheral device, including forming wiring around the display unit, the wiring having a circular shape and connecting the display unit to components of the peripheral device that are around the wiring, the wiring being between the display unit and the components of the peripheral device. Formation of the peripheral device consists of:
    (a) Forming a device layer on a substrate,
    (b) Separating the device layer from the substrate,
    (c) Flattening the first contact lens by pulling the first contact lens in radial directions,
    (d) Transferring the device layer to the flattened first contact lens,
    (e) Forming the wiring to connect the device layer and the display unit, and
    (f) Returning the first contact lens to an original shape.
4. Forming a passivation layer to cover the display unit and the peripheral device, and
5. Forming a material layer on the first contact lens to cover the passivation layer, the material layer making hermetic contact with the first contact lens around the passivation layer wherein the material layer covers only a front surface of the first contact lens in the first contact lens.

The method of operating the smart contact lens consists of (122):

1. Receiving information,
2. Transmitting the information to a display unit, and
3. Projecting the light directly onto a retina using the display unit.

1.10.3 Wearable Smart Contact Lenses

Wearable smart contact lenses have attracted extensive interest because of their ability to monitor physiological information and ambient information directly from eyeball and body fluids (123).

However, conventional smart contact lens systems lack efficient sensor modalities, facile fabrication process, mechanical stability, or biocompatibility. A multifunctional, high-transparency and easy-access smart contact lens system was developed (123).

Here, the serpentine mesh sensor system can be directly mounted onto the lens substrate and maintain direct contact with tears, delivering high detection sensitivity, while being mechanically robust and not interfering with either blinking or vision. This integrated contact lens sensor system and fabrication strategy allows for easy incorporation of other functional components, such as an electrode array for electroretinography, antennas for wireless communication, and power modules for future *in-vivo* exploration (123).

In such a system, MoS_2 transistors were chosen as the core sensing material because of their large surface-to-volume ratio, layered dangling-bond-free surface, tunable bandgap and charge transfer properties, and good biocompatibility (123).

1.10.4 Collimated Light-Emitting Diodes

A design of a contact lens display has been presented, which features an array of collimated light-emitting diodes and a contact lens, for the augmented reality. By building the infrastructure directly on top of the eye, the eye is allowed to move or rotate freely without the need of exit pupil expansion nor eye tracking (124). The resolution of light-emitting diodes is foveated to match with the density of cones on the retina. In this manner, the total number of pixels as well as the latency of image processing can be significantly reduced.

The proposed contact lens display consists of two components, i.e., a contact lens and a collimated light-emitting diode (LED) array. For the sake of symmetry, the contact lens, LED array and eye are center-aligned. Adjacent to the cornea is a thin layer of contact lens for fixing the refractive errors. On top of the contact lens is an array of LEDs, each pixel of which is able to emit a collimated beam of light towards the center of the eye lens. In this regard, this contact lens display is analogous to the said virtual retinal display or retinal scanning display. The major difference is that in this contact lens display, the eye can rotate freely without losing the image, thanks to the surface tension of tears that tightly adheres the whole device to the eye (124).

The idea of contact lens display is validated through the numerical simulation on Code V (Synopsys). The design wavelength was 532 *nm*.

1.11 Siloxane Macromers

Because of the hydrophobic characteristic on the surface of silicone hydrogel contact lenses, it is apt to incur a bacteria breed and eye irritation. Therefore, a composition of contact lenses has been provided that does not show the above disadvantages (125). Such a composition contains a siloxane macromer, a hydrophilic monomer, a crosslinking agent and an initiator.

The preparation of such a siloxane macromer runs as follows (125):

Preparation 1–9: First, 4.44 *g* of isophorone diisocyanate, 0.0025 *g* of dibutyltin dilaurate as the catalyst, and 40 *ml* of methylene chloride were added to a flask, and the solution stirred under a stream of nitrogen. Then, 20 *g* of α-butyl-ω-[3-(2,2-(dihydroxyethyl)butoxy)propyl]poly(dimethyl siloxane) was accurately weighed and added dropwise to the solution over about 1 *h*. After the reaction at room temperature for 12 *h*, another 0.0025 *g* of dibutyltin dilaurate and 7.2 *g* of poly(ethylene glycol) mono methacrylate were accurately weighed and added dropwise to the solution over about 1 *h*. After the reaction is conducted at room temperature for another 12 *h*, the resulting reaction product was washed with a large amount of water, and then dehydrated and filtered to obtain the raw product. Then, the methylene chloride was evaporated to obtain a siloxane macromer.

According to the method presented above, a second similar macromer was synthesized.

The hydrophilic monomer was selected from a group consisting of HEMA, *N*-vinyl-2-pyrrolidone (NVP), methacrylic acid, acrylic acid, glycidyl methacrylate, *N*-methyl acrylamide, *N,N*-dimethylacrylamide (DMA), vinyl carbamate and a combination thereof. Some of these monomers are shown in Figure 1.46

The initiator suitably used in conventional compositions for manufacturing contact lenses can be used in the corn position, such as materials shown in Table 1.28 and in Figure 1.47.

Preferably, the initiator for manufacturing contact lenses is 2,2′-azo-bis(isoheptonitrile).

For the preparation of contact lenses, both siloxane macromers, HEMA and NVP, 2,2′-Azo-bis(isoheptonitrile), and EGDMA were mixed and stirred about 1 *h*.

The contents of the contact lenses are shown in Table 1.29.

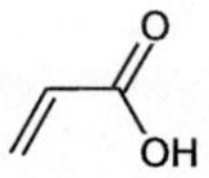

Acrylic acid

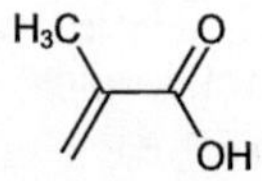

Methacrylic acid

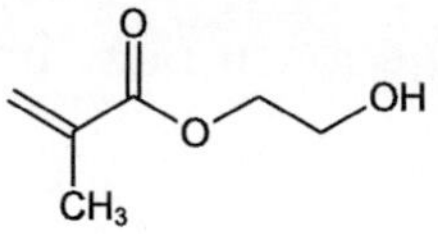

2-Hydroxyethyl methacrylate

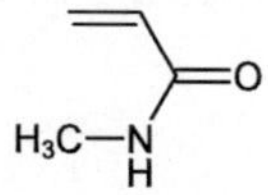

N-Methyl acrylamide

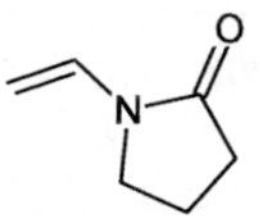

N-Vinyl-2-pyrrolidone

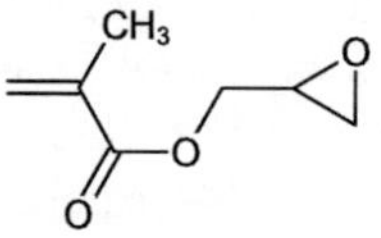

Glycidyl methacrylate

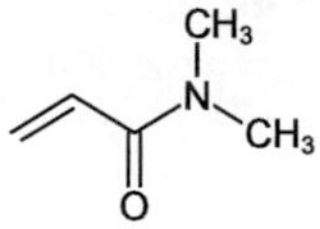

N,*N*-Dimethyl acrylamide

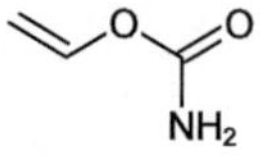

Vinyl carbamate

Figure 1.46 Hydrophilic monomers.

Table 1.28 Initiators.

Initiator
2,2′-Azo-bis(isoheptonitrile)
2,2′-Azo-bis(2,4-dimethylvaleronitrile)
2,2′-Azo-bis(2-methyl-propanenitrile)
2,2′-Azo-bis(2-methyl-butanenitrile)
Benzoyl peroxide

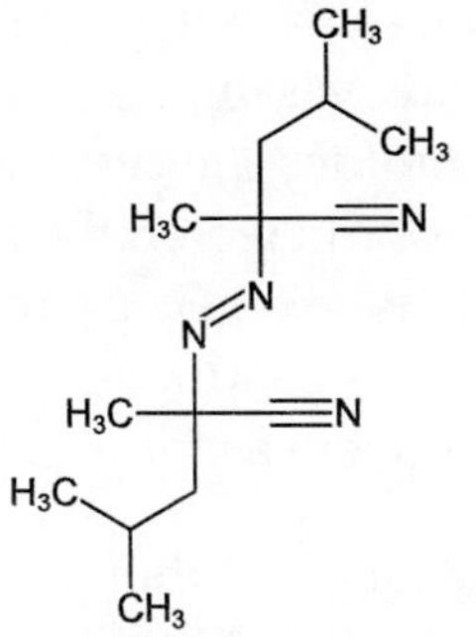

2,2′-Azo-bis(isoheptonitrile)

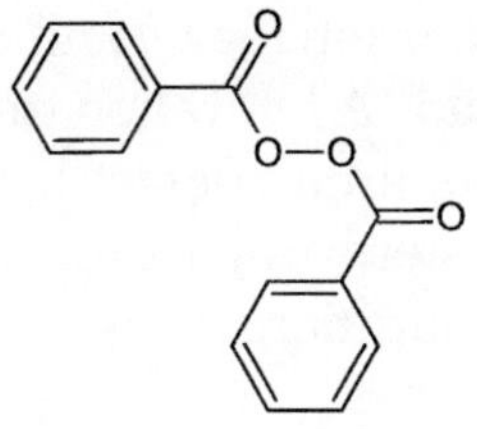

Benzoyl peroxide

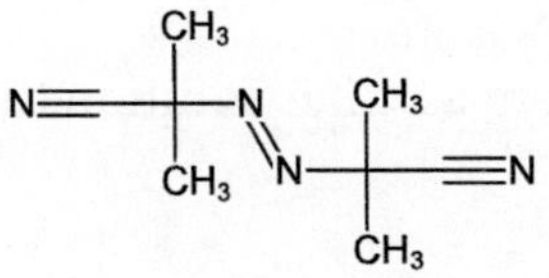

2,2′-Azobis
(2-methyl-propanenitrile)

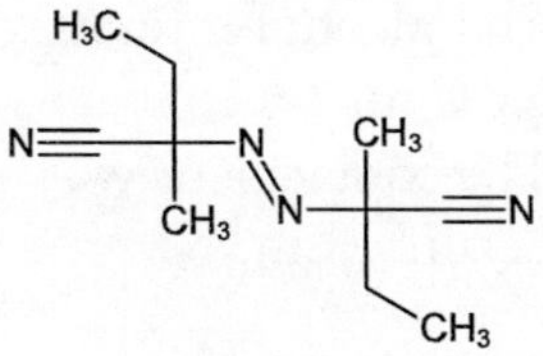

2,2′-Azobis
(2-methyl-butanenitrile)

Figure 1.47 Initiators.

Table 1.29 Contents of the contact lenses (125).

Compound	Amount/[%]
Siloxane macromer (A)	15 ~ 60
Siloxane macromer (B)	0 ~ 30
N-Vinyl-2-pyrrolidone	30 ~ 75
2-Hydroxyethyl methacrylate	0 ~ 10
Ethylene glycol dimethacrylate	0 ~ 10
2,2′-Azo-bis(isoheptonitrile)	0.1 ~ 1

Then the mixtures were injected into a mold of contact lens made of PP and heated to initiate the radical polymerization thereof at 60°C for 1 *h*, at 80°C for 2 *h*, and then at 135°C for 2 *h*. After the polymerization was completed, the mold was immersed in 80% alcohol solution for 1 *h* and the resulting molded lens was taken out of the mold. A hydration treatment was conducted on the resulting lens to obtain a contact lens with excellent oxygen permeability. Finally, a sterilizing treatment on the lens was conducted. The steps and the conditions of hydration treatment were as follows (125):

1. The mold was immersed in 80% alcohol solution for 1 *h* then the resulting molded lens was taken out of the mold.
2. The resulting polymer molded lens was then immersed in 90% alcohol solution for 1 *h*.
3. The alcohol-immersed contact lens was heated in water at 80°C for 1 *h*.
4. The contact lens was immersed in a buffer solution to obtain equilibrium.

The sterilizing treatment was done at 12°C for 30 *min* (125).

1.11.1 Silicone Urethane Polymers

It has been discovered that if polyfunctional high-molecular-weight poly(siloxane)s, whose equivalent weight is not greater than 5000 and which are connected to at least two terminal or pendant polymerizable vinyl groups through bisurethane linkages, are incorporated into a crosslinked vinyl copolymer, hard, stiff and clear products are obtained which have excellent oxygen permeability, which even at a siloxane content of greater than 50% are stiff enough to fulfill the requirements of a hard contact lens (126). Furthermore, it has been found that the siloxane-containing polymers can be made with better wettability than conventional PMMA hard lenses, despite their high poly(siloxane) content.

The poly(siloxane) macromers are obtained conveniently by a 2-step synthesis from the corresponding polyfunctional poly(siloxane)s.

In the first step, the poly(siloxane) is reacted, either in bulk or in solution, with a given amount of a diisocyanate or triisocyanate in the presence of any of the conventional catalysts. These catalysts may be tertiary amino groups containing compounds, such as triethylamine, pyridine or diaminobicyclooctane, or metal-based catalysts like dibutyltin dilaurate or stannous octoate. Some catalysts are shown in Figure 1.48. The reaction is carried out at either ambient or elevated temperatures under a dry nitrogen blanket.

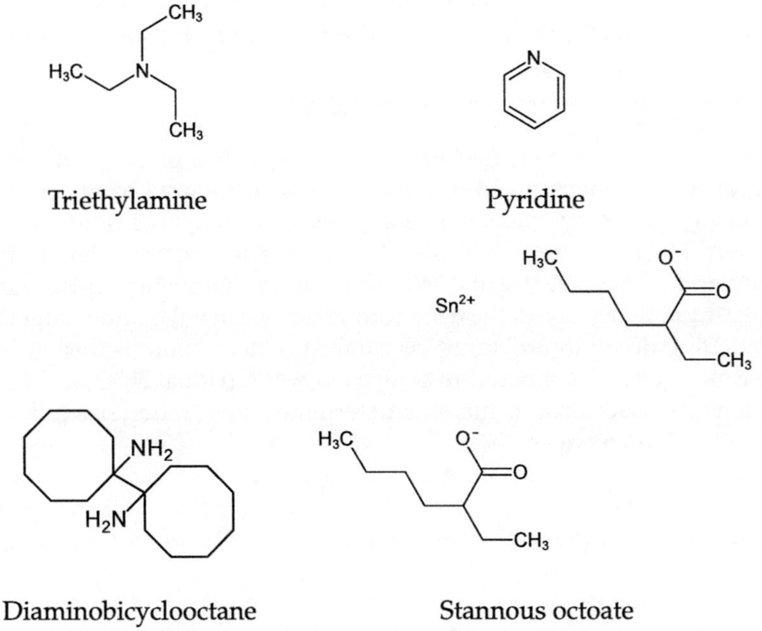

Figure 1.48 Catalysts.

The second step of the reaction consists of end-capping this poly(isocyanate) with a hydroxy or amino-functional vinyl compound, most commonly with 2-hydroxyethyl methacrylate. It is advisable to use at least a small excess of the end-capping monomer. Since it is a preferred practice to incorporate a small amount of a water-soluble monomer into the final polymer in order to achieve good wetting characteristics, a greater excess of the hydroxy or amino-functional monomer is not detrimental. The reaction proceeds at ambient or elevated temperatures over a period of several hours with no additional catalyst necessary.

The transparent, hard and oxygen-permeable polymers are produced in a final synthesis step by free radical copolymerization, either in bulk or in the presence of small amounts of solvents. The polymerization is suitably carried out with a free radical generating initiator at a temperature in the range from about 50°C to about 100°. The here used initiators are preferably peroxides or azo catalysts having a half-life at the polymerization temperature of at least 20 *min*. Also, other free radical generating mechanisms can be employed, such as X-rays, electron-beams and UV radiation.

Typical useful free radical generating initiators are shown in Table 1.30 and in Figure 1.49.

In detail, the preparation runs as follows (126):

Preparation 1–10: A 1-*l* 3-necked flask fitted with a mechanical stirrer, thermometer, condenser and nitrogen inlet is charged with 186.6 *g* (0.03 *mol*) of poly(dimethyl siloxane)-triol (Dow Corning, 1248 fluid), which had been stripped free of volatiles by passing it through a wiped-film evaporator. Then, 21.0 *g* (0.0945 *mol*) 1-isocyanatomethyl-5-isocyanato-1,3,3-trimethylcyclohexane (isophorone diisocyanate) is added together with 0.025 *g* dibutyltin dilaurate as catalyst. The mixture is then stirred under nitrogen in a temperature controlled water bath at 50°C for 5 *h*. At that time the isocyanate content as determined by titration has fallen to 1.94% (2.00% theoretical).

Then, 169.4 *g* of the poly(dimethyl siloxane triisocyanate) prepolymer is diluted with 10.2 *g* 2-hydroxyethyl methacrylate and stirred under nitrogen atmosphere at room temperature until all –N=C=O groups have been reacted as determined by the absence of the isocyanate band from the infrared spectrum. The resulting product consists of more than 99.9% methacrylate-terminated poly(siloxane) and a minor amount of HEMA-capped isophorone diisocyanate, indicating that some chain extension had taken place. This was also confirmed by GPC

Then, the preparation of the polymer samples is done as follows:

Preparation 1–11: First, 30 *g* each of the poly(siloxane) macromer prepared according to preparation 1–10 are mixed with various comonomers, as shown in Table 1.31. Then, 0.06 *g* (0.2%) 1-Hydroxycyclohexyl phenyl ketone, IRGACURE-184, (a Ciba-Geigy UV-initiator) is added and each mixture and is thoroughly degassed and then stored under nitrogen atmosphere. One portion of each mixture is used to prepare 0.1 *mm* thick films between silane-treated glass plates. A 0.1 *mm* thick Mylar film (polyester film from DuPont) is used as a spacer and the mold is held together by clamps. The molds are exposed to UV light from a black light blue lamp (Sylvania) for 3 *h*, after which time the polymer is removed from the mold to be used for oxygen permeability measurements.

Table 1.30 Free radical generating initiators (126).

Peroxides
Isopropyl percarbonate
tert-Butyl peroctoate
Benzoyl peroxide
Lauroyl peroxide
Decanoyl peroxide
Acetyl peroxide
Succinic acid peroxide
Methyl ethyl ketone peroxide
tert-Butyl peroxyacetate
Propionyl peroxide
2,4-Dichlorobenzoyl peroxide
tert-Butyl peroxypivalate
Pelargonyl peroxide
2,5-Dimethyl-2,5-bis(2-ethylhexanoylperoxy)hexane
p-Chlorobenzoyl peroxide
tert-Butyl peroxybutyrate
tert-Butyl peroxymaleic acid
tert-Butyl-peroxyisopropyl carbonate
Bis(1-Hydroxycyclohexyl)peroxide
Azo compounds
2,2-Azo-bis-isobutyronitrile
2,2′-Azo-bis(2,4-dimethylvaleronitrile)
1,1′-Azo-bis(cyclohexane carbonitrile)
2,2′-Azo-bis(2,4-dimethyl-4-methoxyvaleronitrile)
Photoinitiators
Diethoxyacetophenone
1-Hydroxycyclohexyl phenyl ketone
2,2-Dimethoxy-2-phenylacetophenone
Phenothiazine
Diisopropylxanthogen disulfide
Benzoin

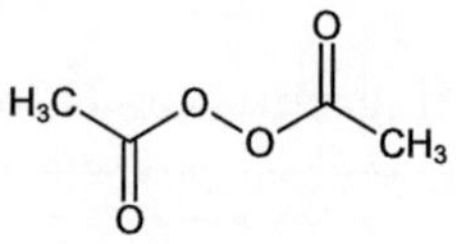

Acetyl peroxide

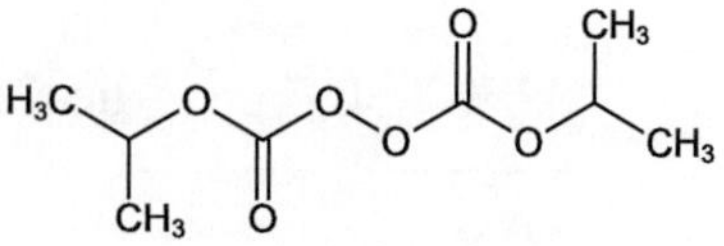

Isopropyl percarbonate

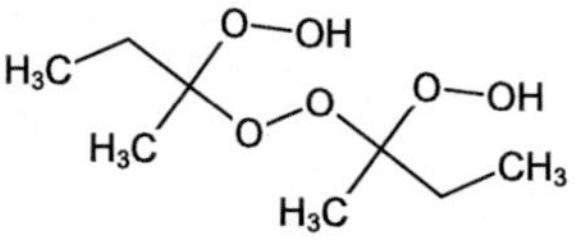

Methyl ethyl ketone peroxide

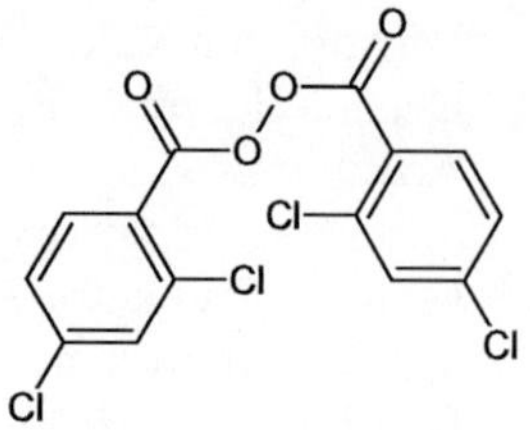

2,4-Dichlorobenzoyl peroxide

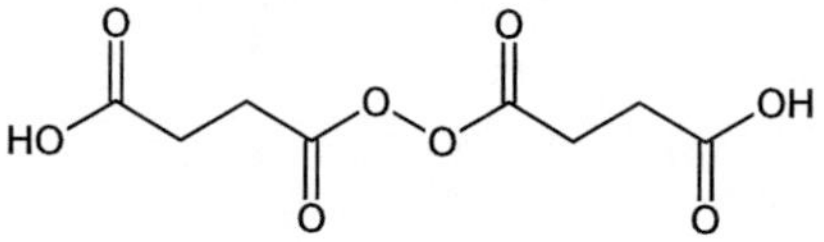

Succinic acid peroxide

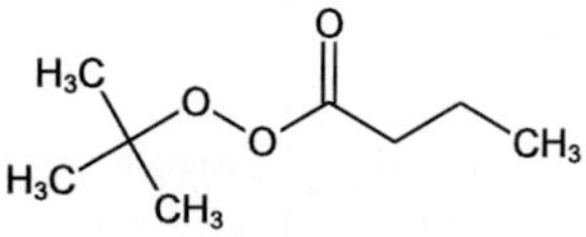

tert-Butyl peroxybutyrate

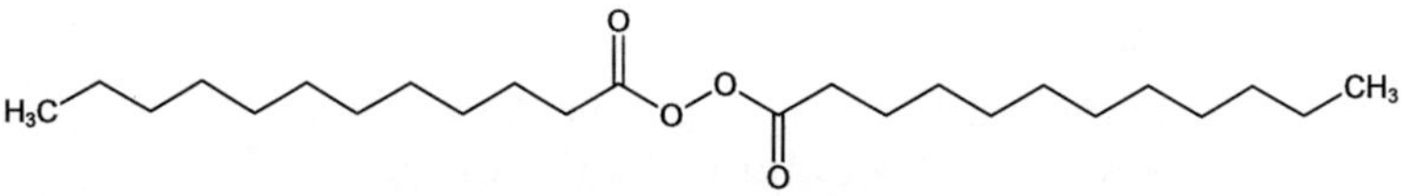

Lauroyl peroxide

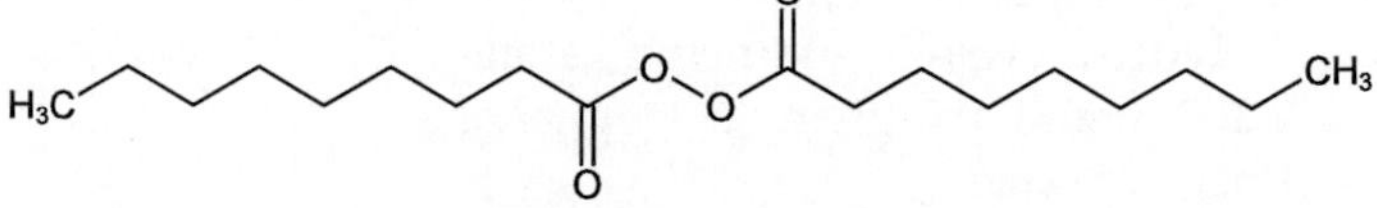

Pelargonyl peroxide

Figure 1.49 Peroxides.

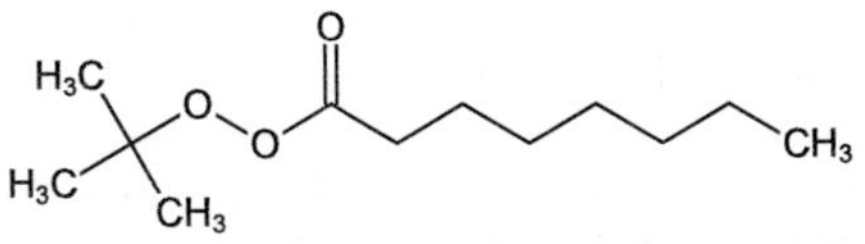

tert-Butyl peroctoate

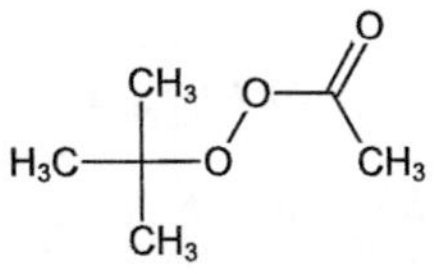

tert-Butyl peroxyacetate

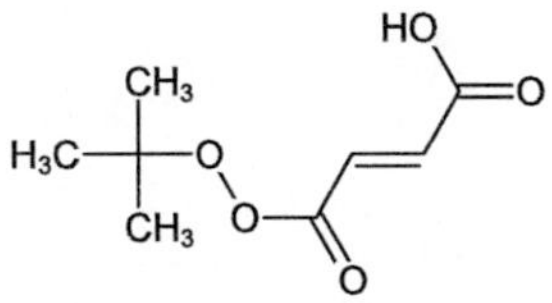

tert-Butyl peroxymaleic acid

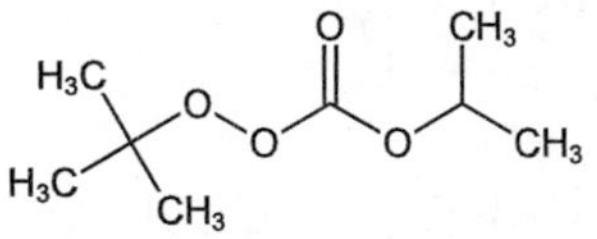

tert-Butyl-peroxyisopropyl carbonate

Figure 1.49 (cont) Peroxides.

Furfuryl methacrylate and Dicyclopentenyl-oxy-ethyl methacrylate are shown in Figure 1.50.

The hardness and clarity of these polymers are a result of two features: first, in the case of the comb-like structure of a high--molecular-weight poly(siloxane), the actual linear chain length of $-SiO(CH_3)_2-$ between crosslinks is relatively short, despite an overall high molecular weight. This short effective chain length between crosslinks restricts the mobility of the poly(siloxane) chains.

Because of their good tissue compatibility and oxygen permeability and strength and elasticity, the polymers are particularly suitable for use as intramuscular and subcutaneous implants in warm-blooded animals and as contact lens material. For the same reasons, these materials may also be fashioned into substituted blood vessels or extracorporeal shunts (126).

1.12 Oxygen-Permeable Lenses

1.12.1 Extended Wear Lenses

Contact lenses have been described that are useful as extended wear contact lenses. The lens is preferably formed by copolymerization

Table 1.31 Synthesis and properties of polymers.

Comonomer	Appearance	H_2O Content	Young's Modulus	Shore D /[*GPa*]	Hardness
Methyl methacrylate	clear	24.3	95	2.0	78
Cyclohexyl methacrylate	clear	31.0	120	1.5	79
Furfuryl methacrylate	opaque	36.3	131	–	65
Isobornyl methacrylate	clear	33.4	119	1.4	82
Methoxy-styrene	clear	30.7	118	–	79
Styrene	clear	33.2	109	1.6	75
Isobutyl methacrylate	clear	31.3	117	1.2	69

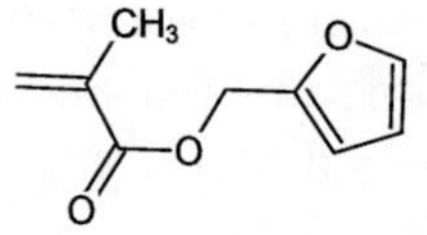

Furfuryl methacrylate

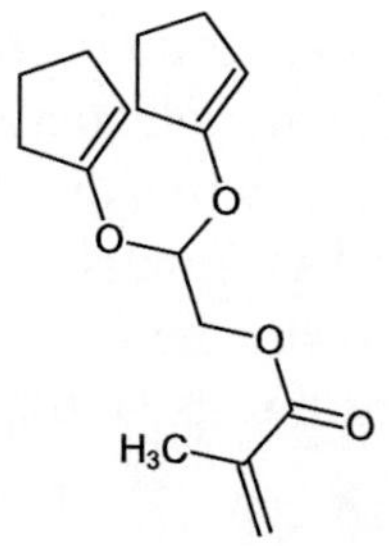

Dicyclopentenyl-oxy-ethyl methacrylate

Figure 1.50 Monomers.

Table 1.31 (cont) Synthesis and properties of polymers.

Comonomer	Appearance	H_2O Content	Young's Modulus	Shore D /[*GPa*]	Hardness
Benzyl methacrylate	clear	52.4	110	1.0	71
Methylene bornenyl methacrylate	clear	29.1	144	1.3	79
Dicyclopentenyl methacrylate	clear	33.8	123	1.6	79
Dicyclopentenyloxy-ethyl methacrylate	clear	37.7	114	1.0	69
Allyl methacrylate	clear	48.4	120	1.3	74
tert-Butyl methacrylate	clear	32.2	115	1.4	79
Methyl methacrylate:*tert*-Octyl methacrylate 1:1	clear	30.5	127	1.4	78
Isopropyl methacrylate	clear	41.0	112	1.2	77

of at least (127):

1. One oxyperm polymerizable material which is capable of polymerizing to form a polymer having a high oxygen permeability, and
2. One ionoperm polymerizable material which is capable of polymerizing to form a polymer having a high ion permeability.

Oxyperm polymerizable materials include a wide range of materials which may be polymerized to form a polymer displaying a relatively high oxygen diffusion rate therethrough. In addition, these materials must be relatively ophthalmically compatible. These oxyperm polymerizable materials include siloxane-containing macromers and monomers, fluorine-containing macromers and monomers, and carbon-carbon triple bond-containing macromers and monomers. The oxyperm macromer or monomer may also contain hydrophilic groups.

Ionoperm polymerizable materials include a wide range of materials which may be polymerized to form a polymer displaying a relatively high ion diffusion rate therethrough. In addition, these materials must be relatively ophthalmically compatible.

Oxyperm polymerizable materials and ionoperm polymerizable materials are listed in Table 1.32.

Table 1.32 Monomers (127).

Oxyperm monomers
Siloxane-containing macromers and monomers
Poly(dimethyl siloxane)s
Fluorine-containing macromers and monomers
Carbon-carbon triple bond-containing macromers
Ionoperm monomers
2-Hydroxyethyl methacrylate
Acrylamide
Methacrylamide
Dimethyl acrylamide
N-Vinyl-2-pyrrolidone

A preferred poly(siloxane) macromer segment is defined by the formula CP-PAO-DU-ALK-PDMS-ALK-DU-PAO-CP, where (127):

PDMS is a divalent poly(disubstituted siloxane),
CP is an isocyanatoalkyl acrylate or methacylate, preferably 2-isocyanatoethyl methacrylate, where the urethane group is bonded to the terminal carbon on the PAO group,
PAO is a divalent poly(oxyalkylene), which may be substituted, and is preferably a poly(ethylene oxide),
DU is a diurethane, preferably including a cyclic structure, where an oxygen of the urethane linkage is bonded to the PAO group and an oxygen of the urethane linkage is bonded to the ALK group, and
ALK is an alkylene or alkylenoxy group having at least 3 carbon atoms, preferably a branched alkylene group or an alkylenoxy group with 3 to 6 carbon atoms, and most preferably a *sec*-butyl group or an ethoxypropoxy group.

The diurethane (DU) group can be formed from a wide variety of diisocyanates or triisocyanates, including aliphatic, cycloaliphatic or aromatic poly(isocyanate)s. Examples are shown in Table 1.33 and in Figure 1.51.

The poly(siloxane) macromer may be synthesized by the following process (127):

Preparation 1–12: At about 20°C–25°C, a poly(dimethyl siloxane) dialkanol having hydroxyalkyl (e.g., hydroxy-*sec*-butyl) or hydroxyalkoxy (e.g., hydroxyethylpropoxy) end groups and having a molecular weight of preferably about 2200 *Da*, i.e., having about 28 repeating siloxane groups, is reacted with isophorone diisocyanate at about a 1:2 molar ratio, using about 0.2% weight percent dibutyltin dilaurate added as a catalyst.

The reaction is carried out for about 36 *h* to 60 *h*. To this mixture poly(ethylene glycol) (PEG) is added having a molecular weight of preferably about 500 *Da* to 700 *Da* molar ratio of about a 2:1 or 2.1:1 molar ratio with respect to the poly(dimethyl siloxane), about 0.4 to 0.5 weight percent dibutyltin dilaurate (based on PEG weight), and chloroform sufficient to ensure substantial mixture homogeneity.

This mixture is agitated for about 12 *h* to 18 *h*, then held at a temperature of about 44°C to 48°C for about 6 *h* to 10 *h*. The excess chloroform is evaporated therefrom at about room temperature to produce a composition having about 50% solids. Then, 2-isocyanatoethyl methacrylate, cf. Figure 1.52, is added to the mixture in about a 2:1 to 2.3:1 molar ratio with respect

Table 1.33 Isocyanates (127).

Diisocyanate Compounds
Ethylene diisocyanate
1,2-Diisocyanatopropane
1,3-Diisocyanatopropane
1,6-Diisocyanatohexane
1,2-Diisocyanatocyclohexane
1,3-Diisocyanatocyclohexane
1,4-Diisocyanatobenzene
Bis(4-isocyanatocyclohexyl)methane
Bis(4-isocyanatophenyl)methane
1,2-Toluene diisocyanate
1,4-Toluene diisocyanate
3,3-Dichloro-4,4′-diisocyanatobiphenyl
1,5-Diisocyanatonaphthalene
1-Isocyanatomethyl-5-isocyanato-1,3,3-trimethylcyclohexane
Isophorone diisocyanate
1,6-Diisocyanato-2,2,4-trimethylhexane
2,2′-Diisocyanatodiethyl fumarate
1,5-Diisocyanato-1-carboxypentane
Diisocyanatonaphthalenes
2,4-Diisocyanato-1-methylnaphthalene
2,7-Diisocyanato-1-methylnaphthalene
1,4-Diisocyanatomethylcyclohexane
1,3-Diisocyanato-6(7)-methylnaphthalene
Diisocyanato phenyl compounds
4,4′-Diisocyanatobiphenyl
4,4′-Diisocyanato-3,3′-dimethoxybisphenyl
3,3′-Diisocyanato-2,2′-dimethylbisphenyl
4,4′-Diisocyanato-2,2′-dimethylbisphenyl
Bis(4-isocyanatophenyl) ethane
Bis(4-isocyanatophenyl ether)
1,2-Toluene diisocyanate
1,4-Toluene diisocyanate
2,4-Toluene diisocyanate
Triisocyanate Compounds
Tris(4-isocyanatophenyl)methane
1,3,5-Tris(6-isocyanatohexyl) biuret

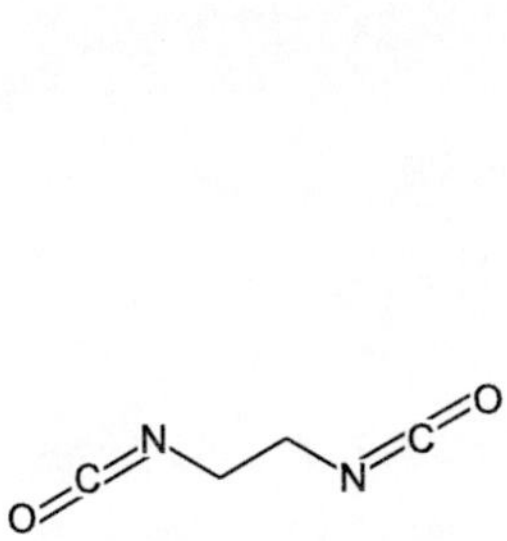

Ethylene diisocyanate

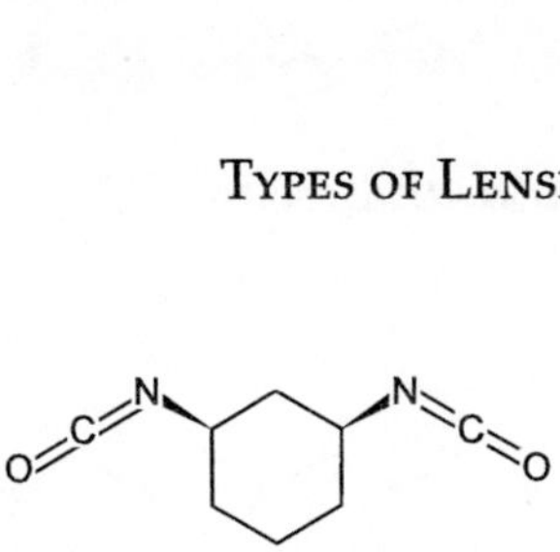

1,3-Diisocyanatocyclohexane

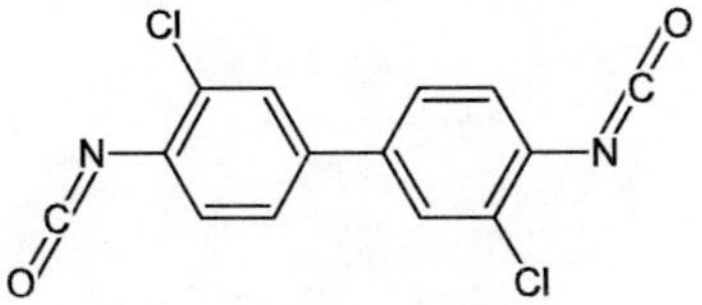

3,3-Dichloro-
4,4′-diisocyanatobiphenyl

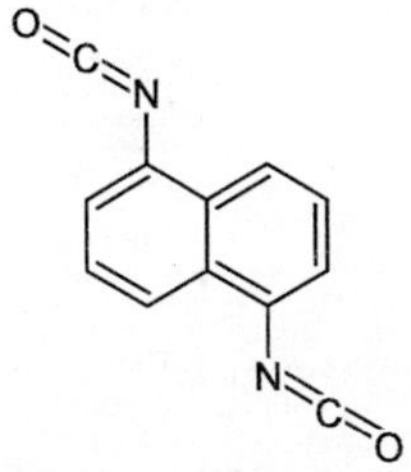

1,5-Diisocyanatonaphthalene

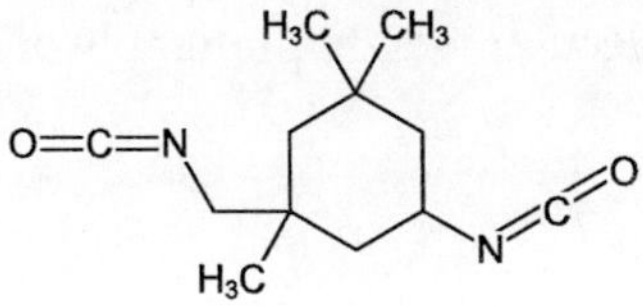

Isophorone
diisocyanate

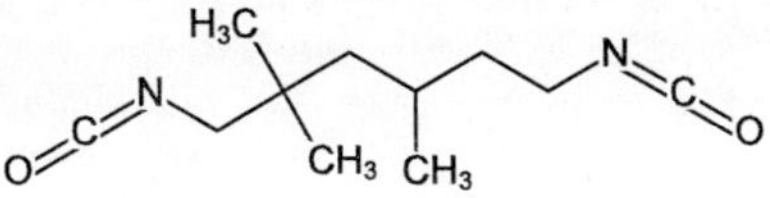

1,6-Diisocyanato-
2,2,4-trimethylhexane

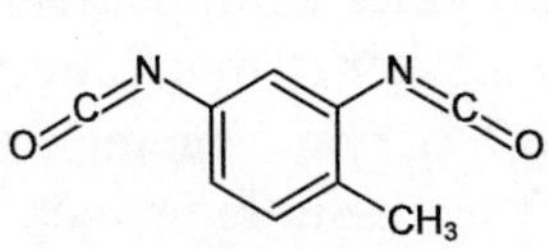

2,4-Toluene diisocyanate

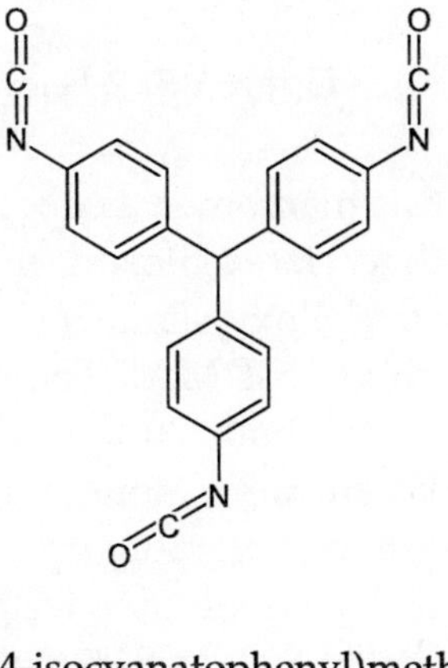

Tris(4-isocyanatophenyl)methane

Figure 1.51 Isocyanates.

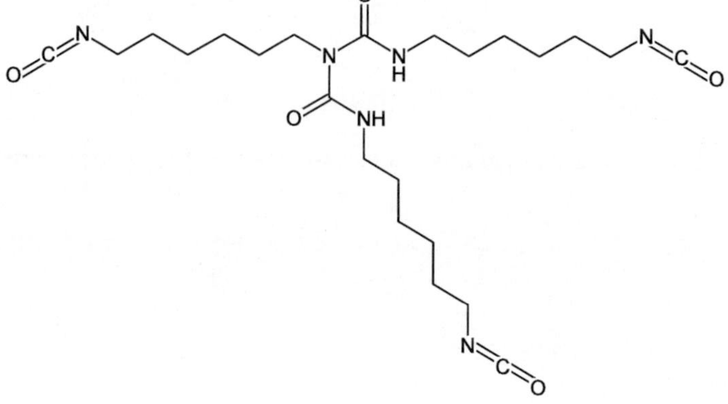

Figure 1.51 (cont) 1,3,5-Tris(6-isocyanatohexyl) biuret.

to the poly(dimethyl siloxane). The mixture is agitated at room temperature for about 15 *h* to 20 *h*. The resulting solution contains a poly(siloxane) macromer having a number average molecular weight preferably of about 3000 *Da* to 5000 *Da*.

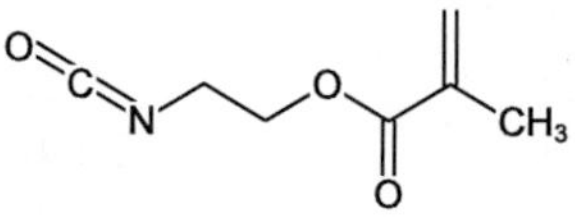

Figure 1.52 2-Isocyanatoethyl methacrylate.

From this macromer, a copolymer can be formed with an acrylated or methacrylated siloxane monomer, 3-(methacryloyloxy)propyltris(trimethylsiloxy)silane (TRIS) or HEMA, and a crosslinking agent such as EGDMA. The final copolymer composition preferably includes about 70% to 90% poly(siloxane) macromer; about 8% to 20% siloxane monomer,1% to 5% acrylate or methacrylate monomer, and preferably up to about 2% crosslinking agent, based on a total dry copolymer weight. A more preferred composition includes about 80% to 84% poly(siloxane) macromer, about 12% to 15% TRIS, about 3% to about 4% 2-hydroxyethyl methacrylate, and about 0.7% to about 1.2% EGDMA.

Then, contact lenses may be prepared from the monomer solution by applying the monomer solution to appropriate lens molds and applying sufficient UV radiation to initiate the polymerization. The UV light may be applied for a period of a few minutes to about 5 *h*, depending on the intensity of light applied. Subsequent to polymerization, the contact lens may be extracted with a solvent, e.g., isopropanol, to remove the unreacted monomers.

In summary, the preparation of the contact lenses runs as (127):

1. Contacting a poly(dialkylsiloxane) dialkanol with a diisocyanate compound in the presence of a first catalyst at conditions sufficient to cause reaction of said dialkanol with said diisocyanate, thereby forming a first mixture,
2. Contacting said first mixture with poly(alkylene glycol), a second catalyst, and sufficient solvent to ensure mixture homogeneity, thereby forming a second mixture,
3. Evaporating sufficient solvent from said second mixture to generate a third mixture having a solids content of about 40% to 60%,
4. Adding isocyanatoalkyl methacrylate to said third mixture, thereby forming a fourth mixture containing a poly(siloxane) macromer,
5. Adding to the said fourth mixture TRIS, a hydrophilic monomer, a crosslinking agent and a photoinitiator, thereby forming a fifth mixture,
6. Placing said fifth mixture into a mold, and
7. Applying sufficient radiation to copolymerize said monomers, thereby forming said polymeric material into a molded polymeric article.

1.12.2 *Structures for Thick Payloads*

Contact lenses that provide refractive vision correction are ubiquitous (128). In addition, therapeutic lenses may be used to treat eye diseases and injuries. For example, scleral contact lenses, which are supported at the periphery of the eye and form a tear-filled vault over the cornea, may be used to treat cornea disorders and severe dry eye syndrome, in addition to providing refractive vision correction.

Due to the lack of blood vessels within the human cornea, the tissue that makes up the cornea must receive oxygen through exposure to air. As such, in order to maintain corneal health, any contact lens disposed over the cornea requires at least a threshold amount of oxygen permeability to allow for a sufficient amount of oxygen from the air to reach the cornea.

Various contact lens structures may be used to perform different functions. In some cases, the contact lens structure may contain active devices, which will be referred to as active payloads. For example, an active contact lens structure may contain a sensor device for monitoring glucose concentration in tear fluid, or for measuring intraocular pressure (128). As another example, a very small projector or camera may be contained in the contact lens structure; for example, a femtoprojector as described by Deering (129, 130).

The projector may project images onto the wearer's retina, thus superimposing virtual objects onto the field of view of the wearer. Thus, when a person is wearing the contact lens display, he may see an augmented reality (128). Other active payloads may include other electronic, optical or micro-electromechanical devices.

In order to embed a payload within a contact lens, the contact lens structure may be made thicker. However, increasing the thickness reduces the oxygen transmission to the cornea. In addition, relatively impermeable materials may be used to provide a mechanical support for the payload, thus further reducing oxygen transmission to the cornea. Insufficient oxygen transmission to the cornea may quickly become intolerable for the wearer and may even lead to eye discomfort.

To avoid such problems, a contact lens structure is constructed using layers of materials with high oxygen transmissibility and low oxygen transmissibility. The low transmissibility layers have sufficient rigidity for providing an mechanical support for the active payloads, and the high transmissibility layers provide adequate oxygen transmission. The ratio of the thicknesses of the two layers changes abruptly at the boundaries between the payload and non-payload regions of the structure.

A contact lens structure is shown in Figure 1.53.

Here, the eye includes a cornea and a sclera. The scleral contact lens structure is designed to contact the sclera and to form a tear-filled vault over the cornea. The contact lens structure also includes

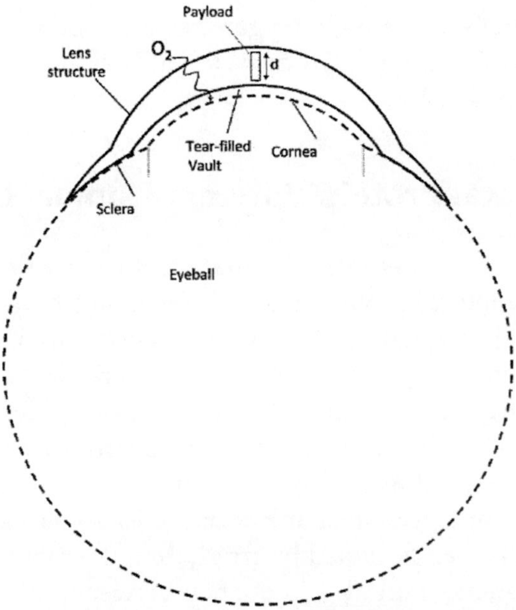

Figure 1.53 Contact lens structure (128).

a payload of thickness *d*, which may be a femtoprojector. Oxygen permeates through the lens structure to the cornea, based upon the oxygen transmissibility properties and thickness of the materials of the contact lens structure. In some embodiments, the contact lens structure may have a thickness of a few hundred microns above or below the payload in order to provide mechanical support for the payload.

In some designs, the low transmissibility material is the inner layer facing the eye. When rigid materials face the sclera, this can reduce potential slippage between the eye and the contact lens structure. Rigid gas-permeable materials may offer a good stiffness for mechanical support with some transmissibility. For example, a contact lens display with a femtoprojector may require some minimum stiffness in order to prevent the femtoprojector from shifting or moving relative to the wearer's eye, particularly if the femtoprojector is intended to always project images to the same part of the user's retina. However, rigid gas-permeable materials thicker than a few hundred microns typically do not transmit enough oxygen to maintain corneal health (128).

Poly(siloxane)s offer a high oxygen transmissibility (126). Plasma treatments may be used to promote the adhesion between the different materials (128).

1.13 Natural Protein Polymer Contact Lenses

A method has been presented for manufacturing a flexible contact lens from a biological protein material, wherein a hydrogel is made by hydrating the proteinous biological material (131). Then, a lens preform is made from the hydrogel at a temperature between ambient temperature and the temperature at which the material liquefies.

The preform is then placed in a mold made from a low-loss dielectric material and in at least two parts which, when locked together, define a three-dimensional shape and a finished lens surface state. The hydrogel is then liquefied by irradiating the mold by means of an electromagnetic field at a frequency between 10^8 and 10^{10} *Hz*. The parts of the mold are then locked together, the hydrogel is then gelified by cooling in the mold and the hydrogel is then crosslinked by contact with a crosslinking agent.

Gelatine hydrogels and collagen hydrogels can be used. A gelatine hydrogel can be prepared as follows (131):

Preparation 1–13: First, 100 *g* of powdered gelatine is swelled in 400 *ml* of deionized water for a period of 2 *h* to 11 *h*. The mixture is then heated to 60°C ± 5°C for 30 *min* to homogenize it. The so produced hydrogel showed a paste-like consistency, and was cast into preforms in the molds.

The liquefaction temperature was found to be around 70°C to 80°C. Two types of preforms were used during the tests.

Some had a central area substantially the same shape as the finished lens and an annular flange approximately 0.3 *mm* thick. They were made by injection molding, in a mold with a shape complementary to that of the preform, a quantity of hydrogel the weight of which exceeded that of the finished lens by 20 to 40%, averaging 30%.

The others were made in substantially the same shape as the finished lens. A quantity of hydrogel exceeding the weight of the finished lens by 2 to 4%, averaging 3%, was injected into a mold similar to the finished lens molds.

The prepared preforms were placed in the finished lens molds, and these molds were placed between the plates of a portable press. The press and the loaded molds were placed in a 2.45 *GHz* microwave oven. The oven was adjusted to deliver an electromagnetic power of 500 *W* and this power was applied to the molds for 30 *s*. After completion of the irradiation, the fluid under pressure was applied to the press to lock the molds. The latter were then removed from the oven and placed in an enclosure cooled to approximately 4°C.

1.14 Ultrathin Coating

Silicone rubber has great advantages as a contact lens material because of its very high oxygen permeability, softness, and excellent mechanical strength and durability (132). However, its practical application is hampered by inherent characteristics of elastomers, i.e., high tackiness and highly hydrophobic surface properties.

By applying a thin layer, e.g., 5 *nm*, of plasma polymer of methane, it was found that all these disadvantages can be eliminated without sacrificing high oxygen permeation rate, e.g., less than 15% reduction. It could be shown that the contact angle of methane plasma polymerized sheets, treated with wet oxygen plasma, decreased to 2.9 times less than that of the uncoated film.

Also, the optimization of the operational parameters to achieve this task has been investigated. It was found that under optimal conditions the coating withstood severe and repeated flexing of the contact lens (132).

The unique technique of glow discharge polymerization is capable of producing a highly crosslinked, pin-hole-free, thin film (10 *nm*) of an organic polymer. It can also be used to widely vary the properties of the polymer surface without changing the bulk properties of the substrate when the plasma polymer film is deposited.

As a cornea contact lens will inevitably be in contact with the corneal epithelium and tear fluid, the high wettability of the lens surface which can be achieved through the plasma technique plays an important role in eliminating irritation of eyes and preventing mucus material from accumulating on the surface of the lens. In addition, the thin, tightly grafted polymer film provides an effective barrier for prohibiting lipids, large molecules, and water vapor from penetrating through the lens without offsetting the optical index and high permeabilities of oxygen and carbon dioxide.

A methane plasma polymer can be formed in an extremely tight network, which not only functions as a good barrier but also provides excellent surface durability (133, 134).

The composite parameter *W/FM* is used to represent the energy supply per unit mass of the monomer, where *W* is the discharge power to maintain glow, *F* is the flow rate of the gas given in cubic centimeters per minute introduced into the system, and *M* is the molecular weight of the monomer. *W/FM* represents the energy input per unit mass of monomer, and its SI units are $J\,kg^{-1}$ (132).

The contact angle of water of a silicone rubber sheet coated by a a methane plasma polymer versus *W/FM* is shown in Figure 1.54.

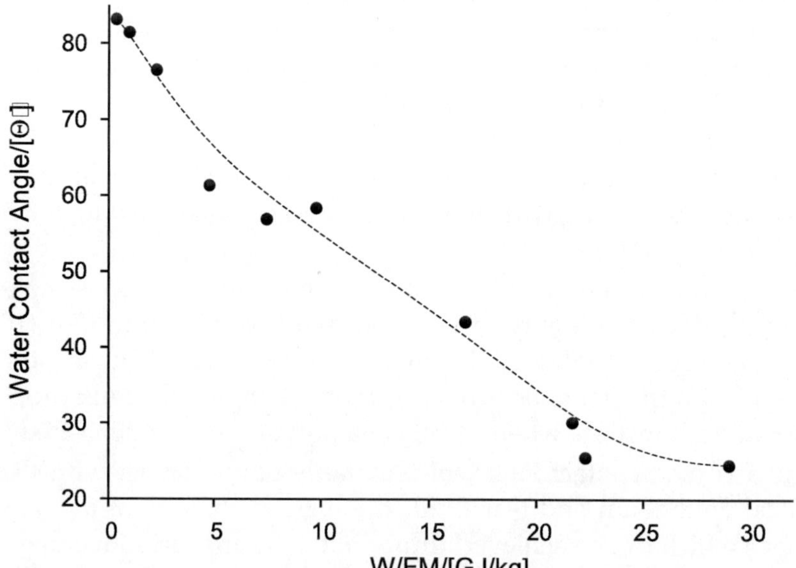

Figure 1.54 Contact angle of water of a silicone rubber sheet coated by a methane plasma polymer versus *W/FM* (132).

1.15 Anti-Biofouling Contact Lenses

1.15.1 *Phosphorylcholine*

Poly(3-trimethoxysilyl propyl methacrylate) and poly(2-methacryloyl oxyethyl phosphorylcholine) with various compositions were synthesized for the surface modification of current commercially available lenses (135).

The properties of these anti-biofouling contact lenses were investigated, which indicated that the modified contact lenses had a significant surface wettability improvement, superior antibacterial adhesion properties and resistance to protein adsorption.

The polymers can be immobilized on current commercially available lenses by a one-step modification while maintaining their excellent clinical performance and biocompatibility. The prepared anti-biofouling contact lenses may be realized in a more convenient and feasible way (135).

1.15.1.1 *Improvement of Properties*

2-Methacryloyloxyethyl phosphorylcholine (MPC) can enhance the adsorption of water molecules and is therefore used for contact lenses. The mechanical strength, anti-protein deposition, and anti-lipid adsorption effects of the addition of MPC to contact lenses was investigated (136). The contact lenses were produced by copolymerizing multiple ratios of MPC to HEMA.

Atomic force microscopy revealed that the addition of MPC increased the surface roughness. The anti-protein deposition and anti-lipid adsorption effects on poly(HEMA-MPC) polymers with various phosphorylcholine quantities were experimentally confirmed (136). Furthermore, the water content of the contact lenses was proportional to the MPC content in the polymer. The hydrated PC moiety of MPC drastically altered the network of the copolymer by inserting water molecules, which were trapped in the concave region of the surface. The addition of MPC had negative effects on all examined strength factors because of structural destabilization of the copolymer through water insertion. The anti-deposition effects of MPC were verified by examining the lysozyme and lipid adsorption abilities of the prepared contact lenses.

The results of the study revealed that MPC enhanced interactions of the poly(HEMA-MPC) copolymer with water molecules. These interactions weakened the mechanical strength of the copolymer but markedly improved the anti-adsorption property of the biomolecules. The optimal proportion of HEMA-MPC for contact lenses is in the range of 14.9% to 28.5% (136).

1.15.1.2 Surface Grafting

Biomimetic phospholipid polymers possess excellent anti-biofouling properties and biocompatibility and have the potential to play a valuable role in the surface modification of a silicone hydrogel (137). A representative phospholipid polymer containing a MPC unit can suppress nonspecific protein adsorption, can increase the cell compatibility and contributes to blood compatible biomaterials.

The synthesis of the monomers MPC and (2-methacryloyloxy)ethyl-[*N*-(2-methacryloyloxy)ethyl] phosphorylcholine is shown in Figure 1.55.

The phospholipid polymer coating on the silicone hydrogel improved its water wettability and biocompatibility, while maintaining high oxygen permeability, compared with the original silicone hydrogel. Furthermore, the prepared phospholipid-type intermolecular crosslinking agent made it possible to synthesize a 100% phospholipid polymer hydrogel that can enhance the anti-biofouling properties and biocompatibility (137).

A silicone hydrogel contact lens material has been designed for long-term ocular performance. An enhancement of this silicone hydrogel contact lens material was achieved through surface modification using a crosslinkable bioinspired 2-methacryloyloxyethyl phosphorylcholine polymer, which creates a soft surface gel layer on the silicone hydrogel base material (138).

The surface properties of this 2-methacryloyloxyethyl phosphorylcholine polymer-modified lens were characterized under hydrated condition revealing, inter alia, its unique polymer structure, excellent hydrophilicity, lubricity, and flexibility. The analysis of the 2-methacryloyloxyethyl phosphorylcholine polymer layer in a hydrated state was performed using a combination of a high-resolution environmental scanning electron microscopy and atomic force microscopy.

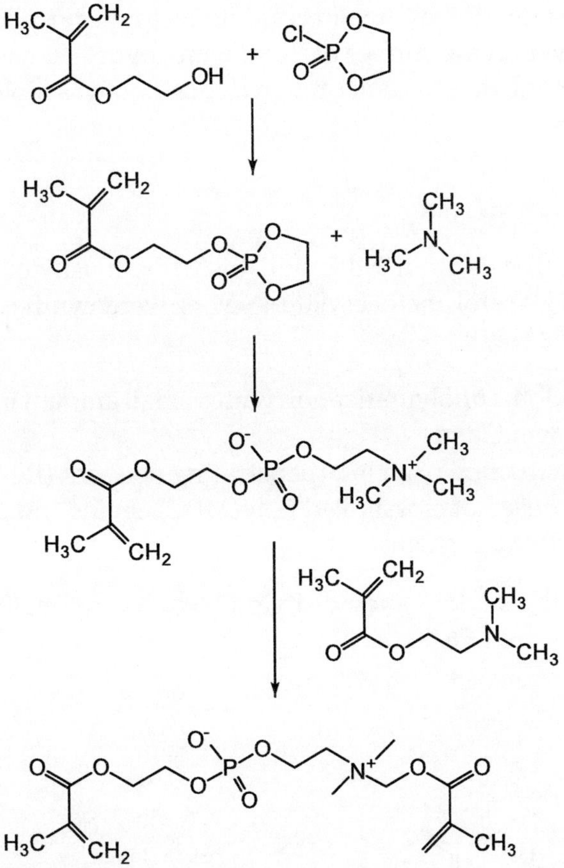

Figure 1.55 Synthesis of 2-methacryloyloxyethyl phosphorylcholine and (2-methacryloyloxy)ethyl-[*N*-(2-methacryloyloxy)ethyl] phosphorylcholine (137).

Compared to the silicone hydrogel base material, this surface had a higher captive bubble contact angle, which corresponds to higher hydrophilicity of the surface. In addition, the hydrated 2-methacryloyloxyethyl phosphorylcholine polymer layer exhibited an extremely soft surface and reduced the coefficient of friction by more than 80%. These characteristics were attributed to the hydration state of the 2-methacryloyloxyethyl phosphorylcholine polymer layer on the surface of the silicone hydrogel base material. Also, the interaction force of protein deposition was lowered on the surface (138).

1.15.1.3 Silicone Hydrogels

Silicone hydrogels from MPC and bis(trimethylsilyloxy) methylsilylpropyl glycerol methacrylate (SiMA) were synthesized using two methods (139):

1. Random copolymerization with a small amount of crosslinking agent, and
2. Construction of an interpenetrating network (IPN) structure composed of crosslinked poly(MPC) chains and crosslinked poly(SiMA) chains.

Bis(trimethylsilyloxy)methylsilylpropyl glycerol methacrylate is shown in Figure 1.56.

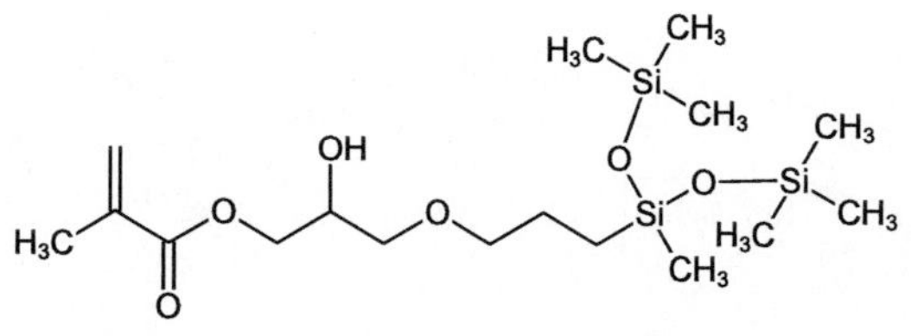

Figure 1.56 Bis(trimethylsilyloxy)methylsilylpropyl glycerol methacrylate.

The polymerization was carried out by photoreaction. The surface hydrophilicity and water absorbability of P(SiMA-co-MPC) increased with an increase in the MPC unit composition.

On the other hand, in the case of the IPN, a superhydrophilic surface was obtained by the surface enrichment of the MPC units.

The optical and mechanical properties of PSiMA-ipn-PMPC are suitable for use as a material for preparing contact lenses. In addition, the oxygen permeability remains high because of the Poly(SiMA) chains. The MPC units at the surface of the hydrogels reduce protein adsorption effectively (139).

1.15.1.4 *Grafted Silicone Hydrogels*

Silicone hydrogel contact lenses permit an increased oxygen permeability through their incorporation of siloxane functional groups (140). However, contact lens biofouling can be problematic with these materials. So, a surface modification to increase the lens compatibility is necessary for acceptable properties.

The creation of an antifouling contact lens surface was tested through a novel grafting method. A polymer incorporating MPC, cf. Figure 1.11, that is well known for its antifouling and biomimetic properties, was grafted onto the model lens surfaces using surface-initiated atom transfer radical polymerization (ATRP). This modification generated a unique double-grafted polymeric architecture designed to resist protein adsorption through the presence of a surrounding hydration layer due to the PC groups and steric repulsion due to the density of the grafted chains. The polymer was grafted from model silicone hydrogel contact lens using a four-step surface-initiated ATRP process (140).

1.15.2 2-Hydroxyethyl methacrylate

Hydrogels based on polymers from HEMA were examined for contact lenses (141).

A study was conducted on how to reduce the adsorption of protein components from tears and bacterial deposition by a surface modification of the hydrogel with different functional groups. These groups included carboxylic acid, primary amine, and quaternary ammonium.

The hydrogel was treated with a solution of sulfuric acid for partial hydrolysis of the poly(2-hydroxyethyl methacrylate) (PHEMA) ester groups to induce acid groups on the surface of the hydrogel. Carboxylic acid groups of the modified PHEMA were converted to primary amine and quaternary ammonium groups via carbodiimide chemistry.

The surface physical and chemical properties of different samples were investigated by atomic force microscopy and X-ray photoelectron spectroscopy, respectively.

A bicinchoninic acid assay was used to evaluate protein deposition from artificial tear fluid on samples. Bicinchoninic acid is shown in Figure 1.57.

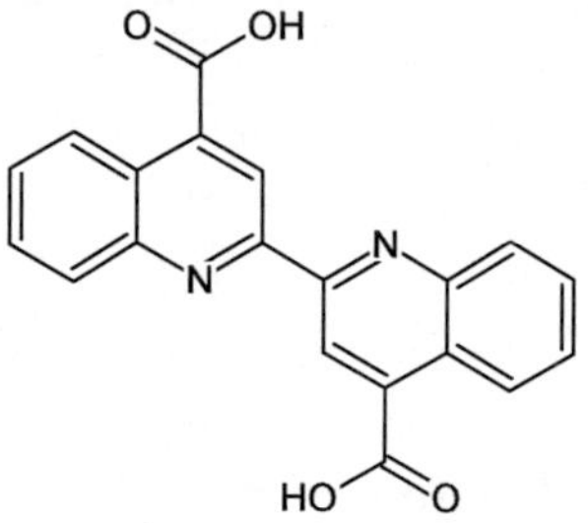

Figure 1.57 Bicinchoninic acid.

Also, the antibacterial properties of the modified hydrogels were investigated with a culture of *Staphylococcus aureus*, one of the major causes of eye infections.

The cytotoxicity test for the modified hydrogels was done by optical microscopy and immunofluorescent staining for corneal epithelial marker cytokeratin (red) and DAPI (blue) for the identification of the nuclei. Cytokeratins are keratin proteins. 4′,6-Diamidin-2-phenylindol (DAPI) is shown in Figure 1.58.

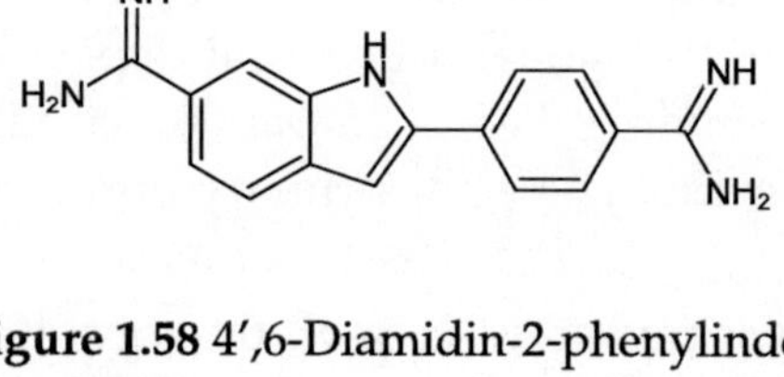

Figure 1.58 4′,6-Diamidin-2-phenylindol.

A biofouling evaluation of hydrogels is shown in Table 1.34.

The number of colony-forming units (CFUs) was determined to

Table 1.34 Protein absorption of artificial tear fluid on the surface of sample groups (141).

Modified hydrogel	Protein amount/[$\mu g\, cm^{-1}$]
Neat	26.5
Acid	22.0
Amine	12.1
Ammonium	7.2

quantify bacterial attachment to the samples. The results are shown in Table 1.35.

Table 1.35 Number of colony-forming units (141).

Modified hydrogel	Colony-forming units
Neat	264.3
Acid	354.8
Amine	57.1
Ammonium	78.6

The data of these tests showed that positively charged amine and ammonium groups efficiently resisted the protein adsorption and the bacterial deposition compared to alcohol and carboxylic acid groups (141).

1.15.3 Chitosan

Chitosan-conjugated PHEMA was used for contact lens application (142), with the aim of increasing the affinity of anionic drugs used in treatment of eye diseases. A part of a chitosan polymer is shown in Figure 1.59.

The delivery of the small molecule anionic drug, ascorbic acid, cf. Figure 1.30, from the chitosan-conjugated PHEMA was evaluated (142). The chitosan immobilization improves the drug loading efficiency and induces a sustained release of ascorbic acid. The chitosan-modified hydrogel also reduces the biofouling of tear fluid components.

The results of this study showed that surface modification by chitosan inhibits protein and bacterial deposition on the contact lens.

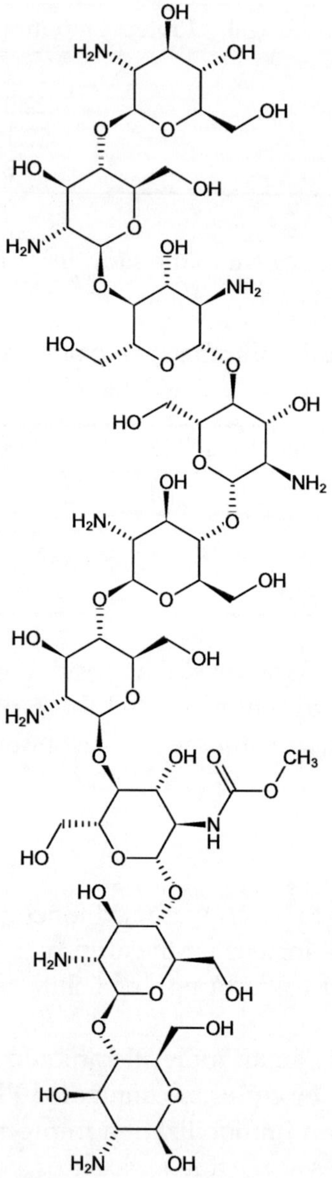

Figure 1.59 Chitosan structure.

Protein absorption analysis revealed that neat PHEMA adsorbed tear proteins at a density of 28.4±4.4 $\mu g\, cm^{-2}$, whereas the chitosan-conjugated hydrogel adsorbed tear proteins at a density of 18.5±1.8 $\mu g\, cm^{-2}$. Moreover, the neat PHEMA bacterial adhesion had a mean CFU value of 273±27. However, a significant decrease in the number of bacterial colonies was observed in the chitosan group with a CFU value of 9±6 (142).

1.16 Drug Delivery via Hydrogel Contact Lenses

1.16.1 Hydrogels with Phosphate Groups

Hydrogels that contain phosphate groups in side chains were studied for their usefulness in drug-loaded soft contact lenses (143). Naphazoline (2-(1-naphthyl methyl)-2-imidazoline nitrate), a model drug having a cationic group, was incorporated into a soft contact lens because of its phosphate groups and was released over a period of about 14 *h*. For the soft contact lense, the naphazoline content was equivalent to the phosphate group content. Naphazoline is shown in Figure 1.60.

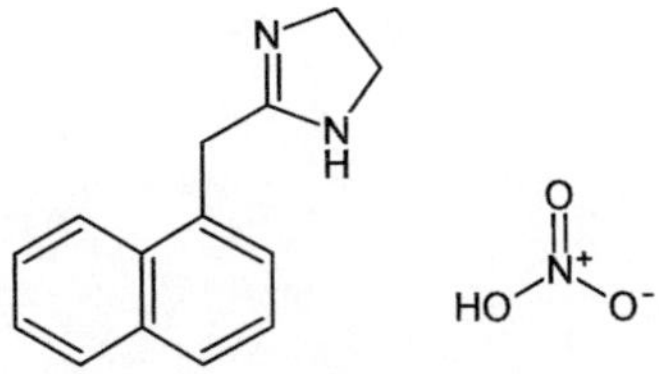

Figure 1.60 Naphazoline.

Drug-loaded soft contact lenses can be designed to contain the needed amount of a drug through the choice of the ionic group for the ligand. Furthermore, the soft contact lens having amide groups and phosphate groups had high transparency and an unchanged shape.

As monomers for the contact lenses, 2-methacryloxyethyl phosphate, cf. Figure 1.61, MA, and EGDMA were used (143). Here, EGDMA acts as crosslinking agent. As initiator, *AIBN* was used for the preparation of the anionic hydrogels. The drugs were introduced into the hydrogel by immersion in a 0.5% naphazoline aqueous solution at 25°C for 2 *d* to allow naphazoline adsorption. Free naphazoline was removed from the hydrogel by consecutive washing with an aqueous solution at 25°C for 24 *h*.

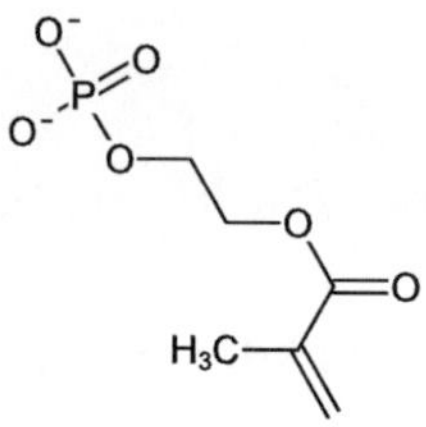

Figure 1.61 2-Methacryloxyethyl phosphate.

The relationship between the MA and 2-methacryloxyethyl phosphate ligand concentration and the naphazoline content of the hydrogel is shown in Figure 1.62.

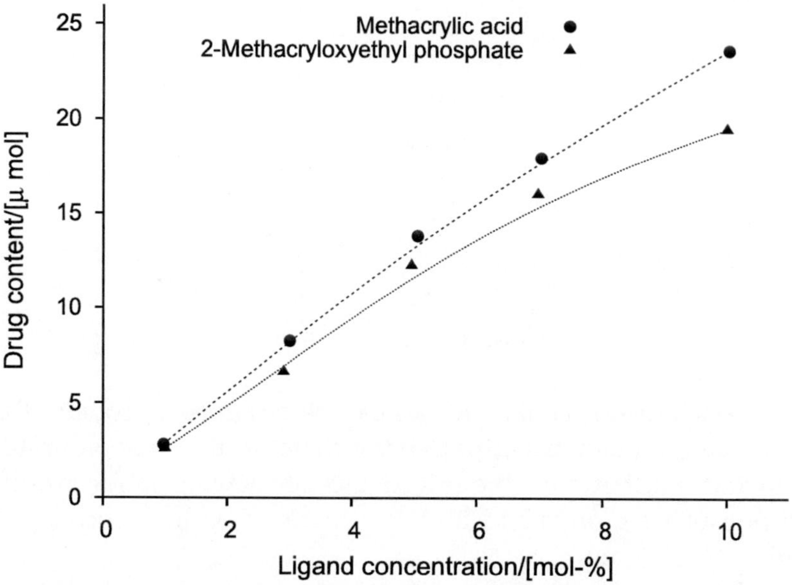

Figure 1.62 Ligand concentrations versus naphazoline content.

For MA hydrogels, naphazoline in the hydrogels was released for over 5 *h*, but for 2-methacryloxyethyl phosphate hydrogels, naphazoline was continuously released for 14 *h*.

It is suggested that amide groups and phosphate groups must be introduced into the polymer in equimolar amounts to give the necessary polymer-drug interaction. Therefore, hydrogels having a drug delivery system were synthesized by the inclusion of a phosphate group and an amide group. These hydrogels are also applicable to soft contact lens materials (143).

1.16.2 *Ophthalmic Drug Delivery*

Polymeric hydrogels for contact lens-based ophthalmic drug delivery systems, their advantages and drawbacks, have been critically analyzed in reviews (144, 145).

Only about 5% of drugs administrated by eye drops are bioavailable, and currently eye drops account for more than 90% of all ophthalmic formulations. The bioavailability of ophthalmic drugs can be improved by a soft contact lens-based ophthalmic drug delivery system. Several polymeric hydrogels have been investigated for soft contact lens-based ophthalmic drug delivery systems (144):

1. Polymeric hydrogels for conventional contact lens to absorb and release ophthalmic drugs,
2. Polymeric hydrogels for piggyback contact lens combining with a drug plate or drug solution,
3. Surface-modified polymeric hydrogels to immobilize drugs on the surface of contact lenses,
4. Polymeric hydrogels for inclusion of drugs in a colloidal structure dispersed in the lens,
5. Ion ligand-containing polymeric hydrogels, and
6. Molecularly imprinted polymeric hydrogels which provide the contact lens with a high affinity and selectivity for a given drug.

Conventional soft contact lenses have the ability to absorb a number of drugs when the lenses are presoaked in the drug solution, subsequently releasing them into the post-lens lacrimal fluid. As an alternative, one can also insert conventional soft contact lenses into eyes then apply eye drops. By this means, drugs can be absorbed and released by the soft contact lens, minimizing clearance and sorption through the conjunctiva (146–148).

HEMA polymers, which are widely used for preparing soft contact lenses, have been investigated for delivery of several ophthalmic drugs (149, 150).

To enhance the potential of the PHEMA hydrogels as an effective biomaterial for a contact lens-based ophthalmic drug delivery system, 4-vinylpyridine and *N*-(3-aminopropyl)methacrylamide were incorporated into the network (151).

Also, copolymer hydrogels of DMA and 2-(*N*-ethylperfluorooctanesulfonamido)ethyl acrylate were investigated for their potential application in contact lens-based drug delivery systems (152).

The abovementioned compounds are shown in Figure 1.63.

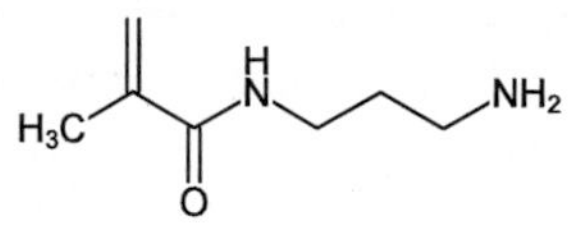

N-(3-Aminopropyl)methacrylamide

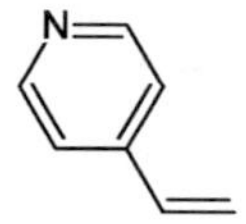

4-Vinylpyridine

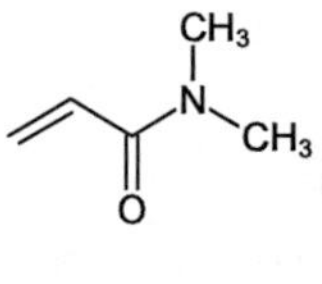

N,*N*-Dimethyl acrylamide

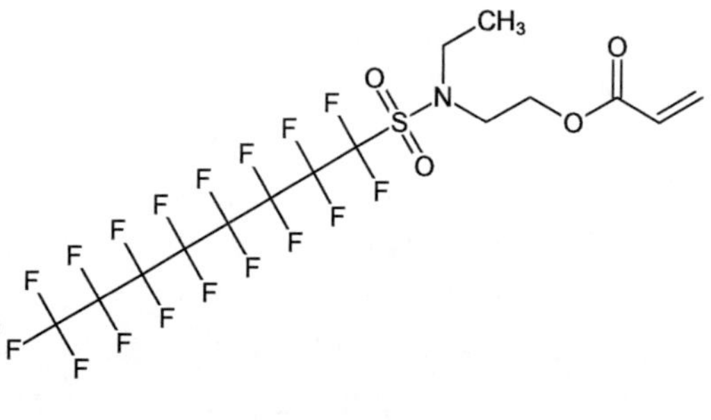

2-(*N*-Ethylperfluorooctanesulfonamido) ethyl acrylate

Figure 1.63 Monomers for an ophthalmic drug delivery system.

2-(*N*-Ethylperfluorooctanesulfonamido)ethyl acrylate can be incorporated into the networks to modify the glass transition temperature and water sorption and desorption kinetics of the hydrogels by changing the structure, location, or concentration of the hydrophobic group.

1.17 Simulation Methods

1.17.1 Ocular Topography Parameters

To evaluate the effect of varying lens and ocular topography parameters on soft contact lens fit, a computer spreadsheet model was used (153). The spreadsheet-based computer model used a ellipto-conical corneal model coupled with population data on the corneoscleral topography obtained in a clinical study. The model calculated the lens edge strain (circumferential elongation) as a predictor of the tightness of the lens. The following parameters were systematically varied (153):

1. Corneal curvature,
2. Corneal diameter,
3. Corneal shape factor,
4. Corneoscleral junction angle,
5. Lens base curve, and
6. Diameter.

The ellipto-conical corneal model showed a closer concordance with the actual measurements of the corneal sagittal height than a simple elliptical model (limits of agreement, ±0.20 vs. ±0.25 *mm*; $p = 0.0015$). For an eye with average ocular parameters wearing a typical soft contact lens design (lens base curve, 8.60; diameter, 14.2 *mm*), the model calculated an edge strain of 2.7%.

For the same soft contact lens, the tightest fit (8.5% strain) was found with the eye showing the combination of smallest, flattest, most aspheric cornea. Conversely, the loosest fit (−2.6%) was found with the eye showing the combination of largest, steepest, least aspheric cornea. A change in the lens base curve of 0.4 *mm* typically resulted in changes in edge strain of less than 2.5%, whereas a change in diameter of 0.5 *mm* resulted in a change of less than 2%. Using the typical soft contact lens design and average corneal model, wide variations in corneoscleral junction angle did not critically affect lens fit. More extreme combinations of soft contact lens and ocular parameters resulted in an edge strain likely to result in a tight (>6%) or loose fit (<0%) (153).

1.17.2 *Rigid Gas-Permeable Lenses*

Multi-view learning has been one of the focuses in medical image analysis in the recent years. The combination of various image properties for medical decision-making has had a high impact on the medical field (154).

The Pentacam-4 refractive map is one of the sources for detecting rigid gas-permeable lens properties for irregular astigmatism patients. A radial-sectoral segmentation approach has been presented to analyze the Pentacam-4 refractive maps individually.

Canonical correlation analysis and a neural network with two hidden layers is applied as a means of multi-view learning and base curve identification. The combination of the segmentation method with canonical correlation analysis combinatory feature vector, results in a 0.970 coefficient of determination in rigid gas-permeable base curve identification.

This result considerably improves the current findings and confirms optometrist findings based on the importance of the image maps. The proposed method has a great impact on reducing patient chair time and optometrist and patient satisfaction (154).

1.17.3 *Computerized Videokeratography*

Computerized videokeratography has become the standard method for measuring the corneal curvature after refractive surgery. However, only a few resources exist on the use of computerized videokeratography data for postoperative contact lens fitting, and no recommendations exist on the selection of the best topographic algorithm relevant to gas-permeable lens fitting.

The optimal use of topographic data was investigated to fit spherical gas-permeable contact lenses on patients who have undergone laser-assisted *in-situ* keratomileusis (LASIK) (155).

LASIK is performed by lifting the front surface of an eye by forming a thin hinged flap under which the shape of the cornea is changed by using an excimer laser or other surgical device (156). A microkeratome is usually used to cut the flap, but a femtosecond laser can also be used to make the flap.

A retrospective analysis of computerized videokeratography maps from eight post-LASIK eyes fitted with spherical gas-permeable lenses was performed in the Contact Lens Service of the Department of Ophthalmology at Case Western Reserve University and University Hospitals of Cleveland (155).

Axial and tangential maps from the Dicon CT 200 (version 3.50) or Humphrey Atlas (version A8) topographer were analyzed (155). Averaged dioptric curvatures from different locations (inferior, superior, and temporal) at various distances (2.0 *mm*, 2.5 *mm*, 3.0 *mm*, 3.5 *mm*, and 4.0 *mm*) from the vertex normal of each eye were compared with the base curves of the prescribed gas-permeable contact lenses.

One-way analysis of variance, Pearson correlation analysis, and paired t-tests showed that the best topographic predictors of a successful gas-permeable base curve were the average curvatures at the 4.0 *mm* distance on the axial maps ($r = 0.8078$, $P=0.05$) and at the 2.0 *mm* distance on the tangential maps ($r = 0.9738$, $P = 0.0002$).

The mean dioptric powers of the gas-permeable base curve, axial map 4.0 *mm* curvature, and tangential map 2.0 *mm* curvature were 41.50 *D* (diopters), 42.65 *D*, and 42.67 *D*, respectively.

So, to simplify and guide gas-permeable fitting after LASIK, the average dioptric curvature 4.0 *mm* from the vertex normal on axial maps or 2.0 *mm* from the vertex normal on tangential maps are the best predictors of accurate gas-permeable base curve selection (155).

References

1. T. Bowden, *Contact Lenses: The Story*, Bower House, 2009.
2. J. Lamb and T. Bowden, The history of contact lenses in A.J. Phillips and L. Speedwell, (Eds.), *Contact Lenses (Sixth Edition)*, chapter 1, pp. 2–17. Elsevier, London, sixth edition, 2019.
3. H.W. Hofstetter and R. Graham, Leonardo and contact lenses, *Optometry and Vision Science*, Vol. 30, 1953.
4. C.-H. Chen, Contact lens fabrication method and tool, US Patent Application 20 090 166 905, assigned to Unicon Optical Co. Ltd., July 02, 2009.

5. N. Efron, History in N. Efron, (Ed.), *Contact Lens Practice E-Book*, chapter 1, pp. 3–9. Elsevier Health Sciences, 3rd edition, 2018.
6. A.E. Fick, Eine Kontaktbrille, *Archiv für Augenheilkunde*, Vol. 18, p. 279, 1888.
7. O. Wichterle and D. Lim, Hydrophilic gels for biological use, *Nature*, Vol. 185, p. 117, 1960.
8. W. Otto and L. Drahoslav, Process for producing shaped articles from three-dimensional hydrophilic high polymers, US Patent 2 976 576, assigned to Wichterle Otto, Lim Drahoslav, March 28, 1961.
9. K. Tanaka, K. Takahashi, M. Kanada, S. Kanome, and T. Nakajima, Copolymer for soft contact lens, its preparation and soft contact lens made thereof, US Patent 4 139 513, assigned to Toyo Contact Lens Co. Ltd., February 13, 1979.
10. B.J. Tighe and A. Mann, Contact lens materials in A.J. Phillips and L. Speedwell, (Eds.), *Contact Lenses*, chapter 2, pp. 18–31. Elsevier, London, sixth edition, 2019.
11. A.G. Sabell, The history of contact lenses, *Contact Lens*, Vol. 1, p. 73, 1980.
12. O. Sitchevska, Contact glasses in keratoconus and in ametropia: Report of cases, *American Journal of Ophthalmology*, Vol. 15, p. 1028, 1932.
13. T.E. Obrig, Molded contact lenses, *Archives of Ophthalmology*, Vol. 19, p. 735, May 1938.
14. C. Musgrave and F. Fang, Contact lens materials: A materials science perspective, *Materials*, Vol. 12, p. 261, January 2019.
15. N. Efron, P.B. Morgan, L.W. Jones, and J.J. Nichols, 21st century citation analysis of the field of contact lenses, *Clinical and Experimental Optometry*, Vol. 0, p. 1, 2021.
16. R. Moreddu, D. Vigolo, and A.K. Yetisen, Contact lens technology: From fundamentals to applications, *Advanced Healthcare Materials*, Vol. 8, p. 1900368, 2019.
17. A.J. Phillips and L. Speedwell, (Eds.), *Contact Lenses*, Elsevier, 6th edition, 2019.
18. C. Geraths and R. Schäfer, Polymer materials for contact lens applications, US Patent 11 008 414, assigned to CIS Pharma AG, May 18, 2021.
19. J.F. Kunzler and G.D. Friends, Polymer compositions for contact lenses, US Patent 5 006 622, assigned to Bausch & Lomb Incorporated (Rochester, NY), April 9, 1991.
20. D. Myung, J. Noolandl, C. Ta, and C.W. Frank, Interpenetrating polymer network hydrogel contact lenses, US Patent 7 857 447, assigned to the Board of Trustees of the Leland Stanford Junior University (Palo Alto, CA), December 28, 2010.

21. E.-P. Lin, W.-Y. Chen, and C.-H. Teng, Multifocal contact lens and contact lens product, US Patent Application 20 190 302 478, assigned to Largan Medical Co. Ltd., October 03, 2019.
22. A. Alli and D. Sinha, Silicone hydrogels comprising *n*-alkyl methacrylamides and contact lenses made thereof, US Patent Application 20 180 011 223, assigned to Johnson & Johnson Vision Care Inc., January 11, 2018.
23. T.L. Maggio, M.C. Turnage, M.R. Clark, K. Fujisawa, and M. Nakamura, Silicone (meth)acrylamide monomer, polymer, ophthalmic lens, and contact lens, US Patent 8 415 405, assigned to Johnson & Johnson Vision Care Inc., April 09, 2013.
24. Standard test method for tensile properties of plastics by use of microtensile specimens, ASTM Standard D1708-18, ASTM International, West Conshohocken, PA, 2018. https://www.astm.org/Standards/D1708.htm.
25. Standard test method for tear-propagation resistance (trouser tear) of plastic film and thin sheeting by a single-tear method, ASTM Standard D1938-19, ASTM International, West Conshohocken, PA, 2019. https://www.astm.org/Standards/D1938.htm.
26. Y. Liu, Polymerizable contact lens formulations and contact lenses obtained therefrom, US Patent 8 820 925, assigned to CooperVision International Holding Company, LP (St. Michael, BB), September 2, 2014.
27. W.E. Becker, Corneal contact lens fabricated from transparent silicone rubber, US Patent 3 228 741, assigned to Mueller Welt Contact Lenses Inc., January 11, 1966.
28. P.L. Valint, Jr., D.M. Ammon, Jr., J.A. McGee, G.L. Grobe, III, and R.M. Ozark, Surface treatment for silicone hydrogel contact lenses comprising hydrophilic polymer chains attached to an intermediate carbon coating, US Patent 6 902 812, assigned to Bausch & Lomb Incorporated (Rochester, NY), June 7, 2005.
29. G.D. Friends and J.F. Kunzler, Polymeric materials with high oxygen permeability and low protein substantivity, US Patent 4 810 764, assigned to Bausch & Lomb Inc., March 07, 1989.
30. Y. Shimamura and Y. Matsuoka, Polyoxyethylene compound having multiple hydroxyl groups at end, and contact lens, US Patent 10 941 311, assigned to NOF Corp, March 09, 2021.
31. L. Yao and X. Niu, Polyolefin contact lens molds and uses thereof, US Patent 8 003 024, assigned to CooperVision International Holding Co. LP, August 23, 2011.
32. Standard test method for melt flow rates of thermoplastics by extrusion plastometer, ASTM Standard D1238-13, ASTM International, West Conshohocken, PA, 2018. https://www.astm.org/Standards/D1238.htm.

33. T.J. Morrill, Method of cast molding contact lenses, US Patent 5 843 346, assigned to Polymer Technology Corp, December 01, 1998.
34. S. Ansell and C. Yin, Molds for producing ophthalmic lenses, US Patent Application 20 060 051 454, assigned to Johnson & Johnson Vision Care Inc., March 09, 2006.
35. H.N. Beck, Heterogeneous nucleating agents for polypropylene crystallization, *Journal of Applied Polymer Science*, Vol. 11, p. 673, 1967.
36. M. Al-Ghazawi and R.P. Sheldon, Heterogeneous nucleation studies on polypropylene, *Journal of Polymer Science: Polymer Letters Edition*, Vol. 21, p. 347, 1983.
37. B.F.M. Wanders and H. Haitjema, Hydrogel contact lens comprising a polymer comprising a carboxy betaine ester monomer, US Patent Application 20 100 069 544, assigned to Procornea Holding BV, March 18, 2010.
38. M.S. Rad, B. Khameneh, Z. Sabeti, S.A. Mohajeri, and B.S.F. Bazzaz, Antibacterial Activity of Silver Nanoparticle-Loaded Soft Contact Lens Materials: The Effect of Monomer Composition, *Current Eye Research*, Vol. 41, p. 1286, 2016.
39. J.C. Yoo, Y.L. Kang, and M.Y. Kong, Transparent hydrogel membrane including hyaluronic acid, and contact lens including same, US Patent Application 20 200 262 985, assigned to JCBio Co. Ltd., August 20, 2020.
40. R.-Y. Ma and D.-S. Xiong, Synthesis and properties of physically crosslinked poly(vinyl alcohol) hydrogels, *Journal of China University of Mining and Technology*, Vol. 18, p. 271, June 2008.
41. S. Gupta, S. Sinha, and A. Sinha, Composition dependent mechanical response of transparent poly(vinyl alcohol) hydrogels, *Colloids and Surfaces B: Biointerfaces*, Vol. 78, p. 115, June 2010.
42. M. Willcox, N. Keir, V. Maseedupally, S. Masoudi, A. McDermott, R. Mobeen, C. Purslow, J. Santodomingo-Rubido, S. Tavazzi, F. Zeri, and L. Jones, CLEAR - contact lens wettability, cleaning, disinfection and interactions with tears, *Contact Lens and Anterior Eye*, Vol. 44, p. 157, 2021.
43. W.G. Deichert, G.C. Niu, and M.F. VanBuren, Water absorbing contact lenses made from polysiloxane/acrylic acid polymer, US Patent 4 277 595, assigned to Bausch & Lomb Incorporated (Rochester, NY), July 7, 1981.
44. R.L. Merker and M.J. Scott, The copolymerization of cyclic siloxanes, *Journal of Polymer Science*, Vol. 43, p. 297, 1960.
45. P. Terry, Bandage contact lenses: Information for patients, Information for Patients OMI 11034P, Oxford Eye Hospital, Oxford, 2017. electronic: https://www.ouh.nhs.uk/patient-guide/leaflets/files/11034Pbandage.pdf.

46. C. Tromans, Therapeutic contact lenses in A.J. Phillips and L. Speedwell, (Eds.), *Contact Lenses*, chapter 26, pp. 477–485. Elsevier, London, sixth edition, 2019.
47. A.K. Vijay, H. Zhu, J. Ozkan, D. Wu, S. Masoudi, R. Bandara, R.N. Borazjani, and M.D. Willcox, Bacterial adhesion to unworn and worn silicone hydrogel lenses, *Optometry and Vision Science*, Vol. 89, p. 1095, 2012.
48. M.L. Read, P.B. Morgan, and C. Maldonado-Codina, Measurement errors related to contact angle analysis of hydrogel and silicone hydrogel contact lenses, *Journal of Biomedical Materials Research Part B: Applied Biomaterials: An Official Journal of The Society for Biomaterials, The Japanese Society for Biomaterials, and The Australian Society for Biomaterials and the Korean Society for Biomaterials*, Vol. 91, p. 662, 2009.
49. M.J. Giraldez, C. Serra, M. Lira, M.E.C.R. Oliveira, and E. Yebra-Pimentel, Soft contact lens surface profile by atomic force microscopy, *Optometry and Vision Science*, Vol. 87, p. E475, 2010.
50. M.J. Giraldez, C.G. Resua, M. Lira, M.E.C.D.R. Oliveira, B. Magariños, A.E. Toranzo, and E. Yebra-Pimentel, Contact lens hydrophobicity and roughness effects on bacterial adhesion, *Optometry and Vision Science*, Vol. 87, p. E426, 2010.
51. A. Yee, R. Rosenzweig, M.N. Dickson, E. Liang, and S.-W. Wang, Novel anti-microbial bandage contact lens with ocular drug delivery, US Patent Application 20 190 101 669, assigned to Regents of the University of California, Oakland (CA), April 4, 2019.
52. H. Gandhi, H. Gao, M. Baig, and R. Chen, Functional contact lens and related systems and methods, WO Patent 2 015 157 855, assigned to Gandhi Harry, Gao Huayi, Baig Maarij, Ray Chen, October 22, 2015.
53. J.T. Baca, D.N. Finegold, and S.A. Asher, Tear glucose analysis for the noninvasive detection and monitoring of diabetes mellitus, *The Ocular Surface*, Vol. 5, p. 280, 2007.
54. N. von Thun und Hohenstein-Blaul, S. Funke, and F.H. Grus, Tears as a source of biomarkers for ocular and systemic diseases, *Experimental Eye Research*, Vol. 117, p. 126, 2013.
55. C. Salvisberg, N. Tajouri, A. Hainard, P.R. Burkhard, P.H. Lalive, and N. Turck, Exploring the human tear fluid: Discovery of new biomarkers in multiple sclerosis, *PROTEOMICS Clinical Applications*, Vol. 8, p. 185, 2014.
56. N. Thomas, I. Lahdesmaki, A. Lingley, Y. Liao, J. Pandey, A. Afanasiev, B. Otis, T. Shen, and B.A. Parviz, Functional contact lenses for remote health monitoring in developing countries, in *2011 IEEE Global Humanitarian Technology Conference*, pp. 212–217, 2011.

57. J.-W. Seok and A.Y. Sung, Physical properties of high functional contact lenses with hydrophilic substance and graphene oxide nanocolloids, *Journal of Nanoscience and Nanotechnology*, Vol. 20, p. 4860, 2020.
58. F.J. Ascaso and V. Huerva, Noninvasive continuous monitoring of tear glucose using glucose-sensing contact lenses, *Optometry and Vision Science*, Vol. 93, p. 426, 2016.
59. D.H. Keum, S.-K. Kim, J. Koo, G.-H. Lee, C. Jeon, J.W. Mok, B.H. Mun, K.J. Lee, E. Kamrani, C.-K. Joo, S. Shin, J.-Y. Sim, D. Myung, S.H. Yun, Z. Bao, and S.K. Hahn, Wireless smart contact lens for diabetic diagnosis and therapy, *Science Advances*, Vol. 6, 2020.
60. W.J. Biederman and D.J. Yeager, Capacitive sensing using a contact lens sensor, US Patent 10 201 297, assigned to Verily Life Sciences LLC, February 12, 2019.
61. H. Gandhi, H. Gao, M. Baig, and R. Chen, Functional contact lens and related systems and methods, US Patent Application 20 170 042 480, assigned to Medella Health Inc., February 16, 2017.
62. D.R. Whikehart, *Biochemistry of the Eye*, Elsevier Inc., 2003.
63. M. Ku, J. Kim, J.-E. Won, W. Kang, Y.-G. Park, J. Park, J.-H. Lee, J. Cheon, H.H. Lee, and J.-U. Park, Smart, soft contact lens for wireless immunosensing of cortisol, *Science Advances*, Vol. 6, 2020.
64. B.E. Lemoff, G.D. Miller, I. Opris, and H.Y. Pang, Adaptive tuning of a contact lens, US Patent 10 673 414, assigned to Tectus Corp., June 02, 2020.
65. R. Winoto, Wireless communication between a contact lens and an accessory device, US Patent 10 602 513, assigned to Tectus Corp., March 24, 2020.
66. L. Jones, A. Hui, C.-M. Phan, M.L. Read, D. Azar, J. Buch, J.B. Ciolino, S.A. Naroo, B. Pall, K. Romond, P. Sankaridurg, C.M. Schnider, L. Terry, and M. Willcox, CLEAR - contact lens technologies of the future, *Contact Lens and Anterior Eye*, Vol. 44, p. 398, 2021.
67. W.F. March and M.F. Mowery-McKee, Ocular analyte sensor, US Patent 6 980 842, assigned to Novartis AG, December 27, 2005.
68. V.L. Alexeev, S. Das, D.N. Finegold, and S.A. Asher, Photonic crystal glucose-sensing material for noninvasive monitoring of glucose in tear fluid, *Clinical Chemistry*, Vol. 50, p. 2353, 2004.
69. C.D. Geddes, R. Badugu, and J.R. Lakowicz, Quaternary nitrogen heterocyclic compounds for detecting aqueous monosaccharides in physiological fluids, US Patent 8 569 502, assigned to Chris Geddes, University of Maryland at Baltimore, October 29, 2013.
70. C.A. Morris, F.P. Carney, and J.D. Lane, Kits for assays of rapid screening of diabetes, US Patent 7 429 462, assigned to Novartis AG, September 30, 2008.

71. J. Zhang and W.G. Hodge, Contact lens integrated with a biosensor for the detection of glucose and other components in tears, US Patent 8 385 998, assigned to Jin Zhang, William Gerald Hodge, February 26, 2013.

72. B.L. Ibey, V.K. Yadavalli, R.M. Rounds, H.T. Beier, G.L. Cote, and M.V. Pishko, Method for glucose monitoring using fluorescence quenching, US Patent 8 088 595, assigned to Texas A&M University System, January 03, 2012.

73. W.F.A. Besling, Flexible eye insert and glucose measuring system, US Patent 9 737 245, assigned to NXP BV, August 22, 2017.

74. T. Kajisa and T. Sakata, Glucose-responsive hydrogel electrode for biocompatible glucose transistor, *Science and Technology of Advanced Materials*, Vol. 18, p. 26, 2017.

75. C.A. Yildirim, A contact lens design sensing tear glucose level, WO Patent 2 017 116 350, assigned to Dokuz Eylül Üniversitesi Rektörlügü, July 06, 2017.

76. M. Elsherif, M.U. Hassan, A.K. Yetisen, and H. Butt, Wearable contact lens biosensors for continuous glucose monitoring using smartphones, *ACS Nano*, Vol. 12, p. 5452, 2018.

77. M. Lamrani, Glucose sensing contact lens, US Patent 10 478 104, assigned to Menicon Co. Ltd., November 19, 2019.

78. K. Aslan, J.R. Lakowicz, and C.D. Geddes, Tunable plasmonic glucose sensing based on the dissociation of Con A-aggregated dextran-coated gold colloids, *Analytica Chimica Acta*, Vol. 517, p. 139, 2004.

79. W. March, D. Lazzaro, and S. Rastogi, Fluorescent measurement in the non-invasive contact lens glucose sensor, *Diabetes Technology & Therapeutics*, Vol. 8, p. 312, 2006.

80. B.M. Cummins, J.T. Garza, and G.L. Cote, Optimization of a Concanavalin A-based glucose sensor using fluorescence anisotropy, *Analytical Chemistry*, Vol. 85, p. 5397, 2013.

81. H. Yao, Y. Liao, A.R. Lingley, A. Afanasiev, I. Lähdesmäki, B.P. Otis, and B.A. Parviz, A contact lens with integrated telecommunication circuit and sensors for wireless and continuous tear glucose monitoring, *Journal of Micromechanics and Microengineering*, Vol. 22, p. 075007, 2012.

82. B. Otis, Y.-T. Liao, B. Amirparviz, and H. Yao, Wireless powered contact lens with biosensor, US Patent 8 608 310, assigned to University of Washington Center for Commercialization, December 17, 2013.

83. Z. Liu, Contact lenses having two-electrode electrochemical sensors, US Patent Application 20 140 194 713, assigned to Google LLC, July 10, 2014.

84. J. Park, J. Kim, S.-Y. Kim, W.H. Cheong, J. Jang, Y.-G. Park, K. Na, Y.-T. Kim, J.H. Heo, C.Y. Lee, et al., Soft, smart contact lenses with integrations of wireless circuits, glucose sensors, and displays, *Science Advances*, Vol. 4, p. aap9841, 2018.
85. L. Zhou, S.Z. Zhao, S.K. Koh, L. Chen, C. Vaz, V. Tanavde, X.R. Li, and R.W. Beuerman, In-depth analysis of the human tear proteome, *Journal of Proteomics*, Vol. 75, p. 3877, 2012.
86. L. Zhou and R.W. Beuerman, The power of tears: How tear proteomics research could revolutionize the clinic, *Expert Review of Proteomics*, Vol. 14, p. 189, 2017.
87. M.P. Molloy, S. Bolis, B.R. Herbert, K. Ou, M.I. Tyler, D.D. Van Dyk, M.D.P. Willcox, A.A. Gooley, K.L. Williams, C.A. Morris, and B.J. Walsh, Establishment of the human reflex tear two-dimensional polyacrylamide gel electrophoresis reference map: New proteins of potential diagnostic value, *Electrophoresis*, Vol. 18, p. 2811, 1997.
88. P.S. Goedegebuure, M.A. Watson, C.T. Viehl, and T.P. Fleming, Mammaglobin-based strategies for treatment of breast cancer, *Current Cancer Drug Targets*, Vol. 4, p. 531, 2004.
89. V. Evans, C. Vockler, M. Friedlander, B. Walsh, and M.D. Willcox, Lacryglobin in human tears, a potential marker for cancer, *Clinical & Experimental Ophthalmology*, Vol. 29, p. 161, 2001.
90. A. Lebrecht, D. Boehm, M. Schmidt, H. Koelbl, R.L. Schwirz, and F.H. Grus, Diagnosis of breast cancer by tear proteomic pattern, *Cancer Genomics-Proteomics*, Vol. 6, p. 177, 2009.
91. A. Lebrecht, D. Boehm, M. Schmidt, H. Koelbl, and F.H. Grus, Surface-enhanced laser desorption/ionisation time-of-flight mass spectrometry to detect breast cancer markers in tears and serum, *Cancer Genomics-Proteomics*, Vol. 6, p. 75, 2009.
92. D. Böhm, K. Keller, J. Pieter, N. Boehm, D. Wolters, W. Siggelkow, A. Lebrecht, M. Schmidt, H. Koelbl, N. Pfeiffer, et al., Comparison of tear protein levels in breast cancer patients and healthy controls using a de novo proteomic approach, *Oncology Reports*, Vol. 28, p. 429, 2012.
93. L. Michaud and S. Vincent, Scleral lenses and hypoxia: A balanced approach, *Contact Lens Spectrum*, Vol. 34, p. 40, 2019.
94. C.B. Nau, J. Harthan, E. Shorter, J. Barr, A. Nau, N.T. Chimato, D.O. Hodge, and M.M. Schornack, Demographic characteristics and prescribing patterns of scleral lens fitters: The SCOPE study, *Eye & Contact Lens*, Vol. 44, p. S265, 2018.
95. L. Michaud, E. van der Worp, D. Brazeau, R. Warde, and C.J. Giasson, Predicting estimates of oxygen transmissibility for scleral lenses, *Contact Lens and Anterior Eye*, Vol. 35, p. 266, 2012.

96. V. Compañ, M. Aguilella-Arzo, T.B. Edrington, and B.A. Weissman, Modeling corneal oxygen with scleral gas permeable lens wear, *Optometry and Vision Science*, Vol. 93, p. 1339, 2016.
97. J.P.G. Bergmanson, D.F. Ezekiel, and E. Van Der Worp, Scleral contact lenses and hypoxia: Theory versus practice, *Contact Lens and Anterior Eye*, Vol. 38, p. 145, 2015.
98. M.M. Schornack, Scleral lenses: A literature review, *Eye & Contact Lens*, Vol. 41, p. 3, 2015.
99. X. He, K.E. Donaldson, V.L. Perez, and P. Sotomayor, Case series: Overnight wear of scleral lens for persistent epithelial defects, *Optometry and Vision Science*, Vol. 95, p. 70, 2018.
100. Wikipedia contributors, Hypoxia (medical) — Wikipedia, the free encyclopedia, https://en.wikipedia.org/w/index.php?title=Hypoxia_(medical)&oldid=992085061, 2020. [Online; accessed 7-December-2020].
101. Y.H. Kim, B. Tan, M.C. Lin, and C.J. Radke, Central corneal edema with scleral-lens wear, *Current Eye Research*, Vol. 43, p. 1305, 2018.
102. W.J. Benjamin, Oxygen transport through contact lenses, 1994.
103. J.A. Legerton and W.E. Meyers, Scleral contact lens and methods for making and using the same, US Patent 8 113 653, assigned to CRT Technology Inc., February 14, 2012.
104. G.-M. Dai, *Wavefront Optics for Vision Correction*, Vol. 179 of *SPIE Press monograph*, SPIE Press, 2008.
105. R.J. Macedo-de Araújo, E. van der Worp, and J.M. González-Méijome, Practitioner learning curve in fitting scleral lenses in irregular and regular corneas using a fitting trial, *BioMed Research International*, Vol. 2019, p. 1, 2019.
106. M. Barnett, Mastering scleral lens fitting, *Contact Lens Spectrum*, November 2019.
107. M. Barnett, Ocular drug delivery systems using scleral lenses, *Contact Lens Spectrum*, p. 1, November 2019.
108. N. N., Eye health data and statistics, Technical report, National Eye Institute, Bethesda, Maryland, USA, 2019. https://www.nei.nih.gov/learn-about-eye-health/resources-for-health-educators/eye-health-data-and-statistics.
109. K. Kalwerisky, B. Davies, L. Mihora, C.N. Czyz, J.A. Foster, and S. DeMartelaere, Use of the Boston ocular surface prosthesis in the management of severe periorbital thermal injuries: A case series of 10 patients, *Ophthalmology*, Vol. 119, p. 516 , 2012.
110. J.B. Ciralsky, K.O. Chapman, M.I. Rosenblatt, P. Sood, A.G.A. Fernandez, M.N. Lee, and K.C. Sippel, Treatment of refractory persistent corneal epithelial defects: A standardized approach using continuous wear prose therapy, *Ocular Immunology and Inflammation*, Vol. 23, p. 219, 2015.

111. M. Lim, D.S. Jacobs, P. Rosenthal, and K.G. Carrasquillo, The Boston Ocular Surface Prosthesis as a novel drug delivery system for bevacizumab, in *Seminars in Ophthalmology*, Vol. 24-3, pp. 149–155. Taylor & Francis, 2009.
112. A.M. Keating and D.S. Jacobs, Anti-VEGF treatment of corneal neovascularization, *The Ocular Surface*, Vol. 9, p. 227, 2011.
113. L. Espandar, D. Caldwell, R. Watson, T. Blanco-Mezquita, S. Zhang, and B. Bunnell, Application of adipose-derived stem cells on scleral contact lens carrier in an animal model of severe acute alkaline burn, *Eye & Contact Lens*, Vol. 40, p. 243, 2014.
114. C. Alvarez-Peregrina, M.A. Sanchez-Tena, M. Martin, C. Villa-Collar, and F.J. Povedano-Montero, Multifocal contact lenses: A bibliometric study, *Journal of Optometry*, pp. 1–7, 2020.
115. C. Wildsmith, M. Widman, and J.P. Adams, Method and apparatus of forming a translating multifocal contact lens having a lower-lid contact surface, US Patent 9 417 464, assigned to Johnson & Johnson Vision Care Inc., August 16, 2016.
116. Center for Devices and Radiological Health, Types of contact lenses, Medical devices, U.S. Food and Drug Administration, Silver Spring, Maryland, 2018. https://www.fda.gov/medical-devices/contact-lenses/types-contact-lenses#scl.
117. Wikipedia contributors, List of soft contact lens materials — Wikipedia, the free encyclopedia, https://en.wikipedia.org/w/index.php?title=List_of_soft_contact_lens_materials&oldid=962467878, 2020. [Online; accessed 14-June-2020].
118. Y. Goto, Y. Sakai, and H. Yamaguchi, Tilted-wear type contact lens, US Patent 8 192 020, assigned to Menicon Co. Ltd., June 05, 2012.
119. H.M. Park, Y.U. Ryu, I.-J. Park, and B.S. Chu, Can tinted lenses be used to manipulate pupil size and visual performance when wearing multifocal contact lenses?, *Clinical Optometry*, Vol. 12, p. 27, March 2020.
120. H. Köse and N. Güner-Yildiz, Augmented reality (AR) as a learning material in special needs education, *Education and Information Technologies*, Vol. 26, p. 1921, 2020.
121. T.L. Owens and H.Y. Pang, Multi-coil field generation in an electronic contact lens system, US Patent Application 20 190 331 937, assigned to Tectus Corp., October 31, 2019.
122. T. Kim, S. Hwang, S. Kim, H. Ahn, and D. Chung, Smart contact lenses for augmented reality and methods of manufacturing and operating the same, US Patent 10 359 648, assigned to Samsung Electronics Co. Ltd., July 23, 2019.
123. S. Guo, K. Wu, C. Li, H. Wang, Z. Sun, D. Xi, S. Zhang, W. Ding, M.E. Zaghloul, C. Wang, F.A. Castro, D. Yang, and Y. Zhao, Integrated

contact lens sensor system based on multifunctional ultrathin MoS_2 transistors, *Matter*, Vol. 4, p. 969, 2021.
124. J. Chen, L. Mi, C.P. Chen, H. Liu, J. Jiang, W. Zhang, and Y. Liu, A foveated contact lens display for augmented reality, in B.C. Kress and C. Peroz, (Eds.), *Optical Architectures for Displays and Sensing in Augmented, Virtual, and Mixed Reality (AR, VR, MR)*, Vol. 11310, pp. 36–46. International Society for Optics and Photonics, SPIE, 2020.
125. F.-D. Jan, Composition for manufacturing contact lenses and method for manufacturing contact lenses by using the same, US Patent Application 20 170 038 498, assigned to BenQ Materials Corp., February 09, 2017.
126. K.F. Mueller, S.J. Heiber, and W.L. Plankl, Strong, silicone containing polymers with high oxygen permeability, US Patent 4 486 577, assigned to Novartis Corp., December 04, 1984.
127. P.C. Nicolson, R.C. Baron, P. Chabrecek, J. Court, A. Domschke, H.J. Griesser, A. Ho, J. Hopken, B.G. Laycock, Q. Liu, D. Lohmann, G.F. Meijs, E. Papaspiliotopoulos, J.S. Riffle, K. Schindhelm, D. Sweeney, W.L. Terry, Jr., J. Vogt, and L.C. Winterton, Extended wear ophthalmic lens, US Patent 6 951 894, assigned to Ciba Vision Corporation (Duluth, GA), October 4, 2005.
128. E.A. Perozziello, Oxygen permeable contact lens structures for thick payloads, US Patent 10 646 282, assigned to Tectus Corp., May 12, 2020.
129. M.F. Deering, Systems using eye mounted displays, US Patent 8 786 675, assigned to Michael Frank Deering, July 22, 2014.
130. M.F. Deering and A. Huang, Eye mounted displays and systems using eye mounted displays, US Patent 9 812 096, assigned to Spy Eye LLC, November 07, 2017.
131. C. Bourset and G. Wajs, Method of manufacturing natural protein polymer contact lenses by molding and cross-linking, US Patent 4 879 072, assigned to Essilor International Cie Générale d'Optique (Cretiel, FR), November 7, 1989.
132. C.-P. Ho and H. Yasuda, Ultrathin coating of plasma polymer of methane applied on the surface of silicone contact lenses, *Journal of Biomedical Materials Research*, Vol. 22, p. 919, 1988.
133. N. Inagaki and H. Yasuda, Adhesion of glow discharge polymers to metals and polymers, *Journal of Applied Polymer Science*, Vol. 26, p. 3333, 1981.
134. H. Yasuda, A.K. Sharma, and T. Yasuda, Effect of orientation and mobility of polymer molecules at surfaces on contact angle and its hysteresis, *Journal of Polymer Science: Polymer Physics Edition*, Vol. 19, p. 1285, 1981.
135. L. Xu, P. Ma, B. Yuan, Q. Chen, S. Lin, X. Chen, Z. Hua, and J. Shen, Anti-biofouling contact lenses bearing surface-immobilized layers of

zwitterionic polymer by one-step modification, *RSC Advances*, Vol. 4, p. 15030, 2014.

136. W.-H. Chang, P.-Y. Liu, C.-J. Lu, D.-E. Lin, M.-H. Lin, Y.-T. Jiang, and Y.-H.H. Hsu, Reduction of physical strength and enhancement of anti-protein and anti-lipid adsorption abilities of contact lenses by adding 2-methacryloyloxyethyl phosphorylcholine, *Macromolecular Research*, Vol. 28, p. 1064, 2020.
137. T. Goda and K. Ishihara, Soft contact lens biomaterials from bioinspired phospholipid polymers, *Expert Review of Medical Devices*, Vol. 3, p. 167, 2006.
138. X. Shi, D. Cantu-Crouch, V. Sharma, J. Pruitt, G. Yao, K. Fukazawa, J.Y. Wu, and K. Ishihara, Surface characterization of a silicone hydrogel contact lens having bioinspired 2-methacryloyloxyethyl phosphorylcholine polymer layer in hydrated state, *Colloids and Surfaces B: Biointerfaces*, Vol. 199, p. 111539, 2021.
139. T. Shimizu, T. Goda, N. Minoura, M. Takai, and K. Ishihara, Super-hydrophilic silicone hydrogels with interpenetrating poly(2-methacryloyloxyethyl phosphorylcholine) networks, *Biomaterials*, Vol. 31, p. 3274, 2010.
140. A. Spadafora, M. Korogiannaki, and H. Sheardown, Antifouling silicone hydrogel contact lenses via densely grafted phosphorylcholine polymers, *Biointerphases*, Vol. 15, p. 041013, 2020.
141. M. Kazemi Ashtiani, M. Zandi, P. Shokrollahi, M. Ehsani, and H. Baharvand, Surface modification of poly(2-hydroxyethyl methacrylate) hydrogel for contact lens application, *Polymers for Advanced Technologies*, Vol. 29, p. 1227, 2018.
142. M. Kazemi Ashtiani, M. Zandi, P. Shokrollahi, M. Ehsani, and H. Baharvand, Chitosan surface modified hydrogel as a therapeutic contact lens, *Polymers for Advanced Technologies*, Vol. 31, p. 741, 2020.
143. T. Sato, R. Uchida, H. Tanigawa, K. Uno, and A. Murakami, Application of polymer gels containing side-chain phosphate groups to drug-delivery contact lenses, *Journal of Applied Polymer Science*, Vol. 98, p. 731, 2005.
144. L. Xinming, C. Yingde, A.W. Lloyd, S.V. Mikhalovsky, S.R. Sandeman, C.A. Howel, and L. Liewen, Polymeric hydrogels for novel contact lens-based ophthalmic drug delivery systems: A review, *Contact Lens and Anterior Eye*, Vol. 31, p. 57, 2008.
145. F.A. Maulvi, T.G. Soni, and D.O. Shah, A review on therapeutic contact lenses for ocular drug delivery, *Drug Delivery*, Vol. 23, p. 3017, 2016.
146. E. Hehl, R. Beck, K. Luthard, R. Guthoff, and B. Drewelow, Improved penetration of aminoglycosides and fluoroquinolones into the aque-

ous humour of patients by means of Acuvue contact lenses, *European Journal of Clinical Pharmacology*, Vol. 55, p. 317, July 1999.

147. R. Peterson, J. Wolffsohn, J. Nick, L. Winterton, and J. Lally, Clinical performance of daily disposable soft contact lenses using sustained release technology, *Contact Lens and Anterior Eye*, Vol. 29, p. 127, 08 2006.
148. S. Schrader, T. Wedel, R. Moll, and G. Geerling, Combination of serum eye drops with hydrogel bandage contact lenses in the treatment of persistent epithelial defects, *Graefe's Archive for Clinical and Experimental Ophthalmology*, Vol. 244, p. 1345, 11 2006.
149. C.-C. Li and A. Chauhan, Modeling ophthalmic drug delivery by soaked contact lenses, *Industrial & Engineering Chemistry Research*, Vol. 45, p. 3718, April 2006.
150. C.-C. Li and A. Chauhan, Ocular transport model for ophthalmic delivery of timolol through p-HEMA contact lenses, *Journal of Drug Delivery Science and Technology*, Vol. 17, p. 69 , 2007.
151. P. Andrade-Vivero, E. Fernandez-Gabriel, C. Alvarez-Lorenzo, and A. Concheiro, Improving the loading and release of NSAIDs from pHEMA hydrogels by copolymerization with functional monomers, *Journal of Pharmaceutical Sciences*, Vol. 96, p. 802, April 2007.
152. M. Mullarney, T. Seery, and R.A. Weiss, Drug diffusion in hydrophobically modified *N,N*-dimethylacrylamide hydrogels, *Polymer*, Vol. 47, p. 3845, 05 2006.
153. G. Young, Mathematical model for evaluating soft contact lens fit, *Optometry and Vision Science*, Vol. 91, p. e167, 2014.
154. S. Hashemi, H. Veisi, E. Jafarzadehpur, R. Rahmani, and Z. Heshmati, A CCA approach for multiview analysis to detect rigid gas permeable lens base curve, in *2019 IEEE Western New York Image and Signal Processing Workshop (WNYISPW)*, pp. 1–5, 2019.
155. L. Szczotka-Flynn and B.R. Jani, Comparison of axial and tangential topographic algorithms for contact lens fitting after LASIK, *Eye & Contact Lens*, Vol. 31, p. 257, 2005.
156. Wikipedia contributors, Keratomileusis — Wikipedia, the free encyclopedia, https://en.wikipedia.org/w/index.php?title=Keratomileusis&oldid=927675058, 2019. [Online; accessed 30-November-2020].

2

Fabrication Methods

2.1 Computer-Aided Contact Lens Design and Fabrication

The fundamentals of lens design have been presented in a monograph (1). Here, the effective use of software design packages is described. Gas-permeable (GP) lens fitting software programs are about to be introduced that will enable the practitioner to fit GP lenses of all types easily and accurately (2). Several programs have been described, such as Focal Point's Professional Quick Fit. Furthermore, there are Keratron contact lens software, OrthoTool software and EyeArt software.

Other commercially available optical design software are Code V™, Zemax™, OSLO™, MSC.Marc™, and Abaqus FEA (3). These software programs are shown in Table 2.1. Also, a list of optical software can be found in Wikipedia (4).

2.1.1 Spline-Based Mathematical Surfaces

A method of computer-aided contact lens design and fabrication has been described that uses spline-based mathematical surfaces without restrictions of their rotational symmetry (5). The spline encompasses any piecewise function with any associated constraints of smoothness or continuity.

The method can be performed by the following steps: Data acquisition, three-dimensional mathematical surface model construction,

Table 2.1 Optical design software.

Name	Company	Address
EyeArt	Eyenuk, Inc.	Woodland Hills, CA
Abaqus FEA	Dassault Systèmes Simulia Corp.	Johnston, RI
Code V	Optical Research Associates (ORA)	Pasadena, CA
OSLO	Sinclair Optical Services	Gloucestershire, UK
Zemax	Zemax Development Corporation	San Diego, CA

posterior surface description, ray tracing for anterior surface, and peripheral edge system design. The steps are detailed below (5):

Data acquisition: Data is obtained about the patient's cornea using a corneal topographic mapping system, sometimes called a videokeratograph. There are, at present, a dozen or so such systems that are commercially available, as well as several others undergoing research and development. They are based on several different principles, but all share the intent to provide corneal shape information.

Three-dimensional mathematical surface model construction: From the data obtained in **Data acquisition**, an accurate three-dimensional mathematical surface model of the patient's cornea is constructed. The mathematical surface model has no requirements or assumptions of symmetry. This model would generally also be a spline-based cornea model although non-spline-based cornea models could also be used.

Posterior surface description: From the mathematical model of the patient's cornea in **Three-dimensional mathematical surface model construction**, a mathematical description representing the posterior surface of the contact lens is developed. The calculation allows the insertion of a tear layer between the cornea surface and posterior surface. This is particularly important in the case of rigid lenses. This is done by adding offset function to the mathematical representation of the anterior surface cornea to yield the mathematical formulation for the posterior surface of the contact lens. As mentioned above, there are also no requirements or assumptions of symmetry, not even that the footprint of the contact lens be circular.

Ray tracing for anterior surface: Given the posterior surface of the contact lens, ray tracing is used to define the anterior surface of the lens such that the lens will provide the optics to correct the patient's refractive error. The ray tracing yields a set of points on the anterior surface, and then a general spline surface (with no assumptions of symmetry) is fit to these points.

Peripheral edge system design: Given the posterior and anterior surfaces of the contact lens, a mathematical formulation of the edge is defined to meet these surfaces with appropriate continuity.

The result of this method is a mathematical or algorithmic description of a contact lens. This can be used for data compression, transfer, exchange, conversion, formatting, etc., and for driving computer numerical control manufacturing devices, including lathes, grinding and milling machines, molding equipment, and lasers (5).

This approach enables patients to have their corneal topography analyzed in one location and a contact lens fabricated simultaneously or subsequently at a remote location. Both the corneal topography and the contact lens design could be displayed on the computer screen (5).

Another important application of spline-based contact lens design is the calculation of a smooth transition zone for the smoothing of the junction between two adjacent zones of the lens. The new approach involves splines, geometric continuity, and shape parameters to control the flattening of the shape of the transition zone of a contact lens.

In practice, this problem of discontinuities at the junction between zones is addressed by polishing. However, this process alters the specifications of the surface shape in an unknown, unpredictable, and unrepeatable way. Instead of this traditional approach, this new spline method replaces the discontinuous junction with a specially designed transition zone inserted between the two zones, with the important property of joining both zones smoothly. Furthermore, the degree of smoothness where the transition zone joins each adjacent zone can be precisely quantified (5).

2.1.2 *Corneal Refractive Therapy Program*

There are potential difficulties in properly fitting a lens for a patient, which in turn could damage the cornea of the patient or cause discomfort (6, 7). To alleviate the burden of wearing eyeglasses or contact lenses, surgical techniques have been developed for altering the shape of the patient's cornea in an attempt to correct refractive errors of the eye. Such surgical techniques include photorefractive keratectomy, laser *in situ* keratectomy, as well as procedures such as automated lamilar keratectomy, or implanted corneal rings, implanted contact lenses, and radial keratotomy. These procedures are intended to surgically modify the curvature of the cornea to reduce or eliminate visual defects.

Alternatives to permanent surgical procedures to alter the shape of the cornea include corneal refractive therapy and orthokeratology, where a contact lens is applied to the eye to alter the shape or curvature of the cornea by compression of the corneal surface imparted by the lens. The reshaping of the cornea in orthokeratology has been practiced for many years, but typically has required a series of lenses and an extensive period of time to reshape the cornea. It is also typical of orthokeratology treatment plans that the lenses used for reshaping of the cornea must be custom designed and manufactured, thereby greatly increasing the cost and complicating general use of such procedures. Furthermore, orthokeratology lenses typically have various deficiencies, particularly relating to properly designing a lens for a particular patient to achieve the best results in the treatment process. Specifically, corneal abrasions from poorly distributed bearing, corneal warpage from decentered lenses, edema from tight-fitting lenses and discomfort from excessive lens edge standoff are problems associated with an improperly fit lens.

Orthokeratology lens designs have not lent themselves to be easily fitted for a particular patient and their needs, requiring a doctor or other practitioner to have significant skill in complex geometric computation to properly mate the lens shape to the patients cornea and a high level of expertise in properly fitting a patient.

Furthermore, even with a high level of expertise, a lens designer many times will design a lens which will not work properly with a patient, and must be redesigned to account for the errors of the original design. Such a process is lengthy and increases the cost of the treatment correspondingly. It would be desirable to provide a lens for corneal refractive therapy which would allow a novice fitter to more easily select and arrive at a final design to simplify the fitting process (6).

A computer program product and methods for designing and fitting a contact lens have been described (6).

The computer program product has a computer usable storage medium having computer readable program code means embodied in the medium. This computer program needs the following inputs (6):

1. Flattest keratometry reading,
2. Manifest refractive sphere error: in minus cylinder form,
3. Target final refractive error, and
4. Horizontal visible iris diameter.

The fifth input varies depending on whether the fitting lenses used had variable-based curves or variable connecting zone depths. In the case of the former, the input identifies the base curve of the lens observed to just give simultaneous apical and tangential touch, or in the case of the latter, the input identifies the connecting zone depth of the lens observed to just give simultaneous apical and tangential touch. The sixth input also depends on which fitting lens set type is used, concentric rings or variable angles. In the case of the former, the input is the diameter of tangential touch by the lens having the concentric rings, or in the case of the latter, the input identified the peripheral angle observed to meet the criteria of touch diameter relative to lens diameter.

The program output by computation is (6):

1. Lens power to order,
2. Base curve to order,
3. Connecting zone depth to order,
4. Peripheral zone angle to order, and
5. Overall diameter to order.

2.2 Contact Lenses with Selective Spectral Blocking

Contact lenses are a convenient eyewear format for either vision correction or cosmetic use (8). As UV radiation is likely a cause of cataracts and senile macular degeneration, UV-blocking contact lenses are desirable (8). The presence of drusen and pigmentary changes within the retina are a characteristic finding of early and intermediate age-related macular degeneration (9). So, contact lenses that block UV by means of absorption are commercially available and finding increasing popularity (8).

However, contact lenses that block visible and infrared light are difficult to manufacture. Typically, light blocking is achieved by either absorbing or reflecting the light of interest. It is difficult to conventionally deposit a multilayer dielectric coating on plastic contact lenses, as their surface typically has a large radius of curvature. In addition, coating deposition on flexible soft contacts, which are the most popular, is challenging, as the so-called hydrogel lens materials contain more than 50% water.

Coating adhesion may be an issue to overcome. The other approach of using absorptive dyes doping may not be easy. The absorbing dyes may leach out in the aqueous environment of the eye or when stored in a saline solution. The safety profile of absorbing dyes could also be a health issue. A viable alternative is to incorporate dyes that can be copolymerized with hydrogel polymers. However, synthesis of such absorbers is technically difficult. In addition, other impacts on the contact lenses, such as durability, flexibility, hydrophilicity and stability to sterilizing regiments, are uncertain. Thus, a need exists for a contact lens with improved performance.

An ophthalmic lens has been developed that consists of an ophthalmic lens body having one or more films having at least one spectral reflection band. The reflection band has spectral reflection properties to reflect right-handed circularly polarized light, left-handed circularly polarized light, or a combination of right-handed circularly polarized light and left-handed circularly polarized light (8).

A polymeric cholesteric liquid crystal film is incorporated on the surface of or within the body of the ophthalmic contact lens.

Cholesteric liquid crystal blends can be formulated to form either a left-handed helix or a right-handed helix with its reflection band tunable anywhere from ultraviolet to infrared. The handedness, or chirality, is set, for example, by the chiral agents in a nematic liquid crystal blend.

The polymeric cholesteric liquid crystal film is incorporated on the surface of or within the body of an ophthalmic contact lens. The body 10 may be formed of conventional ophthalmic lens material, such as poly(methyl methacrylate) (PMMA) and acrylates, or non-conventional materials such as liquid crystal blends as described herein.

Figure 2.1 graphically illustrates a contact lens 10 having an anterior surface 12 and a posterior surface 14 that incorporates one or more polymeric cholesteric liquid crystal films 16′. The light blocking is achieved by bonding a reflective cholesteric liquid crystal film 16′ on the anterior surface 12 of the contact lens body 10, bonding a reflective cholesteric liquid crystal film 16′ on the posterior surface 14 that incorporates one or more polymeric cholesteric liquid crystal films 16.

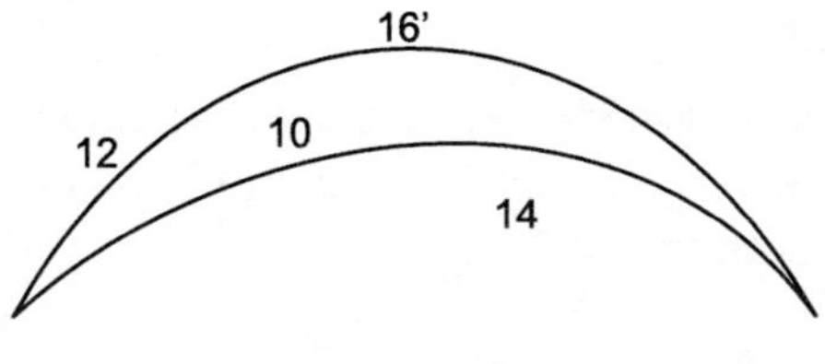

Figure 2.1 Special contact lens (8).

There are two preferred methods to fabricate such films. The first is to utilize curved substrates (10). The second preferred method is to fabricate curved cholesteric liquid crystal films using one substrate. This process is highly advantageous, as the cholesteric liquid crystal film can be directly fabricated on the surface of prefabricated contact lenses. A thick cholesteric liquid crystal film is applied on a curved substrate, either by directly spin coating or knife-edge coating. The surface of the substrate is similarly treated to produce a cholesteric liquid crystal film with Grandjean texture. After annealing, the film is polymerized. The polymerization preferably takes place in an environment without the presence of atmospheric oxygen, which acts as an inhibitor.

This process is used to fabricate a pair of right-handed and left-handed cholesteric liquid crystal films with substantially matched reflection bands in spectral range. The paired films are then stacked and bonded. It is preferable to use the same cholesteric liquid crystal blend as a bonding agent. The bonding layer is polymerized at or above the clearing temperature of the cholesteric liquid crystal blend. The bonding layer is then optically isotropic. The advantage of using the same cholesteric liquid crystal blend for bonding is to achieve matching in the refractive index and porosity. The film stack can be fabricated sequentially.

For example, a right-handed cholesteric liquid crystal film is first fabricated on the curve substrate. Then, a spectrally matched left-handed cholesteric liquid crystal film is fabricated on the right-handed cholesteric liquid crystal film, forming a paired stack. The compound reflecting film can then later be processed to become porous by removing the non-reactive component. The reflecting cholesteric liquid crystal film stack is then integrated with a contact lens.

The same cholesteric liquid crystal material, either of left-handed or right-handed blends, can be used for the lens body. The lens body is polymerized at or above the clearing temperature to be optically isotropic. In addition to close matching in the refractive index through the lens, the entire lens can be porous by removing the non-reactive component (8).

2.3 Colored Contact Lenses

The manufacture of color contact lenses can be done by the pigment application method, the pigment inlay method, the sandwich method, or the binding method (11). The main manufacturing method has been the binding method. At the point of use and manufacture of the color contact lenses, color contacts lenses are classified as tinted and cosmetic types. However, generally coloring of contact lenses is done by the stain method and the staining is manufactured by the thin film methods.

Colored contact lenses are classified into two categories (12). First, there are transparent colored contact lenses. The transparent colored contact lenses have been developed to emphasize transparency or block rays of light, rather than to change the apparent color of the irises. Accordingly, there is a limit to changing the color of the eyes to any desired color using transparent colored contact lenses, and thus they are generally used for identification purposes or for the purpose of blocking ultraviolet rays, rather than for cosmetic purposes.

Second, there are opaque colored contact lenses capable of changing the apparent color of the irises to another color (12). However, since the particle size of an opaque pigment used in the opaque colored contact lenses is generally larger than the pore size of soft contact lenses, it is difficult to directly color contact lenses with the pigment. Such conventional colored contact lenses have pupil portions that make the pupils of the eyes transparent and also have portions that are formed to be larger than the pupils for adding predetermined colors or patterns, and can thus make the eyes appear bigger or have a different color from their original color.

2.3.1 *Hard Colored Contact Lenses*

A colored hard contact lens printing method has been presented that is capable of fabricating a colored hard contact lens having iris designs of various colors and patterns on the front surface thereof (12). Also, a colored hard contact lens printing method has been described, capable of processing a hard contact lens to have a size suited for a user, fabricating a centering jig to have a size suited for the hard contact lens, and preparing a composition capable of maintaining its adherence on the hard contact lens.

The fabrication consists of the following steps (12):

1. A preparation step of preparing a hard contact lens, a centering jig, and a composition for printing so as to print an iris design on the hard contact lens,
2. A printing step of mounting the hard contact lens on the centering jig and printing the iris design by using the composition for printing, and
3. A post-treatment step of post-treating the hard contact lens having the iris design printed thereon.

In another study, a method of fabrication has been shown that consists of (13):

1. Providing a mold that includes a first mold half having a first molding surface defining the anterior surface of a contact lens and a second mold half having a second molding surface defining the posterior surface of the contact lens, wherein the first and second mold halves are configured to receive each other such that a contact lens-forming cavity is formed between the first and second molding surfaces,
2. Applying, by using pad-transfer or inkjet printing technique, at least one pattern selected from a group consisting of outermost starburst pattern and inner starburst pattern onto at least one of the molding surfaces of a lens mold, each of said portions overlapping each other at a plurality of points,
3. Applying, by using pad-transfer or inkjet printing technique, an annular colored pattern together with an outer starburst pattern onto the surface of the mold, where the annular colored pattern and the outer starburst pattern are fused together in a single cliché, wherein the annular pattern is composed of colored dots which are opaque, wherein sizes of the dots and/or amounts of space between the dots of the annular colored pattern are varied in a radially-controlled manner so that local colored dot coverage increases in a radial direction from the inner perimeter of the annular iris section to the outer perimeter of the annular iris section, wherein the dots of the annular pattern cover at least 10% of the iris of an eye to make changes to the color of the eye or enhance the color of the eye, and wherein the combination of the annular colored pattern and the other color patterns enhance or change the apparent color of the iris of the wearer of the lens,
4. Partially or completely curing the ink printed on the mold to convert the colored coat to a colored film,
5. Dispensing a lens-forming material into the lens-forming cavity, and
6. Curing the lens-forming material within the lens-forming cavity to form a colored contact lens, whereby the colored film detaches from the molding surface and becomes integral

> with the body of the contact lens, wherein the colored film becomes part of one of the anterior and posterior surfaces of the colored contact lens and has a good adhesion to the lens.

Colorants that can be used for colored contact lenses have been collected (14).

Representative examples of possible inks and pigment levels are shown in Table 2.2.

Table 2.2 Inks and pigment levels (13).

	Composition/[%]											
Ink Paste	Ethyl lactate	Binder sol	PCN blue	PCN green	TiO_2	IOB	IOR	IOBR	IOY	Cr_2O_3	CAV	HIO
Green	28.53	63.85	0.03							7.59		
Turquoise	30.00	58.16	0.63	2.25	8.88						0.08	
Orange	30.00	58.00				6.00						6.00
Blue	30.55	61.15	1.21		7.09							
Gray	30.75	59.84		0.23	7.34	1.83						
Brown	30.00	55.10				5.70	3.45	5.75				
Black	23.98	64.04				11.98						
Hazel	30.00	63.49	0.06		0.61		1.54		4.30			
IOB	Iron oxide black											
IOR	Iron oxide red											
IOBr	Iron oxide brown											
IOY	Iron oxide yellow											
CAV	Carbazole violet											
HIO	Hydrophobic iron oxide											

The color binding mechanism for contact lenses has been detailed (15).

2.4 Decentered Contact Lenses

There are contact lenses in which the near-sight region and the far-sight region are formed in concentric circles in relation to the lens geometric center (16).

However, in a worn state where the contact lens overlaps on the cornea of the eye, the pupil center which is positioned on the center axis of the eye optical system is often shifted from the geometric center of the contact lens. A possible reason for this is that since the curvature distribution of the corneal surface of the human eye is not uniform, it is easy for the contact lens to stabilize and shift to the ear side, or for the pupil center to be in an eccentric position to the nose side in relation to the geometric center of the cornea.

So, in a worn state, when the pupil center is shifted from the geometric center of the contact lens, with a contact lens of a conventional structure for which a near-sight region and a far-sight region are provided concentrically with the lens geometric center, obtaining a sufficient quality of vision is a problem. Therefore, a decentered type contact lens was proposed for which the optical center axis of the optical region is made to deviate from the nose side from the lens geometric center (16). With such a contact lens it is possible to suppress the distance between the pupil center and optical center axis in a worn state, and to obtain an improved quality of vision.

There are two types of contact lenses; the soft type and hard type. For a soft contact lens, it is possible to use a non-hydrated material, such as an acrylic rubber or a silicone, in addition to a hydrated material, such as poly(2-hydroxyethyl methacrylate) or poly(vinyl pyrrolidone). It is also possible to use this material for a hard contact lens consisting of a rigid gas-permeable lens or the like made of PMMA or a SiMA/MMA polymer. Furthermore, it is also possible to use a two material contact lens having the features of both hard-type and soft-type lenses, and it is also possible to use a compound material formed from the respective materials for these types of lenses (16).

The construction of such a contact lens is shown in Figure 2.2.

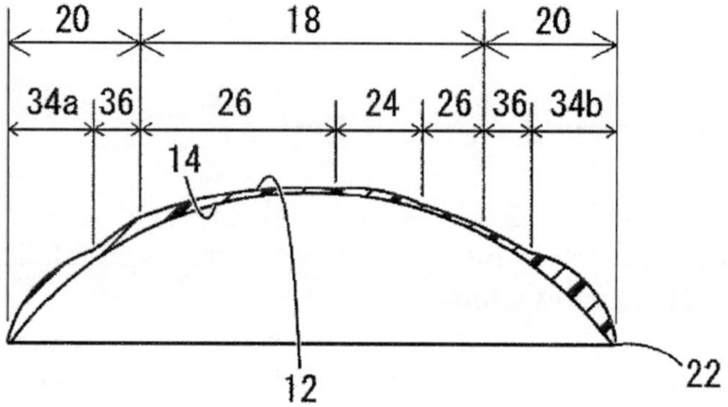

Figure 2.2 Decentered contact lens structure (16).

The contact lens 10 has a circular shape, a roughly convex spherical lens front surface 12, and a roughly concave spherical lens back surface 14. Also, it has an optical zone 18 that expands in roughly a circle from a lens geometric center with a front view at the center part, a peripheral zone 20 that expands roughly in a ring shape with a front view surrounding the optical zone 18, and an edge part 22 that connects the lens front and back surfaces 12 and 14 and is positioned at the lens outermost circumference edge part in the periphery of the peripheral zone 20. The thick parts 34a and 34b in the circumferential direction are used as a transition region 36 for a smooth change of the lens thickness (16).

2.5 Stabilized Contact Lenses

Correction of certain optical defects can be accomplished by imparting nonspherical corrective aspects to one or more surfaces of a contact lens such as cylindrical, bifocal, or multifocal characteristics (17). These lenses must generally be maintained at a specific orientation while on the eye to be effective.

The maintenance of the on-eye orientation of a lens typically is accomplished by altering the mechanical characteristics of the lens. Prism stabilization, including decentering of the lens' front surface relative to the back surface, thickening of the inferior lens periphery, forming depressions or elevations on the lens' surface, and truncating the lens edge, are examples of stabilization approaches. Additionally, dynamic stabilization has been used in which the lens is stabilized by the use of thin zones, or areas in which the thickness of the lens' periphery is reduced. Typically, the thin zones are located at two regions that are symmetric at either the vertical or horizontal axis of the lens from the vantage point of its on-eye placement (17).

Lenses can be designed using the coefficients of a Bézier curve, describing the upper portion of the angular thickness profile such that the sag values are negative (17). When the stabilization zone is added to the lens periphery the thickness of the upper portion of the lens is reduced instead of being increased. Reducing the thickness in the upper portion of the stabilization allows reducing the maximum thickness and still keeping the same thickness differential. Slopes around the location of maximum thickness are not affected too much by this profile change.

The area containing negative sag values is applied on the upper and lower portion of the stabilization zones. Also, the maximum thickness of the stabilization zones differs between the left and the right side. The ramp of the thickness profile toward the positive and/or the negative angles can be adjusted to increase or decrease the ramp angle. Thus, lenses made according to the design method have an improved stabilization.

A front or object view of a stabilized contact lens is shown in Figure 2.3.

The lens has an optical zone. The periphery of the lens surrounds the optical zone. Two thick regions are located in the periphery and act as stabilization zones.

2.6 Additive Manufacturing

Additive manufacturing (3D printing) has the ability to architect structures at microscale, giving rise to the development of functional contact lenses with inbuilt sensing capabilities (18). The 3D printing technology enables the fabrication of contact lenses without surface geometry restrictions.

Spherical, nonspherical, symmetric, and asymmetric lenses can be manufactured in an integrated production process. The advantages

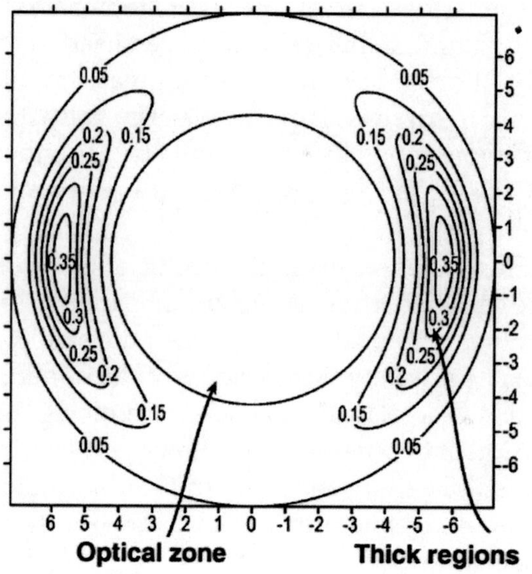

Figure 2.3 Front of a stabilized contact lens (17).

of 3D printing over conventional techniques include fast and easy production, one-step manufacturing, and no post processing such as grinding or polishing.

In addition, and most significantly, 3D printing can create chambers within the wall of the lenses by taking advantage of computer-aided modeling and layer-by-layer deposition of the materials. These inbuilt chambers can be used for loading drugs and sensing elements. The computer-aided design modeling can allow for manufacturing of patient-specific contact lenses. The 3D-printing approaches and the challenges faced in fabricating contact lenses are focused on in an article (18).

2.7 Mold Process

2.7.1 *Injection Molding*

A process for the manufacture of contact lenses has been described (19). A mold insert for an injection mold for the manufacture of the female mold half is shown in Figure 2.4.

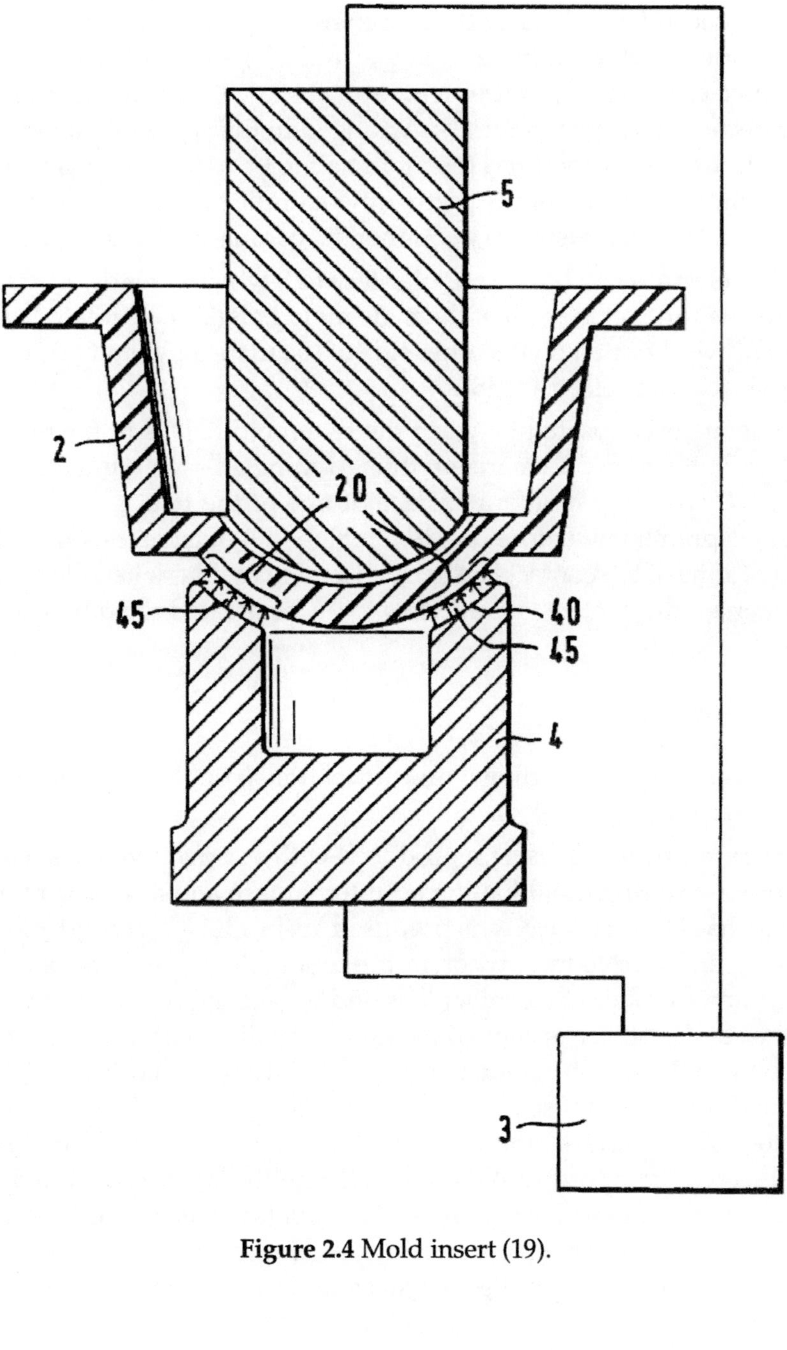

Figure 2.4 Mold insert (19).

Here, a polymerizable contact lens material is dispensed into a mold half (1) (19). The mold is subsequently closed by means of the second mold half (2). A generator (3) is connected to an electrode (4) which supplies that electrode (4) with high voltage. A counter-electrode (5) is arranged at a distance from the electrode connected to the generator (3). Arranged in the space (45) between the electrodes (4) and (5) is the mold half to be treated, in this case a male mold half (2). For the pretreatment of the male mold half (2) it is possible to use customary commercial corona-discharge devices.

The electrode (4) has an annular face (40) which extends substantially over the region (20) of the male mold half (2) to be treated and is concave. Located on the other side of the male mold half (2) is the convex counter-electrode (5).

The material located between the two mold halves in the molding cavity is then polymerized, thus forming an as yet unhydrated contact lens. The molding surface of one of the two mold halves (1, 2) is pretreated, before use, in a region (20) outside the optically active zone of the contact lens in such a manner that, when the mold is opened, the contact lens adheres to the pretreated mold half (19).

2.7.2 *Cast Molding*

A method for cast molding a multifocal translating contact lens has been presented (20, 21).

Here, a first mold insert is produced with a surface which is used to produce a first mold having an internal face and a second mold insert having a surface which is used to produce a second mold having an external face, wherein the first mold represents a shape of an anterior face of a contact lens and the second mold represents a shape of a posterior face of a contact lens, wherein the first and second molds are brought together with the external face of the second mold juxtaposed with the internal face of the first mold so as to define a volume therebetween, the volume between the first and second juxtaposed molds being filled with contact lens material, allowing the contact lens volume in the molds to cure to produce the cast-molded contact lens, wherein the volume defined by the first and second molds is configured so as to form a contact lens with a lower truncation.

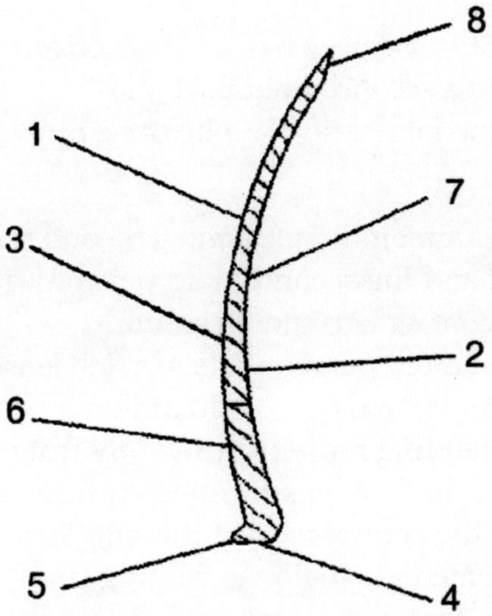

Figure 2.5 Side elevation of a contact lens (21).

Figure 2.5 shows the side elevation of a produced contact lens. A typical contact lens 1 cast-molded is shown in Figure 2.5 showing a posterior face 2 and an anterior face 3 (21). There is also shown a lower truncation 4, a forwardly projecting ledge 5 and the close and distance vision segments 6 and 7 respectively. It is found that the ledge 5 adds bulk to the lower end of the lens 1, so allowing good lid action on the contact lens 1 and the truncation 3 provides a relatively wide surface for resting on a lower eyelid. Furthermore, an upper end of the posterior face 2 is provided with a peripheral lenticulation 8 to facilitate translocation of the lens 1 on the eye.

2.7.3 *Two-Part Mold Assembly*

A contact lens mold assembly has been described that consists of a first mold part and a second mold part (22).

A method for the fabrication can be done by the following steps (22):

1. Providing a first mold part and a second mold part, the first mold part and the second mold part physically engageable to form a contact lens mold assembly,

   The first mold part consists of a first lens-forming surface having a central axis and a circumferential edge, a first stop surface extending radially outwardly from the circumferential edge of the first lens-forming surface in a plane perpendicular to the central axis of the first lens-forming surface, a first intermediate region extending from the first stop surface, and a first alignment surface extending from the first intermediate region in a direction parallel to the central axis of the first lens-forming surface,

   The second mold part consists of a second lens-forming surface having a central axis and a circumferential edge, a second stop surface extending radially outwardly from the circumferential edge of the second lens-forming surface in a plane perpendicular to the central axis of the second lens-forming surface, a second intermediate region extending from the second stop surface, and a second alignment surface extending from the second intermediate region in a direction parallel to the central axis of the second lens-forming surface, and

In the contact lens mold assembly, the first stop surface of the first mold part is in continuous contact with the second stop surface of the second mold part, around the circumferential edge of the second lens-forming surface, and the first alignment surface of the first mold part is in contact with the second alignment surface of the second mold part,

2. Applying a contact lens precursor material to the first lens-forming surface of the first mold part, or to the second lens-forming surface of the second mold part,
3. Placing the first mold part and the second mold part together such that the first alignment surface of the first mold part is in contact with the second alignment surface of the second mold part, and such that the first stop surface of the first mold part is in continuous contact with the second stop surface of the second mold part, around the circumferential edge of the second lens-forming surface of the second mold part.
4. Curing the contact lens precursor material to form an unfinished contact lens,
5. Separating the contact lens from the first mold part and the second mold part to form a separated contact lens, and
6. Placing the separated contact lens in a contact lens package.

Such a contact lens mold assembly is shown in Figure 2.6.

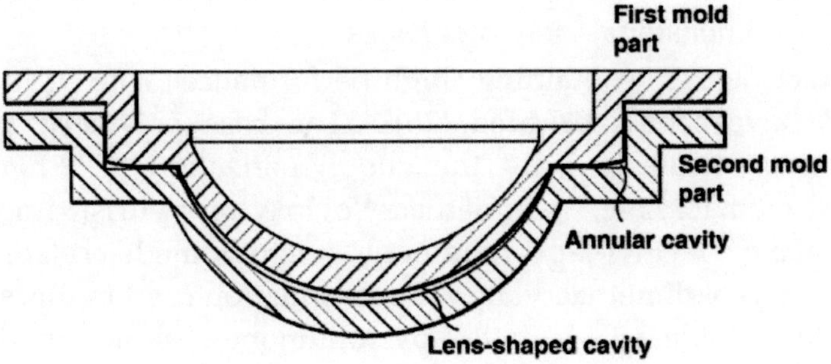

Figure 2.6 Contact lens mold assembly (22).

The contact lens mold assembly contains a first mold part, a second mold part, a lens-shaped cavity, and an annular cavity. In use, contact lens precursor material, such as a polymerizable material or a contact lens formulation, fills the lens-shaped cavity, and excess contact lens precursor material passes into the annular cavity.

The lenses can be fabricated in an automated system. The automated system includes a component for forming a contact lens mold assembly. The automated system can further consists of an injection molding machine, an apparatus for applying the contact lens precursor material, and an apparatus for curing or polymerizing the contact lens precursor material, an apparatus for separating the unfinished contact lens, and an apparatus for placing the separated contact lens in a contact lens package (22).

In order to improve the efficiency of lens manufacturing by thermal curing of a precursor material, a tray for holding contact lens mold assemblies during the thermal curing has been developed (23). The tray contains a plurality of plates and a frame supporting the plates. The frame is configured to cooperate with other identical frames so that a plurality of the trays can be stacked vertically to form a tray stack.

Also, a demolding apparatus has been found to be particularly effective for demolding a two-part contact lens mold assembly (24).

2.8 Reactive Ion Etching

Polarizers are essential components of many electronic devices and are used in a variety of applications such as in liquid crystal displays and three-dimensional viewing glasses.

Contact lenses containing high-performance wire grid polarizers have been fabricated (25). The base polymeric membrane was synthesized by the copolymerization of 2-hydroxyethyl methacrylate, 3-(methacryloyloxy)propyltris(trimethylsiloxy)silane, 1-vinyl-2-pyrrolidinone, methyl methacrylate and ethylene glycol dimethacrylate. The formulation used in this study is shown in Table 2.3. 1-Vinyl-2-pyrrolidinone is shown in Figure 2.7.

All of the components in Table 2.3 were mixed thoroughly, and the photopolymerization was carried out using UV irradiation on a Teflon mold (1.50×1.50 *cm*). The thickness of the membrane was controlled to 50±2 μm after polymerization was completed. Then, nanoimprinting was carried out on this membrane using an epoxy

Table 2.3 Formulation of contact lens (25).

Compound	Weight/[*g*]
2-Hydroxyethyl methacrylate	17.0
N-Vinyl-2-pyrrolidone	0.900
Methyl methacrylate	0.200
3-(Methacryloyloxy)propyltris(trimethylsiloxy)silane	1.80
Ethylene glycol dimethacrylate	0.100
2-Hydroxy-2-methyl-propiophenone	0.100

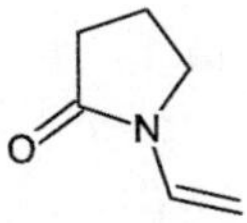

Figure 2.7 1-Vinyl-2-pyrrolidinone.

resin at a mixing ratio of 85:15 (YDF-170:R-1309), which was selected due to its high adhesive strength. The original silicon oxide mold (1.10 *cm* × 1.10 *cm*) used for nanoimprinting featured a nanopattern with a 180 *nm* period, a 110 *nm* line width and a 200 *nm* height. Before the nanoimprinting, Silquest A-187 silane was vapor-coated on the membrane to increase the adhesive strength between the membrane and the nanopattern.

Two consecutive angled aluminium evaporations were performed on the nanopattern, followed by reactive ion etching to form the wire grid polarizer (25). The wire grid polarizer on the membrane was then covered by another layer of the base polymeric material to form the final contact lens.

This membrane demonstrated a high performance as a polarizer, confirmed by measuring transmittance of transverse magnetic polarized light and transverse electric polarized light. This membrane also demonstrated good performance as a contact lens in terms of modulus, water content and oxygen permeability (25).

2.9 Electrospinning

When the polymers for contact lenses are created as a solid or as semi-permeable solid structures, the available oxygen to the corneal surface is reduced (26). Also, tear and aqueous transport through the lens is minimized. The manufacture of a contact lens with a high oxygen permeability has been described. A high degree of oxygen permeability is important, as the cornea is an avascular membrane and receives its oxygen supply directly through the air. Any impediment that obstructs the corneal surface with direct contact with the surrounding air would be detrimental.

It is possible to create a contact lens structure that is made out of varying layers of differing polymer materials, with the possibility of interdispersement of trapped drug layers to maintain a localized point of contact with the desired drug or medication and the corneal surface. The degree of surface hydrophobicity and hydrophilicity could be engineered into the surface, along with the ability to restrain lipid transport into the lens structure from degrading optical clarity.

Here, the base surface side (eye contact surface) of the contact lens could be made of a completely different material than there is on the outside surface of the contact lens. For instance, the base surface side (cornea contact surface) could be made hydrophilic to provide superior wetting while the outside (air contact surface) could be made hydrophobic and prevent the problem of ordinary contact lenses from having a degraded oxygen permeability. Materials that are generally incompatible with the eye could still be used to construct a contact lens, since they will not be coming into actual contact with the eye surface.

2.9.1 *Creating Electrospun Contact Lens Structures*

Transparent contact lens structures can be fabricated that can be placed onto a recipient (26). In order to realize a suitable lens structure, fibrils of a suitable polymer, preferably 2-hydroxyethyl methacrylate (HEMA), must be created and layered to form the basis of a mat which exhibits the transparency and diffusion characteristics of corneal stromal tissue.

Preferably, an electrospinning process produces the polymer fibrils. the polymer under consideration, e.g., collagen, is dissolved by a suitable solvent and injected under hydrostatic pressure into a conductive needle or capillary. A DC potential of preferably 4 *kV* to 12,000 *kV* is maintained between the injection needle and a suitable target located at a distance away from the needle sufficient to preclude production of a coronal discharge or arc (26).

The voltage is adjusted according to the distance and the desired fiber diameter and its structure. The voltage difference between the injection needle and target suited to the given solvent conductivity, polymer, and flow rate, and the resulting electrostatic field at the needle tip, results in the formation of a Taylor cone from the tip of which issues a jet of a micron-sized jet that is attracted to, and impacts with, the ground cathode target.

The applied voltage on the needle can be either positive or negative depending on the situation. Additionally, the voltage does not have to be a constant polarity.

An alternating voltage prevents the charge buildup on electrospun fibers that contributes to a whipping instability. By simply alternating the applied needle voltage from a positive to a negative polarity, the electrospun fibers can be deposited at precise intervals to enable the construction of a precise electrospun mat of polymer material. This electrospun mat of polymer fibers could be constructed in such a way as to maintain mean fibril distance of approximately 200 *nm*.

When the evaporation of the solvent occurs from the electrospray jet, the result is fine micrometer to nanometer diameter polymer strands. The accumulation of such strands creates a mat of media having a diameter ranging from tens of microns or more down to tens of nanometers or less, depending on the concentration and nature of solute, the conductivity and viscosity of liquid, and the potential difference between the needle and target (26).

Collagen mats produced by this process can have diameters up to tens of millimeters and thickness of up to hundreds of microns, depending on deposition time. Similarly, it has been found that a variety of polymers for creating suitable lens structures as part of this invention can be derived from a variety of sources.

It should be noted that extrusion rather than electrospinning of the polymer is an alternative in certain instances, along with laser ablation and chemical etching, to form the lens curvature. Laser cutting is often employed since fibril terminations must be severed and should not be excessively frayed or tangled. Tangling or fraying can affect bonding to native collagen and can vary optical transparency. While the resulting collagen mat consists of disorganized fibrils, this does not interfere with the required transparency or diffusive characteristics.

The general theory of corneal transparency has to do with the diameter of the collagen fibers in reference to the wavelength of the incident light. Organization of the fibers appears to be of less importance. This conclusion is supported by the fact that shark cornea exhibits regions of disorganized fibers and random interfibrillar distances while yet exhibiting a high degree of optical transparency. Use of microspun collagen fibers allows the control of the fibril diameter, and the deposition rate determines the interfibrillar spacing.

Traditional methods of making a contact lens permeable require that an existing solid lens be subjected to various processes that cause the creation of holes to be used. The described invention has these controllable holes throughout each fibril mat of material. The hole infrastructure is built into the lens right from the start, not as a last step in the production line (26).

2.9.2 *Electrospinning Controlled Polymer Fibril Matrices*

A modification of the electrospinning process to yield a crosshatch pattern can be achieved by maintaining either the needle anode at a fixed distance and moving the cathode target, or vice versa (26). Under normal conditions, the electrospun fiber is splayed about by the interplay of mechanical, hydrodynamic, and electrical forces so as to cause the polymer strand to accumulate on the target in a random pattern. While ordinarily this is not a problem in stromal scaffold mat construction, since the fiber diameter is the principal factor in transparency, there are instances where a regular matrix of stromal collagen is desired.

By rapidly moving the needle in a linear direction for a fixed distance and then reversing such motion with respect to the target, while at the same time indexing the target utilizing a stepper motor drive or piezo stack or other such precision positioner, a series of relatively straight, parallel fibers may be laid down on the target surface. After the desired pattern has been achieved in one axis, the target may be rotated ninety degrees and the process can be repeated.

The outer fringes of a mat matrix so created will be less organized than the central axis as the outer edge is where target position reversal occurs. This area can be trimmed away and discarded with a suitable laser. The resulting central scaffold area exhibits a structure, pattern, and diameter that closely mimics natural stromal collagen. If even greater accuracy is required in fibril spacing, the distance the fiber is deposited across a moving target can be increased and the jet shut down at the point of maximum travel. The target is then indexed to the next position, the electrospinning jet reestablished, and the target rapidly moved to the opposite extreme, where the process is repeated until the maximum linear coverage area of fibers in one axis of orientation is achieved.

The target may then be rotated preferably ninety degrees as before and the spinning procedure repeated. The intent is to create a grid of horizontal and vertical fibers (26).

2.9.3 *Electrospinning of a Prepolymer Solution*

Electrospun polymer fibers provide a material with a variety of favorable characteristics that may be tailored to fit various applications. It is therefore desirable to provide an ophthalmic drug delivery system utilizing electrospun polymer fibers. The system may utilize an improved contact lens incorporating electrospun fibers with desired characteristics, and a system and method for delivering ophthalmic drugs from the improved contact lens to an eye over an extended period of time while maintaining the concentration of the drug in the eye at an efficacious level throughout the period of drug delivery.

Electrospinning of a prepolymer solution has been documented. The there described devices and methods overcome many of the limitations inherent in the conventional contact lens design and production, including (27):

1. Providing means of producing contact lenses that exhibit the optical and diffusive characteristics of natural corneal tissue,

2. Providing a scaffold lens structure that can permit the absorption or adsorption of specific chemical species for the purpose of drug delivery to treat specific eye conditions,
3. Providing a scaffold lens structure that can permit the absorption or adsorption of specific chemical species for the purpose of minimizing or eliminating protein deposits,
4. Reducing or eliminating corneal dry eye condition by permitting increased diffusion of tear fluids and by delivering selected compounds to natural tear components,
5. Producing a viable collagen polymer refractive correcting contact lens whose characteristics duplicate natural tissue,
6. Promoting corneal health and reducing the possibility of conventional lens-caused infections, since the diffusive characteristics promote antimicrobial agent distribution natural to the eye,
7. Reducing abnormal blood vessel growth which occurs when long-term contact lens wear reduces the average oxygen transport to the corneal surface,
8. Providing a scaffold lens structure that can permit the absorption or adsorption of various chemical species for the purposes of drug delivery to precise portions of the cornea, thereby keeping a regulated, time-lapse drug delivery confined to not only the cornea, but specific regions of the cornea, and
9. Manufacturing a contact lens with the ability to control the location and the amount of surface hydrophobicity and hydrophilicity tailored to the application, as required.

Electrospinning is used to produce a permeable contact lens composed of micro strands that approximate the nanometer-size fibrils of natural human corneal stromal collagen. The fibril diameter is regarded as the principal factor in achieving corneal transparency. The fibril strands are deposited onto an appropriate target, which allows a suitable polymer fibril scaffold mat to develop. The density and configuration of this mat determine the permeability of the structure to aqueous fluids, lipids, and gases. The density and orientation of these fibrils can be controlled in order to achieve the desired diffusive and optical parameters compatible with natural tissue.

The drug delivery system that can be used utilizes both raw electrospun fibers and an improved contact lens as the means of drug delivery. The fibers and the improved contact lens provide a drug delivery system composed of a drug-releasing scaffold formed from a mat of electrospun fibers and methods for incorporating various therapeutic drugs into the mat.

Therapeutic drugs may be loaded into the drug delivery system by soaking the electrospun mats in a solution containing the drug, or by providing the drugs in the solution feeding the electrospinning process, thus incorporating the drug into the fibers in the electrospun mat. Various processes for treating the electrospun mats after loading with therapeutic drugs are also described for improving the drug delivery characteristics, such as coating the mats in a polymer and crosslinking the electrospun fibers.

Some polymers that can be used for forming the mat are listed in Table 2.4. The monomeric acids are shown in Figure 2.8.

Table 2.4 Polymers for mat production (27).

Polymer compound	Polymer compound
Poly(vinyl ethyl ether)	Poly(acrylic acid)
Poly(methacrylic acid)	Poly(*N*-vinyl pyrrolidone)
Poly(vinyl alcohol)	Poly(methyl methacrylate)
Poly(glycerol methacrylate)	Silicone hydrogels
Fluorocarbon hydrogels	Poly(acrylamide)
Poly(fumaric acid)	Poly(itaconic acid)
Poly(mesaconic acid)	Poly(methyl acrylate)
Poly(ethyl acrylate)	Poly(propyl acrylate)
Poly(isopropyl acrylate)	Poly(isobutyl acrylate)
Poly(isooctyl acrylate)	Poly(isodecyl acrylate)
Poly(cyclohexyl acrylate)	Poly(2-ethylhexyl acrylate)
Poly(ethyl methacrylate)	Poly(propyl methacrylate)
Poly(butyl acrylate)	Poly(vinyl acetate)
Poly(vinyl propionate)	Poly(vinyl butyrate)
Poly(vinyl valerate)	Poly(chloroprene)
Poly(vinyl chloride)	Poly(vinylidene chloride)
Polybutadiene	Poly(vinyl toluene)
Poly(2-hydroxyethyl methacrylate)	Poly(isobornyl methacrylate)

Examples of suitable hydrophobic comonomers are shown in Table 2.5. Some compounds are shown in Figure 2.9.

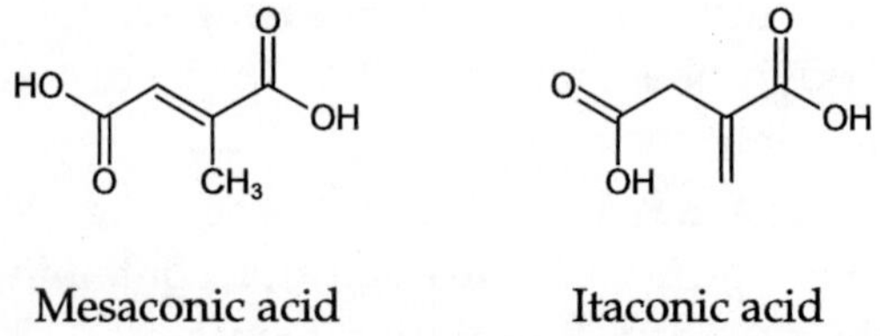

Figure 2.8 Monomeric acids for mat-forming polymers.

Table 2.5 Comonomers for mat production (27).

Comonomer compound	Comonomer compound
Methyl acrylate	Ethyl acrylate
Propyl acrylate	Isopropyl acrylate
Isobutyl acrylate	Isooctyl acrylate
Isodecyl acrylate	Cyclohexyl acrylate
2-Ethylhexyl acrylate	
Methyl methacrylate	Ethyl methacrylate
Propyl methacrylate	Butyl acrylate
Vinyl acetate	Vinyl propionate
Vinyl butyrate	Vinyl valerate
Styrene	Chloroprene
Vinyl chloride	Vinylidene chloride
Acrylonitrile	1-Butene
Butadiene	Methacrylonitrile
Vinyl toluene	Vinyl ethyl ether
Isobornyl methacrylate	Trifluoroethyl methacrylate
Hexafluoroisopropyl methacrylate	Hexafluorobutyl (meth)acrylate
Tris-trimethylsilyloxy-silyl-propyl methacrylate	
Perfluorohexylethylthiocarbonylaminoethyl methacrylate	
3-Methacryloxypropylpentamethyldisiloxane	
Bis(methacryloxypropyl) tetramethyl disiloxane	

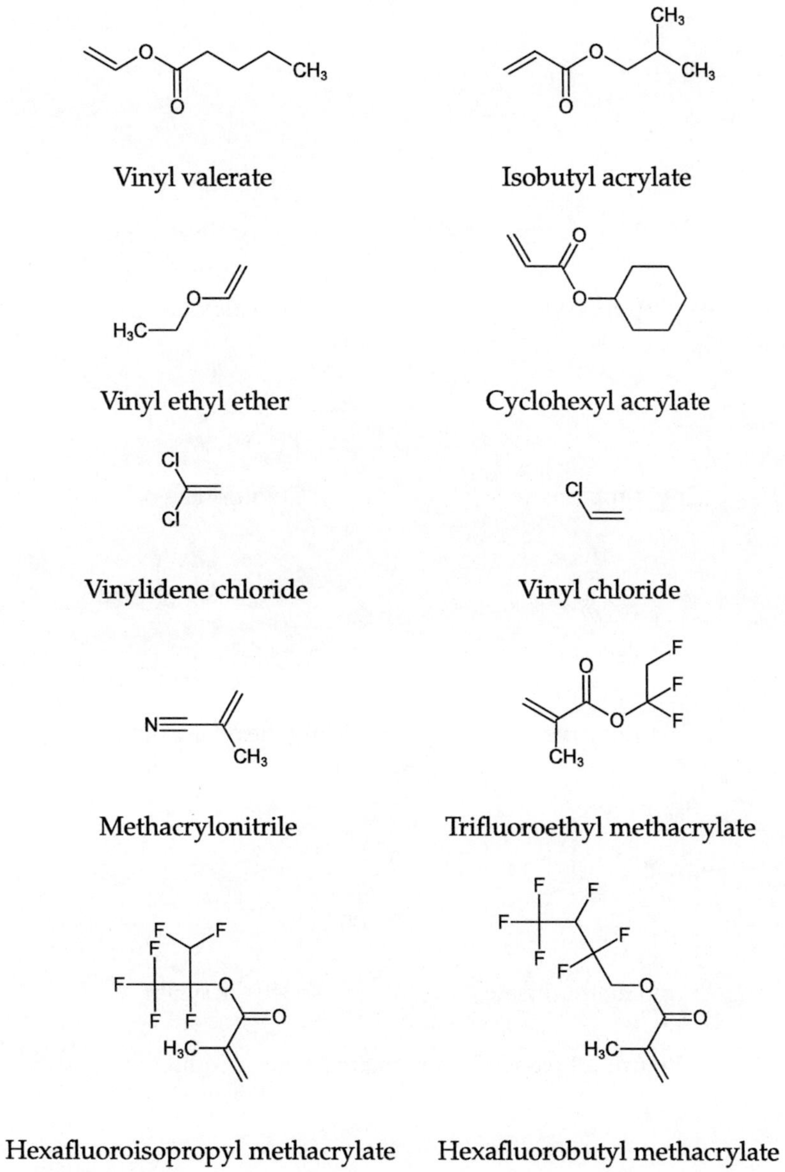

Figure 2.9 Comonomers for mat production.

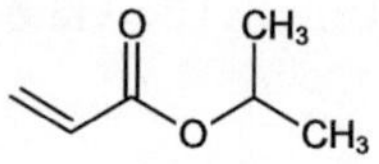

Isopropyl acrylate

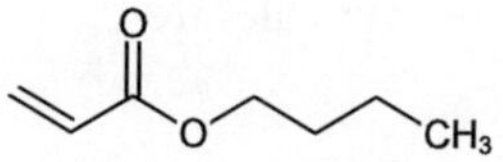

Butyl acrylate

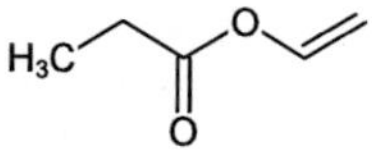

Vinyl propionate

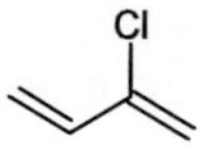

Chloroprene

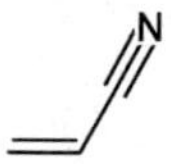

Acrylonitrile

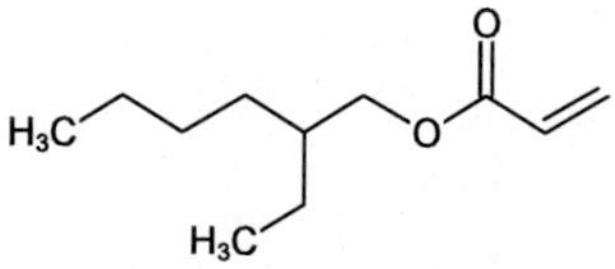

2-Ethylhexyl acrylate

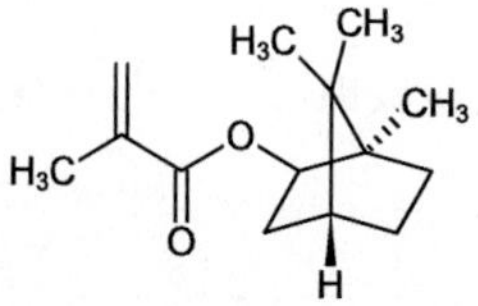

Isobornyl methacrylate

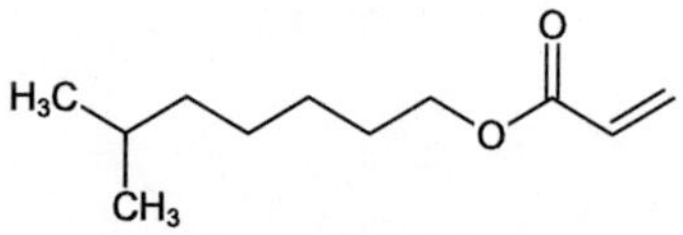

Isooctyl acrylate

Figure 2.9 (cont) Comonomers for mat production.

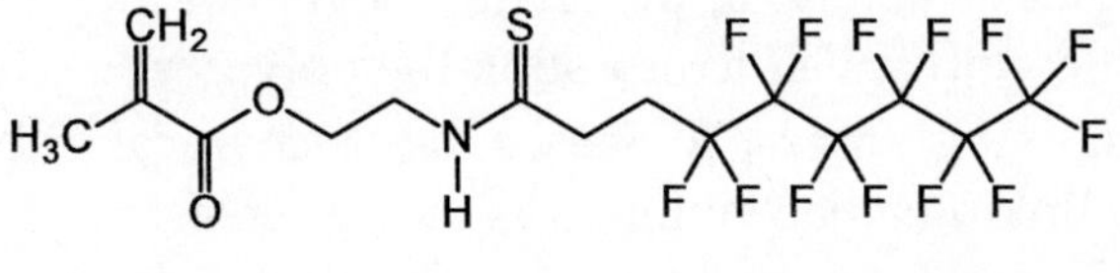

Perfluorohexylethylthiocarbonylaminoethyl methacrylate

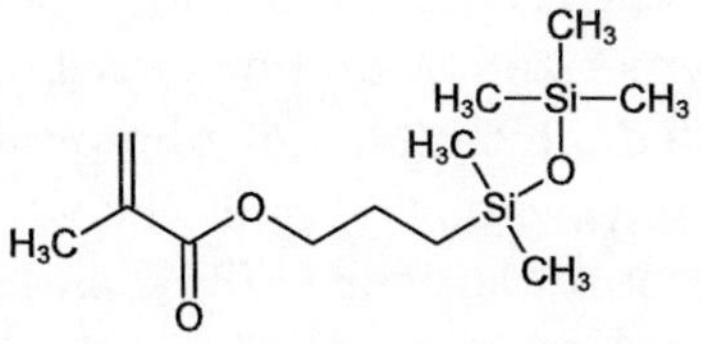

3-Methacryloxypropylpentamethyldisiloxane

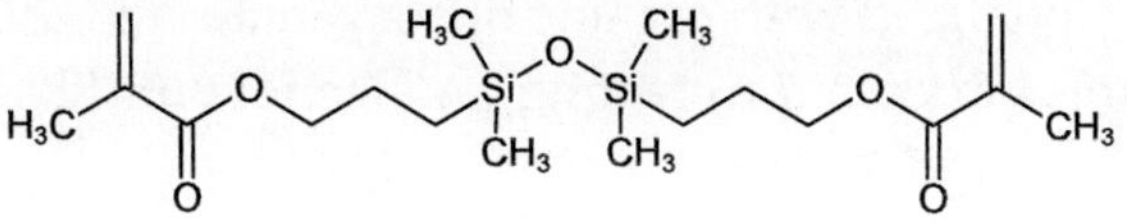

Bis(methacryloxypropyl) tetramethyl disiloxane

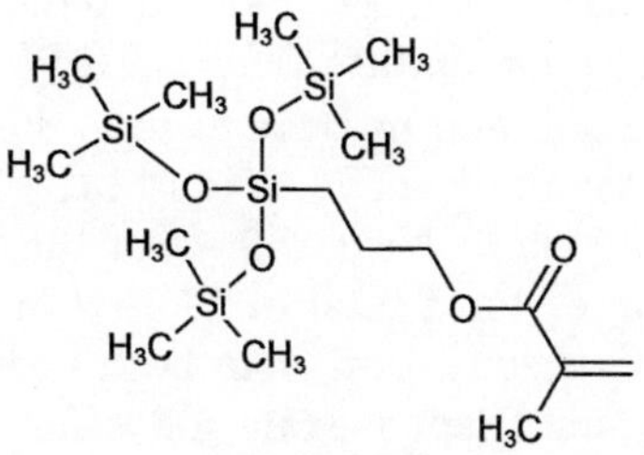

Tris-trimethylsilyloxy-silyl-propyl methacrylate

Figure 2.9 (cont) Comonomers for mat production.

The fiber mats may also be processed by exposing them to a crosslinking agent such as ethylene glycol dimethacrylate (EGDMA), tetraethylene glycol dimethacrylate, divinylbenzene, divinyl acrylamide, or any triallyl crosslinking agent when there is at least one active alkene in the chain. Methanol may be added to poly(vinyl alcohol) (PVA) to crosslink the polymer.

The crosslinking process increases the mechanical stability of the fiber mat by linking adjacent fibers as they intersect randomly in the fiber mat (27).

The polymerization reaction can be carried out using a photoinitiator. For photopolymerization, a photoinitiator which can initiate free radical polymerization and/or crosslinking by the use of light is suitably added. Examples of photoinitiators are benzoin methyl ether, 1-hydroxycyclohexyl phenyl ketone and Darocur and Irgacure types, preferably Darocur 11738® and Darocur 29590®.

Also, reactive photoinitiators, which can be incorporated into a macromer, or can be used as a special comonomer, are also suitable. Examples of these are α-aminoacetophenones containing hydroxyl groups functionalized with organic diisocyanates (28, 29).

An example process for creating an electrospun fiber mat is as follows (27):

Preparation 2–1: The following materials should be combined, mixed, placed over heat and stirred inside a round-bottom flask with an attached condenser for 6.5 *h*: 11.363 *g* PVA, 2.277 *g* Triton X-100, and 27.539 *g* highly purified water is added to the mixture. This is the PVA polymer mixture.

Without allowing the polymer mixture to cool, the following steps are performed: 2.000 *ml* of Vigamox is added to 14.141 *g* of the PVA polymer mixture and stirred for 1 *min*. Next, 7.0 *ml* of the PVA/Vigamox solution is added to 2 syringes for a total of 14.0 *ml* of solution. Then the PVA/Vigamox solution is electrospun from both needles simultaneously at the following parameters: Dispense rate: 1.8 $ml\,hr^{-1}$ 18 gauge blunt-end needles. Voltage: 30 kV. Travel distance: 4 in total time: 2.5 *h*.

After electrospinning, the resulting mat is cut into approximately 3.0 *mg* squares. If crosslinking is desired, the squares are soaked in methanol for 7 *h* and allowed to air dry under ambient conditions overnight. The squares are coated in the remaining PVA polymer solution created in the first step.

Before coating the squares, the PVA polymer solution is heated in a round-bottom flask with attached condenser for 2 *h*. After coating the squares in the polymer solution, they are allowed to air dry under ambient conditions overnight. If a second crosslink is desired, the squares are soaked in methanol for 7 *h* and then air dried under ambient conditions overnight.

Vigamox eye drops from Alcon contain moxifloxacin, cf. Figure 4.49.

A good fit from a contact lens can most easily be achieved from a flexible hydrogel contact lens that drapes easily over the cornea and has minimal interaction with the eyelids during blinking. This fit, achieved by high levels of flexibility, is offset by a reduction in durability. Also, the rigidity of a material affects the flexure of a lens as well as the movement on the eye and tear exchange. The ease of manufacturing of a contact lens, along with the reliability of the quoted parameters and dimensional stability, will also be influenced by the mechanical properties of the lens (27).

2.10 Rigid Plastic Lenses

2.10.1 Rigid Gas-Permeable Contact Lenses

Rigid gas-permeable contact lenses provide a higher oxygen permeability and tear exchange rate than soft contact lenses. However, their wettability needs to be improved to enhance the wearing comfort (30).

A UV laser with a wavelength of 355 *nm* was used to modify the surface properties of rigid gas-permeable contact lenses with materials of Boston XO (Bausch & Lomb Incorporated). The mesh pattern was fabricated on the rigid gas-permeable contact lens surface by using the laser and smoothed by using an oxygen plasma. The enhanced hydrophilic efficiency was analyzed using a contact angle measurement.

The results of this study indicated that the contact angle of the lens material decreased by approximately 10° to 20° when the pitch of mesh pattern was <50 μm under a 500 $mm\,s^{-1}$ scanning speed. The oxygen plasma enhanced the surface wettability with a decreased contact angle of 40°. The hydrophilic characteristic of the UV laser and oxygen plasma-treated surface was twice that of oxygen plasma-treated and untreated surfaces. So, rigid gas-permeable contact lens edges can be treated with UV laser and oxygen plasma to enhance the tear wettability and the wearing comfort (30).

2.11 Soft Plastic Lenses

2.11.1 *Layer-by-Layer Deposition*

2.11.1.1 *Wettable Coating*

A cost-effective method for making a silicone hydrogel contact lens which has a good wettable coating with a good durability has been described (31).

Soft contact lenses conform closely to the shape of the eye, so oxygen cannot easily circumvent the lens. They must allow oxygen from the surrounding air, i.e., oxygen, to reach the cornea because the cornea does not receive oxygen from the blood supply like other tissues. If sufficient oxygen does not reach the cornea, a corneal swelling occurs. Extended periods of oxygen deprivation cause the undesirable growth of blood vessels in the cornea. By having high oxygen permeability, a silicone hydrogel contact lens allows sufficient oxygen to permeate through the lens to the cornea and to have minimal adverse effects on corneal health (31).

However, a silicone hydrogel material typically has a surface or at least some areas of its surface which is hydrophobic. Hydrophobic surface or surface areas will uptake lipids or proteins from the ocular environment and may adhere to the eye. Thus, a silicone hydrogel contact lens will generally require surface modification.

A known method for modifying the hydrophilicity of a relatively hydrophobic contact lens material can be done through the use of a plasma treatment (31). However, a plasma treatment of silicone hydrogel contact lenses may not be cost-effective, because the preformed contact lenses must be dried before the plasma treatment.

Another method for modifying the hydrophilicity of a relatively hydrophobic contact lens material is a layer-by-layer polyionic material deposition technique. This technique can provide a cost-effective process for rendering a silicone hydrogel material wettable. However, such a layer-by-layer coating may be less durable than a plasma coating for extended wear purpose (31).

Another method proposed for modifying the surface hydrophilicity of a silicone hydrogel contact lens is the incorporation of wetting agents into a lens formulation (32, 33).

This method may be cost-effective, because after cast-molding of silicone hydrogel contact lenses, there is no additional posterior process required for modifying the surface hydrophilicity of the lens. However, the wetting agents may not remain effective over time and may not provide a durable wettable surface. In addition, there may be hydrophobic surface spots which can be extremely susceptible to lipid/protein adsorption and deposition (31).

A method for making a silicone hydrogel contact lens consists of the following steps (31):

1. Obtaining a mold having a first mold half and a second mold half, wherein the first mold half includes a first molding surface and the second mold half includes a second molding surface, wherein the first and second mold halves are configured to receive each other such that a lens-forming cavity is formed between the first molding surface and the second molding surface,
2. Applying a first transferable layer-by-layer coating to the first molding surface and a second transferable layer-by-layer coating to the second molding surface, wherein each of the first and second transferable layer-by-layer coatings consists of at least one layer of a first polyionic polymeric material and optionally at least one layer of a second polyionic material or a non-charged hydrophilic polymer with a hydrophobic backbone, wherein the first and second polyionic material each have a hydrophobic backbone and multiple ionizable or charged pendant groups, wherein the first and second polyionic materials have charges opposite to each other,
3. Dispensing a silicone hydrogel lens-forming fluid material into the lens-forming cavity of the mold with the first and second transferable layer-by-layer coatings on their molding surfaces, wherein the silicone hydrogel lens-forming material is a non-crosslinkable hydrophilic polymer and at least one member selected from the group consists of a silicone-containing vinylic monomer, a silicone-containing macromer with ethylenically unsaturated groups, a crosslinkable silicone-containing prepolymer, and mixtures thereof, wherein the non-crosslinkable hydrophilic polymer is capable of forming an interfacial film at the interface between the coated molding surfaces and the lens-forming fluid material,

4. Soaking the transferable layer-by-layer coatings with the lens-forming fluid material for a time period sufficient to both allow the non-crosslinkable hydrophilic polymer in the interface film to penetrate into the transferable layer-by-layer coatings and to entangle with coating materials in the transferable layer-by-layer coatings, and
5. Curing the lens-forming material within the lens-forming cavity to form the silicone hydrogel contact lens, whereby the transferable layer-by-layer coatings detach from the molding surfaces and reattaches to the formed silicone hydrogel contact lens such that said silicone hydrogel contact lens becomes coated with the transferable layer-by-layer coatings, wherein the non-crosslinkable hydrophilic polymer has a molecular weight or structure that promotes entanglement of the non-crosslinkable hydrophilic polymer in the interfacial film with the polymer matrix of the formed lens so as to obtain a wettable surface coating with a good coating durability characterized by surviving at least five consecutive digital rubbing tests.

Any suitable siloxane-containing macromer with ethylenically unsaturated groups can be used to produce a silicone hydrogel material. Preferred siloxane-containing macromers have been detailed and the synthesis procedures have been described (34).

Macromers that contain two or more vinyl groups can also serve as crosslinking agents. Diblock and triblock macromers consisting of poly(dimethyl siloxane) and poly(akyleneoxide)s could also be of use. Such macromers could be mono- or difunctionalized with acrylate, methacrylate or vinyl groups. For example, one might use methacrylate end-capped poly(ethyleneoxide) block poly(dimethyl siloxane)-block-poly(ethyleneoxide) to enhance the oxygen permeability (31).

The silicone hydrogel lens-forming material can also contain a hydrophilic vinylic monomer. Nearly any hydrophilic vinylic monomer that can act as a plasticizer can be used in the fluid composition. The here preferred hydrophilic monomers are shown in Table 2.6. Some compounds are shown in Figure 2.10.

By incorporating a certain amount of a hydrophobic vinylic monomer in a polymerizable fluid composition, the mechanical

Table 2.6 Hydrophilic monomers (31).

Monomer	Shortcut
N,N-dimethyl acrylamide	DMA
2-Hydroxyethyl methacrylate	HEMA
2-Hydroxyethyl acrylate	
2-Hydroxypropyl acrylate	
2-Hydroxypropyl methacrylate	HPMA
Trimethylammonium 2-hydroxy propyl methacrylate hydrochloride	
2-Dimethylamino ethyl methacrylate	DMAEMA
Dimethylamino ethyl methacrylamide	
Acrylamide	
Methacrylamide	
Allyl alcohol	
Vinylpyridine	
Glycerol methacrylate	
N-(1,1-Dimethyl-3-oxobutyl)acrylamide	
N-Vinyl-2-pyrrolidone	NVP
Acrylic acid	
Methacrylic acid	
N,N-Dimethyl acrylamide	DMA

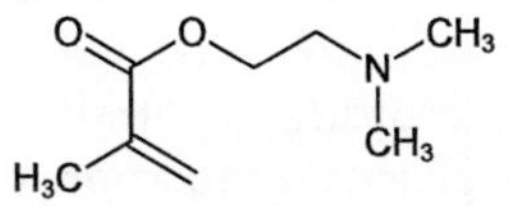

2-Dimethylamino ethyl methacrylate

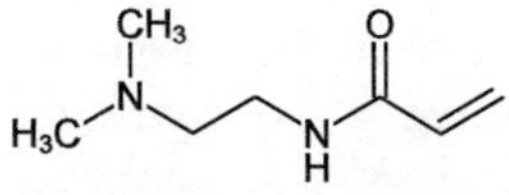

Dimethylamino ethyl methacrylamide

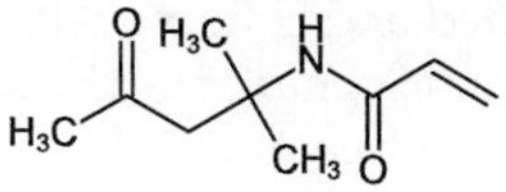

N-(1,1-Dimethyl-3-oxobutyl) acrylamide

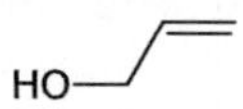

Allyl alcohol

Figure 2.10 Hydrophilic monomers.

properties, e.g., modulus of elasticity, of the resultant polymer may be improved.

Crosslinking agents may be used to improve the structural integrity and mechanical strength. Examples of crosslinking agents include allyl(meth)acrylate, divinyl ether, divinyl sulfone, divinyl benzene, trivinylbenzene, trimethylol propane tri(meth)acrylate, pentaerythritol tetra(meth)acrylate, bisphenol A di(meth)acrylate, methylenebis(meth)acrylamide, triallyl phthalate, or diallyl phthalate. Some of these compounds are shown in Figure 2.11. A preferred crosslinking agent is ethylene glycol dimethacrylate.

The synthesis of a macromer has been described as follows (31):

Preparation 2–2: First, 51.5 *g* (50 *mmol*) of the perfluoropolyether Fomblin® Zdol (from Ausimont S.p.A., Milan) having a mean molecular weight of 1030 $g\,mol^{-1}$ and containing 1.96 $meq\,g^{-1}$ of hydroxyl groups according to end-group titration is introduced into a three-neck flask together with 50 *mg* of dibutyltin dilaurate. The flask contents are evacuated to about 20 *mbar* with stirring and subsequently decompressed with argon. This operation is repeated twice. Then, 22.2 *g* (0.1 *mol*) of freshly distilled isophorone diisocyanate kept under an argon atmosphere is subsequently added in a counterstream of argon. The temperature in the flask is kept below 30°C by cooling with a water bath. After stirring overnight at room temperature, the reaction is complete. Isocyanate titration gives an NCO content of 1.40 $meq\,g^{-1}$ (theory: 1.35 $meq\,g^{-1}$).

Next, 202 *g* of the α,ω-hydroxypropyl-terminated poly(dimethyl siloxane) KF-6001 from Shin-Etsu having a mean molecular weight of 2000 $g\,mol^{-1}$ (1.00 $meq\,g^{-1}$ of hydroxyl groups according to titration) is introduced into a flask. The flask contents are evacuated to approx. 0.1 *mbar* and decompressed with argon. This operation is repeated twice. The degassed siloxane is dissolved in 202 *ml* of freshly distilled toluene kept under an argon atmosphere, and 100 *mg* of dibutyltindilaurate is added. After complete homogenization of the solution, all the perfluoropolyether reacted with isophorone diisocyanate is added under argon. After stirring overnight at room temperature, the reaction is complete. The solvent is stripped off under a high vacuum at room temperature. Microtitration shows 0.36 $meq\,g^{-1}$ of hydroxyl groups (theory 0.37 $meq\,g^{-1}$).

Next. 13.78 *g* (88.9 *mmol*) of 2-isocyanatoethyl methacrylate is added under argon to 247 *g* of the α,σ-hydroxypropyl-terminated poly(siloxane)-perfluoropolyether-poly(siloxane) three-block copolymer (a three-block copolymer on stoichiometric average, but other block lengths are also present). The mixture is stirred at room temperature for three days, after which microtitration no longer shows any isocyanate groups (detection

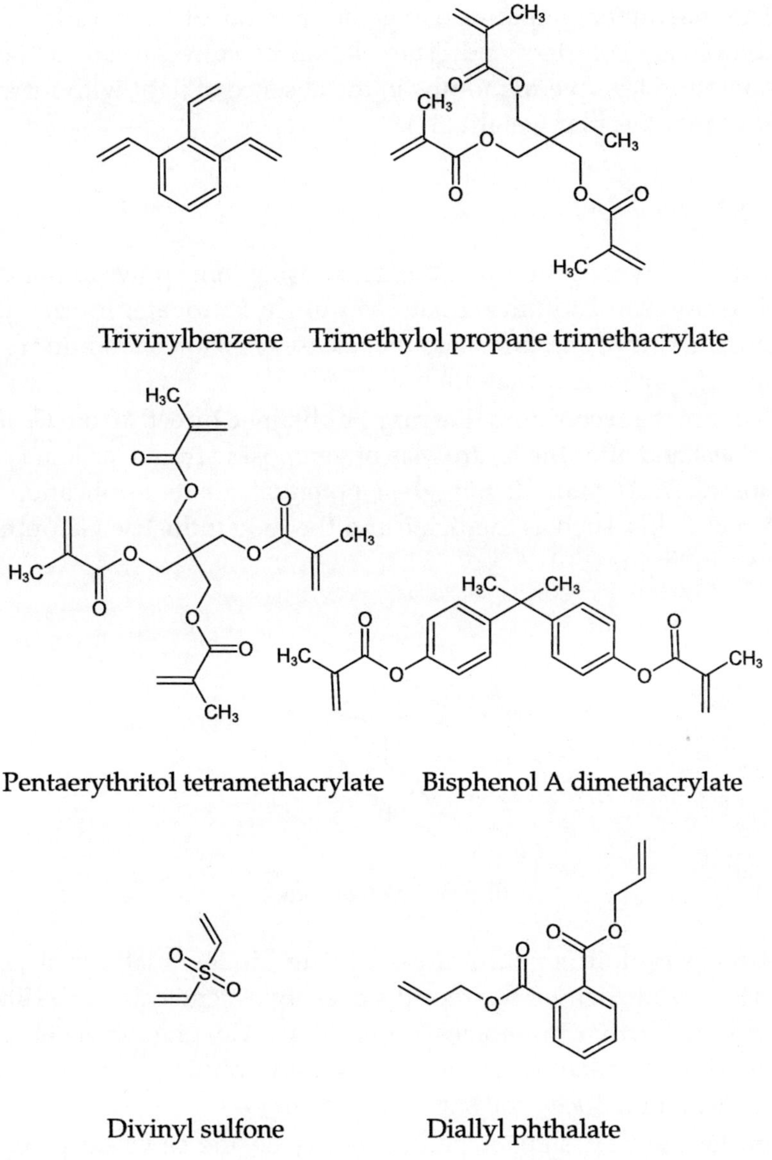

Figure 2.11 Crosslinking agents.

limit 0.01 $meq\,g^{-1}$) and 0.34 $meq\,g^{-1}$ of methacryl groups is found (theory 0.34 $meq\,g^{-1}$).

The macromer prepared using the method of Preparation 2–2 is completely colorless and clear. It can be stored in air at room temperature for several months in the absence of light without any change in molecular weight (31).

2.11.1.2 *Material Release*

A layer-by-layer coating was designed using ionic polysaccharides such as chitosan, sodium alginate, sodium hyaluronate, and genipin as crosslinking agent, to sustain the release of diclofenac sodium salt from soft contact lens materials (35).

Genipin is a secoiridoid that may be obtained directly from *Genipa americana* and after the hydrolysis of geniposide from Gardenia jasminoides fruits (36). It has great potential for its application in different fields, such as medicine and the food industry. Genipin is shown in Figure 2.12.

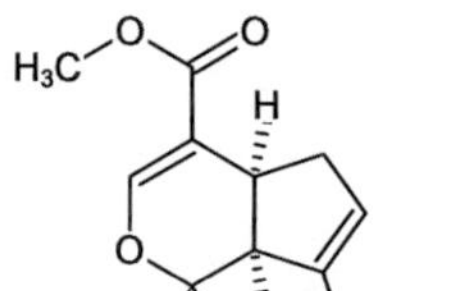

Figure 2.12 Genipin.

Because genipin is a naturally occurring, biodegradable molecule with low cytotoxicity, it has recently been investigated as a crosslinking material in many biological applications. Coatings with genipin as crosslinking agent were found to be hydrophilic, biocompatible, nontoxic, and reduced the bacterial growth (37).

Furthermore, it showed minor effects on the physical properties of the material, such as wettability, ionic permeability, refractive index and transmittance, which remained within the recommended values for soft contact lenses. Such a coating was applied on a silicone-based hydrogel and also on commercial SofLens and

PureVision soft contact lenses (35). The coating attenuated the initial drug burst and extended the therapeutic period for at least two weeks. Relevantly, the problems of sterilizing drug-loaded soft contact lenses coated with biopolymers, using classic methods that involve high temperature or radiation, were successfully solved through high hydrostatic pressure sterilization (35).

2.11.2 *Electron-Beam Irradiation Polymerization*

The polymerization of HEMA, which can be used in soft contact lenses, has been performed by using electron-beam irradiation (38). Also, the best conditions for the polymerization reaction were examined.

Comparing the physical properties of the contact lenses to the one fabricated by thermal polymerization method, the possible use of electron-beam irradiation for the fabrication of a soft contact lens was studied. The degree of polymerization of the HEMA was investigated with respect to the composition of the monomer, the additive ratio and the dose of electron-beam (0 120 kGy).

The degree of polymerization depending on the electron-beam dose was measured to assess the best synthetic conditions under electron-beam irradiation. The physical properties of the contact lens, such as percent of water content, oxygen transmissibility and the optical transmittance, were analyzed by using the results of Fourier transform infrared spectroscopy (FTIR) and comparing the two different polymerization methods (thermal and electron-beam polymerization) with the same additive ratio (38).

When the dose of electron-beam was above 100 kGy, the degree of polymerization of HEMA was above 99% regardless of the crosslinking agent and the initiator. The water content of the lens fabricated by electron-beam method was 10% higher than the one by the thermal method, which was 40%. The lens fabricated by electron-beam method also showed a higher oxygen transmissibility with the same water content, and showed a higher value that was twice that of the lens fabricated by pure HEMA.

According to the FTIR studies, the hydrophilic property of the lens fabricated by electron-beam method was increased due to increasing the intermolecular hydrogen bonding. It showed above 90% optical transmittance in the visible range of wavelength on the contact lenses fabricated by both of the two different polymerization methods.

The polymerization of HEMA without crosslinking agent and initiator was successful above 100 *kGy* of electron-beam irradiation. Moreover, the lens fabricated from the polymer synthesized by pure HEMA with 100 *kGy* of electron-beam showed the highest water content and oxygen transmissibility. Therefore, electron-beam irradiation is a possible method to synthesize a polymer that can be used for soft contact lenses (38).

2.11.3 *Shaping and Cutting*

A method of shaping and cutting a soft contact lens can be done as follows (39):

1. Casting a slurry in an open cylindrical mold and polymerizing at a temperature of 40°C to 60°C to form a hard, self-supporting mass which is hygroscopic and swells anisotropically in a water medium,
2. Cutting away about 90% to 95% of the material from the planar face of the cylinder and from the circular outer periphery of the cylinder to leave the inner concave surface of the casting as the last surface to be cut as a lens blank having an arc of about 120° and in a diameter broad enough to cover the cornea and at least several millimeters of the limbus,
3. Cutting a bevel edge at the periphery of the lens blank to form a lens having a semi-scleral flap which is adapted to be lifted up by tears in the scleral portion of the eye adjacent to the outer edge of the flap while simultaneously forming a circular tear vesicle in the interior edge of the bevel which is spaced inwardly from said flap and which provides a circular well for tears in the eye at the limbal area, while the inner central portion of the lens is relatively flat to contact the cornea without any tear layer therebetween, and
4. Removing the mass and polymerizing at a temperature of 90°C to 120°C to polymerize unreacted material from the polymerization with the first free radical initiator and to complete the hardening of said mass in its self-supporting condition outside of the mold.

In detail, the preparation can be done as follows (39):

Preparation 2–3: To 120 parts of distilled HEMA containing up to 0.2 percent of EGDMA and less than 1% percent of methacrylic acid as impurities were added 40 parts of powdered poly(*N*-vinyl-2-pyrrolidone) (PVP) (Plasdone C Grade, supplied by GAF Corporation) having a Fikentscher K value of 33 and a number molecular weight of M_n 37,000 *Da*. This PVP polymer is hygroscopic and had a moisture content of about 3 percent, but picked up 1% or 2% additional moisture from the atmosphere in the plant.

A 40 part portion of the liquid HEMA methacrylate was mixed with a catalyst, e.g., 0.2 *g* of benzoyl peroxide in powdered form and 0.2 *g* of di-*sec*-butyl peroxy dicarbonate, available under the trade name of Lupersol 225 from Lucidol Chemical Corporation, Buffalo, New York. This compound is shown in Figure 2.13.

The catalyst-liquid mixture, 40 parts, was added to the PVP-HEMA mixture, 120 parts, and was mixed carefully to provide 160 parts of monomer with 40 parts of polymer dispersion or slurry.

These proportions cut down the shrinkage as compared with liquid HEMA alone. The amount of di-*sec*-butyl peroxy dicarbonate catalyst, which is particularly effective at a temperature of 40°C to 60°C, and of benzoyl peroxide catalyst, which is particularly effective at a temperature of 90°C to 120°C, is 0.2 part of each catalyst per 200 parts of liquid PVP mixture containing 160 parts of liquid monomer and 40 parts of PVP, e.g., a proportion of about 0.1% for each of these catalysts.

The dispersion was de-aerated to permit air bubbles to escape, and then the mold was filled. The tray of molds was then placed in an air circulating oven for 20 *h* at a temperature of 40°C. At the end of this time, the molds were removed from the oven and taken apart by using a small arbor press against the flat end of the Teflon core at the bottom of the mold unit. This forced the cast blank out of the other end of the sleeve. The cast blanks were placed on aluminum sheets and returned to the oven where they were post-cured at a temperature of 110°C for 1 *h*. When the trays were removed from the oven, the finished cast plastic blanks were a polymer consisting of PVP to which poly-HEMA had been grafted.

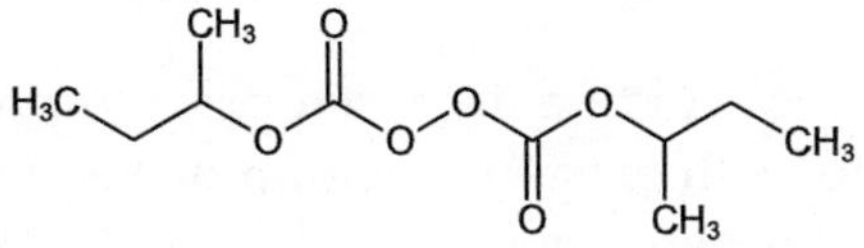

Figure 2.13 Di-*sec*-butyl peroxy dicarbonate.

A dimensionally stable contact lens composition can be obtained by carefully controlling the ingredients of the formulation, the polymerization processes, and the molding techniques (40).

A corrective hydrated lens or an eye bandage can be obtained by utilizing from 0 to 4 *ppm* of a hydroquinone polymerization inhibitor and from 50 to 250 *ppm* of methyl ether of hydroquinone polymerization inhibitor, based on the amount of the HEMA monomer, in the polymerization mix. The polymerization is started at a low temperature using a free radical initiator, degassing the polymerization mix prior to polymerization to substantially remove all oxygen, and conducting the initial polymerization reaction from 23°C to 30°C for 16 to 36 *h* during which time the reaction exotherm is carefully controlled. As initiators, acetyl peroxide, di-*sec*-butyl peroxy dicarbonate, and cyclohexanone peroxide are suitable to initiate the polymerization, because they operate between 23°C to 80°C. A closed casting mold, lined with a polyester film material, is utili zed for polymerizing and shaping the composition.

A preferred formulation, for preparing an improved contact lens composition is shown in Table 2.7.

Table 2.7 Formulation for preparing contact lenses (40).

Compound	Amount/[%]
2-Hydroxyethyl methacrylate	75.7
Poly(*N*-vinyl pyrrolidone)	19.4
Methacrylic acid	1.2
Ethylene glycol dimethacrylate	0.54
Di-*sec*-butyl peroxy dicarbonate	0.02
Water	3
Compound	**Amount/[*ppm* per parts HEMA]**
Hydroquinone	<4
Methyl ether of hydroquinone	100–200

The formulation should be degassed prior to polymerization to substantially remove all oxygen. Vacuum degassing, using known techniques, has been found effective when performed on the polymerization mix in the casting mold just prior to polymerization. Preferably, the degassing operation is performed twice: Once on the polymerization mix after the addition of the polymerization initiator and again after the polymerization mix has been poured into the casting mold.

After the second degassing, the mold is back flushed with an inert gas such as dry nitrogen, and the casting mold is immediately closed to prevent further contamination with atmospheric oxygen.

The polymerized product obtained is subjected to cutting and polishing operations. A contact lens composition is obtained, which is then hydrated in a buffered saline solution maintained at a pH of 7.0 to 7.1 (40).

2.12 Coating Methods

2.12.1 *Zwitterionic Coating*

Ocular dryness and contact lens-related microbial keratitis are two major risks of wearing contact lenses (41). The development of multifunctional surface coating for contact lenses with excellent hydrating and antimicrobial properties is a practical strategy to improve the comfort of contact lens wearers and to prevent corneal infection.

A zwitterionic and antimicrobial metal-phenolic network was developed based on the coordination of copper ions (CuII) and the poly(carboxylbetaine-*co*-dopamine methacrylamide) (PCBDA) copolymer, which can be easily prepared in one step on contact lenses due to the near-universal adherent properties of catechol groups (41).

The zwitterionic and antifouling carboxy betaine groups of the CuII-PCBDA coating can significantly increase the wettability of contact lenses and reduce their protein adsorptions, resulting in a lens surface that is more water retentive and with lower protein binding to prevent tear film evaporation and eye dryness. In addition, since the immobilized copper ions in the metal-phenolic networks impart them with ion-mediated antimicrobial activity, the CuII-PCBDA coating exhibits strong and broad spectrum antimicrobial activity against microbial keratitis-related pathogenic microbes, including bacteria such as *Escherichia coli*, *Pseudomonas aeruginosa*, and *Staphylococcus aureus*, and fungi such as *Candida albicans*. Compared with pristine contact lenses, the CuII-PCBDA-coated contact lenses effectively inhibited biofilm formation even after daily exposure to the above microbial environment for 14 *d*.

Notably, the CuII-PCBDA coating developed in this study is not only biocompatible with 100% cell viability following direct contact with human corneal epithelial cells for 48 *h* but also maintains the optical clarity of the native contact lenses. Thus, the CuII-PCBDA coating has great application potential for the development of a multifunctional surface coating for contact lenses for increased contact lens comfort and prevention of microbial keratitis (41).

2.12.2 Antibacterial Nanocoating

The problem of bacterial infections in general, and in medical devices in particular, has led to extensive research to produce antibacterial coatings (42).

A unique technique for imparting antibacterial properties to contact lenses has been presented (42). The coating consists of nanoparticles of zinc-doped copper oxide. In the coating process, active nanoparticles are formed and immediately deposited onto the surface of the contact lens. The coating thus formed is homogeneous and stable, without leaching of the nanoparticles. The antibacterial activity was evaluated against Gram-positive and Gram-negative bacteria. The optimization of the coating process has led to a smaller particle size and good antibacterial activity (42).

2.13 Disinfection of Contact Lenses

The primary standard to test microbiocidal disinfection efficacy of contact lens care products is ISO 14729 (43). This standard calls out the testing against 5 organisms, two Gram-negative bacteria, *Pseudomonas aeruginosa* and *Serratia marcescens*, a Gram-positive bacteria, *Staphylococcus aureus*, a yeast, *Candida albicans*, and a mold, *Fusarium solani*. During the development of this standard in the 1990s, a discussion was included because *Acanthamoeba* was not included as a part of this test protocol. In 2014 a second standard, ISO 18259 (44), was put in place under ISO testing care products in the presence of lenses and cases. This new standard includes the same five organisms as ISO 14729. But *Acanthamoeba* is not included as a test organism in this standard (43).

2.13.1 *Hydrogen Peroxide and Fibrous Catalyst*

A method for disinfecting contact lenses has been described (45). This is done by immersing the contact lenses in a volume of cleaning agent with about 3% hydrogen peroxide for up to 4 *h*, and immersing up to 0.7 *g* of a fibrous catalyst enhancer material in the volume of cleaning agent for up to 4 *h*. The fibrous catalyst enhancer material is immersed simultaneously with the contact lenses.

Any fabric that includes poly(acrylonitrile) (PAN) fibers can be used as a fibrous catalyst. The fabric that contains PAN fibers is a knitted fabric, such as a fibrous knitted mesh. Thus, in this aspect, the PAN fibers/yarn are capable of being knitted. The knitted fabric may be prepared by any suitable method known in the art.

A fibrous catalyst can be prepared using a process that includes the steps of (45):

1. Treating a fabric made up of PAN fibers with a hydrazine salt selected from dihydrazine sulfate and hydroxylamine sulfate in the presence of a base to provide a modified fabric,
2. Treating the modified fabric with a base, and
3. Treating the modified fabric with an aqueous solution consisting of a sulfate salt of an iron cation and a sulfate salt of a second metal cation, wherein the second metal cation is selected from a lithium, sodium, potassium, magnesium, calcium and zinc cation, and mixtures thereof.

Dihydrazine sulfate and hydroxylamine sulfate are shown in Figure 2.14.

2.13.2 *Hydrogen Peroxide and Metal Catalyst*

A disinfection system for a contact lens using hydrogen peroxide has been described, where the neutralization efficiency of the hydrogen peroxide is increased to reduce the amount of metal used in a metal catalyst, thereby advantageously saving resources (46).

The metal catalyst which carries out the neutralization treatment, in which the hydrogen oxide is detoxified to eliminate an adverse effect on the eye by contacting and decomposing the hydrogen peroxide contained in the disinfecting solution, is appropriately selected from various known metal catalysts which have hitherto been

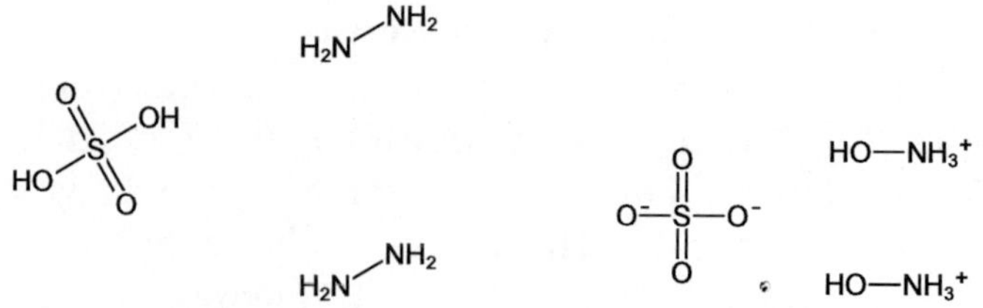

Dihydrazine sulfate Hydroxylamine sulfate

Figure 2.14 Hydrazine salts.

used for the decomposition and neutralization treatment of the hydrogen peroxide. For example, platinum is preferably used as a metal catalyst. In addition, metals such as palladium, silver, copper, manganese, cobalt and aluminum or oxides of such metals can also be used (46).

Also, a chelating agent is present in the composition. The chelating agent improves the stability of the disinfecting agent to advantageously achieve a long-term reservation. The chelating agent is at least one of those selected from the group consisting of ethylenediamine tetraacetic acid (EDTA), or a salt of EDTA, etidronic acid ((1-Hydroxy-1,1-ethanediyl)bis(phosphonic acid)), and a salt of etidronic acid. Etidronic acid is shown in Figure 2.15.

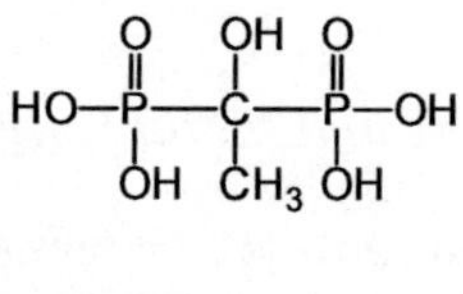

Figure 2.15 Etidronic acid.

In addition, a tonicity agent is added, so that the disinfecting solution after the neutralization treatment has an osmotic pressure of 250 to 350 *mOsm*. The adjustment of the osmotic pressure of the disinfecting solution after the neutralization treatment allows the osmotic pressure of the disinfecting solution to be almost equivalent to the osmotic pressure of the tear fluid, so that it is possible to wear the contact lens after the disinfection and neutralization treatments on the eye as it is (46).

2.13.3 *Removing Hydrogen Peroxide*

Soft contact lenses are generally prepared from certain hydrophilic polymers. While these lenses are not actually perforate, they do have a sufficient degree of molecular porosity to permit water, oxygen and tear fluids to permeate the lens structure (47).

In order for the cleaning of these lenses to be effective after they have been worn, it is important that all contaminants be removed from both surfaces and the interior of the lens. Hydrogen peroxide has been reported to be an effective agent to use on contact lenses in order to kill any contaminating microorganisms.

Hydrogen peroxide penetrates the lens in about 30 *s*, oxidizes any mucoprotein that exists on the surface of the lens and is simultaneously an effective sterilant for any microorganisms present in the eye (47).

However, before being inserted into the eye, a hydrogen peroxide treated soft contact lens must be rinsed repeatedly in isotonic buffered saline in order to remove any residual hydrogen peroxide. Isotonic buffered saline is a 0.85% solution of sodium chloride buffered to a pH of 6.9 to 7.1 and preserved with thimerosal 0.001% and disodium edetate. Thimerosal and disodium edetate are shown in Figure 2.16.

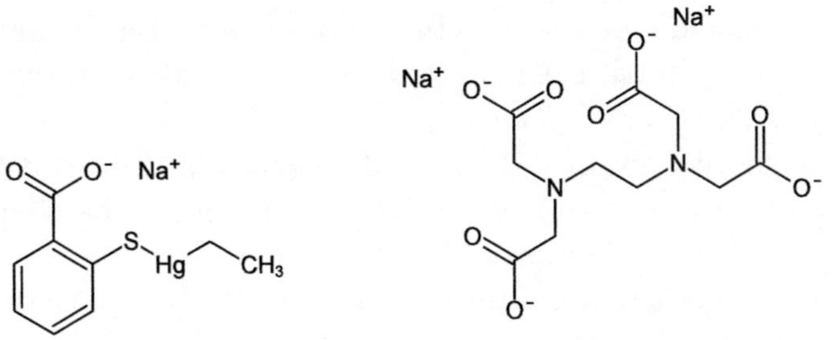

Thimerosal

Disodium edetate

Figure 2.16 Compounds in isotonic buffered saline solution.

Hydrogen peroxide, even in minute amounts such as 10 *ppm*, can cause some irritation of the eye in cases of particular sensitivity. Repeated soaking and rinsing in isotonic buffered saline does not always effectively remove all of the hydrogen peroxide present because rinsing merely acts to serially dilute the hydrogen peroxide to a lower concentration.

Consequently, a rinsed soft contact lens can still retain a sufficient concentration of hydrogen peroxide irritating to the wearer. A method for removing hydrogen peroxide from soft contact lenses which have been sterilized with hydrogen peroxide has been described (47).

The practice of this method is effected and the treatment of the soft contact lenses is carried out by soaking, immersing or contacting the soft contact lens in an aqueous hydrogen peroxide system containing a hydrogen peroxide decomposition catalyst in the form of a catalytic amount of metal from the periods 4, 5 and 6 of the periodic chart of the elements and the lanthanide elements. Thus, the metals are Pt, Pd, Ir, Rh, Re, Au, Ag, Cu, Cr, Os, Co, Fe, Mo, W, Mn, Ce, or Th. These catalysts are most effective in a form presenting the maximum surface for catalytic activity. Platinum, gold or palladium are generally preferred because of their availability. The catalysts are usually supported on a carrier when in use. For example, platinum black is mounted in platinum or on other carriers such as alumina, carbon, stainless steel or any other carriers which are commonly employed as catalyst supports for these catalysts.

The soft contact lens is thus effectively treated and sterilized by the exposure to the hydrogen peroxide action over the course of about 10 *min*. The treated lens need not be removed from the container in which the treatment has been effected since the catalyst present will then decompose (47).

The lens should not fit tightly on the cornea, but instead there should be some movement of the lens on the eye. The shape of the posterior surface should not be identical to that of the cornea, but there should be a lens-cornea relationship involving a mismatch between the corneal surface and the back surface of the lens so as to have a tear layer between the cornea and contact lens.

For a rigid lens, the tear layer varies from 10 μm to 20 μm at the center and 50 μm to 100 μm at the edge. It is much thinner and there is less movement in the case of soft lenses compared to rigid lenses.

The movement of the lens and the volume of the tear layer play important roles in helping provide oxygen to the cornea during the wearing of a rigid contact lens.

The thickness of the tear layer varies at different points under the contact lens. The optimal posterior surface shape depends on many factors, including eyelid forces, surface tension, and tear viscosity.

This involves the complex issues of how the contact lens moves and where it will rest on the eye. For a rigid lens, there is oscillation from an extremum position at the upper eyelid during a blink to an equilibrium position where the lens comes to rest after the eye has been open for at least 5 *s*. After the blink, the lens slowly drifts back to a balance-of-forces position. For a soft lens, there is less movement, a fact which can be exploited in creating soft lenses whose posterior surfaces more closely correspond to the corneal contour (5).

2.14 Integrated Microtubes

Drug delivery is a difficult task in ocular therapeutics due to the physiological and anatomical constraints of the eye (48). The correct therapeutic concentration of a drug at the required site of action is difficult to obtain. For example, only <1% of a topically administered drug reaches the aqueous humor.

A contact lens device with integrated microtubes as drug containers was reported which can provide a simple, noninvasive, extended drug release up to 40 *d* with a higher bioavailability and a lower risk for adverse effects (48).

2.15 Injection Molding

2.15.1 *Aspheric Contact Lenses*

A method to reduce the shrinkage error of shell molds in the injection molding process has been proposed (49). The shell molds are used for casting bi-aspheric soft contact lens with HEMA material. Moldex3D R13.0 was used to simulate and analyze the shrinkage of the front contact lens curve on the front shell mold in Z-axis direction.

First, the experiment method design is applied to obtain the optimal setting parameters such as melt temperature, injection velocity, and packing pressure.

The amount of the shrinkage error is used to compensate the original design curve to improve the shrinkage error in the next simulations. The simulation result after compensation showed that the shrinkage error is reduced as 80.8%. Adding value to compensate the original design curve should be optimized to minimize the shrinkage error.

These results can effectively improve the shrinkage error before fabricating the shell molds of the soft aspheric contact lens (49).

2.16 Handling Tools

The major reasons why those who wear eyeglasses do not use contact lenses is the discomfort of directly touching the eye with their fingers, the fear of infecting or damaging their eye, and the inability to remove or lubricate the lenses when they do not have access to disinfection equipment (50). If unhygienic methods or processes were used, then ocular diseases can develop, such as dry eye, eye infections, etc. For these reasons, there exists a need for a hygienic method to apply, remove, and lubricate contact lenses without direct finger and eye contact.

2.16.1 *Insertion Tool*

For aesthetic reasons and because of their increased effectiveness compared to glasses, contact lenses enjoy a substantial portion of the market for corrective lenses (51). Unfortunately, for a great many contact lens users, the insertion of the lens into the eye can require a great deal of effort and can cause significant discomfort. Furthermore, the risk of contamination to the lens is very great during insertion.

An improved contact lens insertion tool has been developed. The contact lens insertion tool consists of (51):

1. An elongated handle section having a top surface, a bottom surface, and two side surfaces,

2. An intermediate section angularly displaced from the handle section at an obtuse angle, and
3. A lens supporting portion angularly displaced from the intermediate section at a different obtuse angle that is greater than the first obtuse angle, and having a substantially circular cross-sectional land area for engaging the contact lens.

The design of the contact lens insertion tool minimizes the need to blink, which complicates insertion and proper positioning of a lens. The land area may be smooth or roughened and flat, convex, or concave depending upon the desired degree of adhesiveness between the lens and the land area. A faceted ball configuration, emanating from and integral to the lens supporting section of the contact lens insertion tool, provides a multi-land area device suitable for picking up and maneuvering a contact lens. Each facet or land area of said faceted ball construction can be smooth, roughened, concave, convex, or any combination of the foregoing as desired.

A perspective view of the step of depositing a contact lens edge first to the central lower area of the sclera of the eye with the insertion tool is shown in Figure 2.17.

Here, a right-handed user is shown picking up the contact lens insertion tool so that the edge of the lens is brought in contact with the bottom central area of the visible sclera. It may be necessary for the user to pull down gently on the cheek directly beneath the eyelid with the free hand to facilitate the contact between the lower sclera and the edge of the lens. Although Figure 2.17 demonstrates one finger pulling down on the cheek directly beneath the eyelid, it may sometimes be necessary to use two fingers to perform this task. It should be noted that when the edge of the lens is brought up to the user's eye, that based on the unique angle of the contact lens insertion tool, neither the contact lens insertion tool nor the user's hand impedes the user's vision. The angle of the edge of lens relative to the eye when initial lens edge contact with the eye is made, can range from not greater than 90° to approximately 20° depending upon the preference of the user (51).

Upon inserting the lens into the eye, the lens is often not in the correct position over the cornea. In such instances, the lens can be moved into the correct position over the cornea by means of a gentle

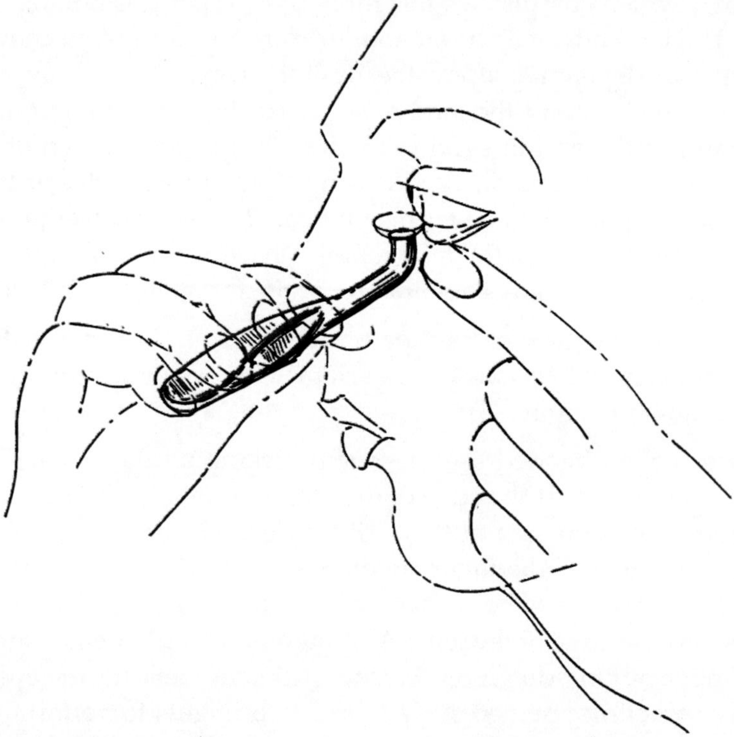

Figure 2.17 Method of inserting a contact lens (51).

nudge with the contact lens insertion tool, or by merely blinking a few times.

2.16.2 *Insertion Tool*

A contact lens handling device has been described (50). This device can be used for contact lens removal, lubrication, storage, and application to the eye without the need for direct contact with the fingers or skin of a subject applying the lenses.

The components of this device include a lens handling tip, a lubrication fluid container, two detachable storage chambers, and, optionally, a detachable ultraviolet disinfection system.

References

1. R. Kingslake and R.B. Johnson, *Lens Design Fundamentals*, Academic Press, Burlington, MA, 2nd edition, 2009.
2. A. Cannella, Virtual fitting of GP lenses: A new frontier, *GP News and Information from Bausch & Lomb*, Vol. 16, p. 3, May 2005.
3. P.F. Jubin, L. Jones, and J.L. Perez, Contact lenses and methods for their design, US Patent 7 862 169, assigned to Johnson & Johnson Vision Care Inc., January 04, 2011.
4. Wikipedia contributors, Category:optical software — Wikipedia, the free encyclopedia, https://en.wikipedia.org/wiki/Category:Optical_software, 2020. [Online; accessed 11-September-2020].
5. B.A. Barsky, Polymer compositions for contact lenses, US Patent 6 241 355, assigned to Brian A. Barsky, June 5, 2001.
6. J.A. Legerton and W.E. Meyers, Contact lens and methods of manufacture and fitting such lenses and computer program product, US Patent 7 270 412, assigned to CRT Technology Inc., September 18, 2007.
7. J.A. Legerton and W.E. Meyers, Contact lens and methods of manufacture and fitting such lenses and computer program product, US Patent 8 794 759, assigned to CRT Technology Inc., August 05, 2014.
8. B. Fan and M. Chang, Contact lenses with selective spectral blocking and method of fabrication thereof, US Patent Application 20 070 052 886, assigned to Bunsen Fan, Michael Chang, March 08, 2007.
9. F.G. Schlanitz, S. Sacu, B. Baumann, M. Bolz, M. Platzer, M. Pircher, C.K. Hitzenberger, and U. Schmidt-Erfurth, Identification of drusen characteristics in age-related macular degeneration by polarization-sensitive optical coherence tomography, *American Journal of Ophthalmology*, Vol. 160, p. 33544, 2015.

10. J.-C. Lee and S. Jacobs, Gradient index liquid crystal devices and method of fabrication thereof, US Patent 5 061 046, assigned to University of Rochester, October 29, 1991.
11. H.-J. Park, Review on the fabrication method and characteristics of colored contact lens, *Journal of Korean Ophthalmic Optics Society*, Vol. 10, p. 127, 2005.
12. N.J. Park and J.S. Park, Colored hard contact lens printing method, US Patent Application 20 180 117 864, assigned to Happy Vision Corp., May 03, 2018.
13. S. Corti and L.A. Creech, Colored contact lens, US Patent 8 770 747, assigned to Novartis AG, July 08, 2014.
14. D.M. Marmion, *Handbook of US Colorants: Foods, Drugs, Cosmetics, and Medical Devices*, John Wiley & Sons, 3rd edition, 1991.
15. M.H. Quinn, Color binding mechanism for contact lenses, US Patent 5 272 010, assigned to Wesley Jessen Inc., December 21, 1993.
16. Y. Goto and M. Nakada, Decentered type contact lens and decentered type contact lens set, US Patent 10 444 542, assigned to Menicon Co. Ltd., October 15, 2019.
17. P. Gerligand, Method for producing stabilized contact lenses, US Patent 8 439 499, assigned to Johnson & Johnson Vision Care Inc., May 14, 2013.
18. F. Alam, M. Elsherif, B. AlQattan, M. Ali, I.M.G. Ahmed, A. Salih, D.S. Antonysamy, A.K. Yetisen, S. Park, and H. Butt, Prospects for additive manufacturing in contact lens devices, *Advanced Engineering Materials*, Vol. 23, p. 2000941, 2021.
19. K. Boneberger, L. Haase, H. Schafer, W. Steffan, and P. Zang, Process and apparatus for the manufacture of a contact lens, US Patent 5 894 002, assigned to Ciba Vision Corp, April 13, 1999.
20. D.F. Ezekiel, Method of cast moulding a translating multifocal contact lens, US Patent 9 676 125, assigned to Ezekiel Nominees Pty Ltd., June 13, 2017.
21. D.F. Ezekiel, Method of cast moulding a translating multifocal contact lens, US Patent 9 943 994, assigned to Ezekiel Nominees Pty Ltd., April 17, 2018.
22. J.R. Gibson and G.D.S. Payne, Contact lens mold parts, contact lens mold assemblies, and methods of making contact lenses, US Patent 9 764 501, assigned to CooperVision International Holding Co. LP, September 19, 2017.
23. J.R. Gibson and G.D.S. Payne, Tray for use in manufacturing contact lenses, US Patent 10 029 430, assigned to CooperVision International Holding Co. LP, July 24, 2018.
24. J.R. Gibson, T.M. Cook, and J.B. Cook, Method and apparatus for demolding contact lens, EP Patent 3 233 446, assigned to CooperVision International Holding Co. LP, October 25, 2017.

25. Y.J. Shin, M.J. Shin, L.J. Guo, and J.S. Shin, Fabrication of contact lens containing high-performance wire grid polarizer, *Polymer International*, Vol. 66, p. 1269, 2017.
26. R. Fuerst, J. Bango, J. Fenn, and M. Dziekan, Fabrication of improved contact lens utilizing polymer electrospinning, US Patent 7 563 396, assigned to Ocugenics LLC, July 21, 2009.
27. K. Davis, M. Reuter, A. Kammerich, A. Tangonan, K. Vedantham, and A. Kelley, Extended release drug-delivery contact lenses and methods of making, US Patent 9 956 168, assigned to Mercy Medical Research Institute, May 01, 2018.
28. P. Chabrecek and D. Lohmann, Functionalised photoinitiator, macromeres and their use, EP Patent 0 632 329, assigned to Ciba-Geigy AG, January 04, 1995.
29. P. Chabrecek, K. Dietliker, and D. Lohmann, Functionalized photoinitiators, derivatives and macromers therefrom and their use, US Patent 6 204 306, assigned to Novartis AG, March 20, 2001.
30. H.-Y. Tsai, Y.-C. Hsieh, Y.-H. Lin, H.-C. Chang, Y.-H. Tang, and K.-C. Huang, Fabrication of hydrophilic surface on rigid gas permeable contact lenses to enhance the wettability using ultraviolet laser system, *Micromachines*, Vol. 10, p. 394, Jun 2019.
31. L.C. Winterton, Method of making silicone hydrogel contact lenses, US Patent 7 858 000, assigned to Novartis AG, December 28, 2010.
32. A.C. Maiden, D.G. Vanderlaan, D.C. Turner, R.N. Love, J.D. Ford, F.F. Molock, R.B. Steffen, G.A. Hill, A. Alli, and K.P. McCabe, Hydrogel with internal wetting agent, US Patent 6 367 929, assigned to Johnson & Johnson Vision Care Inc., April 09, 2002.
33. K.P. McCabe, F.F. Molock, G.A. Hill, A. Alli, R.B. Steffen, D.G. Vanderlaan, and K.A. Young, Biomedical devices containing internal wetting agents, US Patent 6 822 016, assigned to Johnson & Johnson Vision Care Inc., November 23, 2004.
34. P.C. Nicolson, R.C. Baron, P. Chabrecek, J. Court, A. Domschke, H.J. Griesser, A. Ho, J. Hopken, B.G. Laycock, Q. Liu, D. Lohmann, G.F. Meijs, E. Papaspiliotopoulos, J.S. Riffle, K. Schindhelm, D. Sweeney, J. Wilson Leonard Terry, J. Vogt, and L.C. Winterton, Extended wear ophthalmic lens, US Patent 5 760 100, assigned to Commonwealth Scientific and Industrial Research Organization CSIRO, Ciba Vision Corp., June 02, 1998.
35. D. Silva, H.C.M.H.G. de Sousa, L.F. Santos, G.M. Moutinho, M. Salema-Oom, C. Alvarez-Lorenzo, A.P. Serro, and B. Saramago, Diclofenac sustained release from sterilised soft contact lens materials using an optimised layer-by-layer coating, *International Journal of Pharmaceutics*, Vol. 585, p. 119506, 2020.
36. A.M. Ramos-de la Peña, C.M.G.C. Renard, J. Montañez, M. de la Luz Reyes-Vega, and J.C. Contreras-Esquivel, A review through recovery,

purification and identification of genipin, *Phytochemistry Reviews*, Vol. 15, p. 37, 2016.
37. B. Vaandering, Genipin, Project, Western Oregon University, Monmouth, EUA, 2006.
38. K.-H. Hwang, J.-H. Shin, Y.-J. Sung, K.-S. Jeong, and J. Jun, Polymerization of HEMA by electron beam irradiation and fabrication of soft contact lens, *Journal of Korean Ophthalmic Optics Society*, Vol. 17, p. 135, 2012.
39. K.F. O'Driscoll and A.A. Isen, Fabrication of soft plastic contact lens blank, US Patent 3 700 761, assigned to Griffin Laboratories Incorporated, Buffalo, NY., October 24, 1972.
40. A.R.L. Boeuf and W.R. Grovesteen, Fabrication of soft contact lens and composition therefor, US Patent 4 045 547, assigned to Warner-Lambert Co. LLC, August 30, 1977.
41. G. Liu, K. Li, H. Wang, L. Ma, L. Yu, and Y. Nie, Stable fabrication of zwitterionic coating based on copper-phenolic networks on contact lens with improved surface wettability and broad-spectrum antimicrobial activity, *ACS Applied Materials & Interfaces*, Vol. 12, p. 16125, 2020.
42. R. Tuby, S. Gutfreund, I. Perelshtein, G. Mircus, M. Ehrenberg, M. Mimouni, A. Gedanken, and I. Bahar, Fabrication of a stable and efficient antibacterial nanocoating of Zn–CuO on contact lenses, *ChemNanoMat*, Vol. 2, p. 547, 2016.
43. Ophthalmic optics — Contact lens care products — Microbiological requirements and test methods for products and regimens for hygienic management of contact lenses, ISO Standard 14729, International Organization for Standardization, Geneva, Switzerland, 2001. https://www.iso.org/standard/25382.html.
44. Ophthalmic optics — Contact lens care products — Method to assess contact lens care products with contact lenses in a lens case, challenged with bacterial and fungal organisms, ISO Standard 18259, International Organization for Standardization, Geneva, Switzerland, 2014. https://www.iso.org/contents/data/standard/06/19/61901.html.
45. L. Winterton, Method for disinfecting contact lenses, US Patent 10 478 518, assigned to Better Vision Solutions LLC, November 19, 2019.
46. O. Mori and Y. Kojima, Disinfection system of contact lens, US Patent 10 137 218, assigned to Menicon Co, Ltd., November 27, 2018.
47. C.A. Gaglia, Jr., Method for removing hydrogen peroxide from soft contact lenses, US Patent 3 912 451, assigned to Warner-Lambert Co LLC, October 14, 1975.
48. X. Ding, C. Song, and L. Que, Fabrication of contact lens device with integrated microtubes for in situ extended drug delivery for ocular

disease treatment, in *2019 20th International Conference on Solid-State Sensors, Actuators and Microsystems*, pp. 306–309, 2019.
49. C.-C.A. Chen, L.T. Vu, and Y.-T. Qiu, Study on injection molding of shell mold for aspheric contact lens fabrication, *Procedia Engineering*, Vol. 184, p. 344, 2017. Advances in Material & Processing Technologies Conference.
50. X. Basañez, A.H. Molina, A.V. Berain, and D. Zhang, Contact lens handling device, US Patent 9 642 744, assigned to University of Texas System, May 09, 2017.
51. D.A. Selick, Contact lens insertion tool, US Patent 5 348 358, assigned to David A. Selick, September 20, 1994.

3

Properties

The visual experience is critical for many aspects of human life and visual development is essential (1).

The process of emmetropization leads to myopia when the visual input is suboptimal (2).

Being able to perform tasks and navigate safely, particularly for the elderly (3), enhances the quality of life (4).

Correcting vision with glasses can overcome visual impairment due to refractive error. However, wearing glasses can be inconvenient due to related issues such as the experience of the pressure of the frame of the glasses on the skin, the limitation of the field of view, the image magnification (especially for higher refractive errors, reducing the visual acuity of myopes), the steaming up of lenses, the reflections from the lens surfaces, and the increased accommodative and convergence demands for myopes (5).

3.1 Ophthalmic Compatibility Requirements

One ophthalmic compatibility requirement for contact lenses is that the lens must allow oxygen to reach the cornea in an amount which is sufficient for long-term corneal health (6). The contact lens must allow oxygen from the surrounding air to reach the cornea because the cornea does not receive oxygen from the blood supply like other tissue. If sufficient oxygen does not reach the cornea, corneal swelling occurs. Extended periods of oxygen deprivation causes the undesirable growth of blood vessels in the cornea. Soft contact lenses conform closely to the shape of the eye, so oxygen cannot easily circumvent the lens. Thus, soft contact lenses must allow oxygen to diffuse through the lens to reach the cornea.

Another ophthalmic compatibility requirement for soft contact lenses is that the lens must not strongly adhere to the eye. Clearly, the consumer must be able to easily remove the lens from the eye for disinfecting, cleaning, or disposal. However, the lens must also be able to move on the eye in order to encourage tear flow between the lens and the eye. Tear flow between the lens and eye allows for debris, such as foreign particulates or dead epithelial cells, to be swept from beneath the lens and, ultimately, out of the tear fluid. Thus, a contact lens must not adhere to the eye so strongly that adequate movement of the lens on the eye is inhibited (6).

In order to balance the ophthalmic compatibility and consumer comfort requirements, polymers and copolymers of 2-hydroxyethyl methacrylate were developed. These hydrophilic polymers move well on the eye and provide sufficient oxygen permeability for daily wear.

Certain soft contact lenses have been approved by the FDA for extended wear periods of up to about 6 nights of overnight wear and 7 *d* of daily wear. However, the consumer cannot safely and comfortably wear these poly(2-hydroxyethyl methacrylate) lenses for extended periods of seven days or more, because the oxygen permeability is insufficient. True extended wear (i.e., 7 *d* or more) of these lenses may result, at a minimum, in corneal swelling and development of surface blood vessels in the cornea.

In order to improve the oxygen permeability, polymers containing silicone groups were developed (6).

3.2 Standards

Standards for testing contact lenses are collected in Table 3.1. The special issues are subsequently described.

Other ISO standards can be found on the home page of the International Organization for Standardization (7).

3.2.1 Tensile Properties of Plastics

The ASTM-D 1708 standard (8) method covers certain material specifications for which a history of data has been obtained using the

Table 3.1 Standards for testing contact lenses.

Number	Title	Reference
ASTM D1708	Standard Test Method for Tensile Properties of Plastics by Use of Microtensile Specimens	(8)
ASTM D1938	Standard Test Method for Tear-Propagation Resistance (Trouser Tear) of Plastic Film and Thin Sheeting by a Single-Tear Method	(9)
ASTM C1648-12	Standard Guide for Choosing a Method for Determining the Index of Refraction and Dispersion of Glass	(10)
ASTM F803-19	Standard Specification for Eye Protectors for Selected Sports	(11)
ASTM F659-10	Standard Specification for Ski and Snowboard Goggles	(12)
ASTM F2879-19	Standard Specification for Eye Protective Devices for Airsoft Sports	(13)
ASTM F1776-19	Standard Specification for Eye Protective Devices for Paintball Sports	(14)
ASTM D3985-17	Standard Test Method for Oxygen Gas Transmission Rate Through Plastic Film and Sheeting Using a Coulometric Sensor	(15)
ASTM F981-04	Standard Practice for Assessment of Compatibility of Biomaterials for Surgical Implants with Respect to Effect of Materials on Muscle and Insertion into Bone	(16)

Table 3.1 (cont) Standards for testing contact lenses.

Number	Title	Reference
ISO 11978	Ophthalmic optics — Contact lenses and contact lens care products — Labelling	(17)
ISO 7708	Air quality — Particle size fraction definitions for health-related sampling	(18)
ISO 9337-1	Contact lenses — Determination of back vertex power — Part 1: Method using focimeter with manual focusing	(19)
ISO 19045	Ophthalmic optics — Contact lens care products — Method for evaluating Acanthamoeba encystment by contact lens care products	(20)
ISO 14729	Ophthalmic optics — Contact lens care products — Microbiological requirements and test methods for products and regimens for hygienic management of contact lenses	(21)
ISO 14730	Ophthalmic optics — Contact lens care products — Antimicrobial preservative efficacy testing and guidance on determining discard date	(22)
ISO 18259	Ophthalmic optics — Contact lens care products — Method to assess contact lens care products with contact lenses in a lens case, challenged with bacterial and fungal organisms	(23)

standard microtensile specimens.

The test method covers the determination of the comparative tensile strength and elongation properties of plastics in the form of standard microtensile test specimens when tested under defined conditions of pretreatment, temperature, humidity, and testing machine speed. This method is applicable when using specimens of any thickness up to 3.2 *mm*.

3.2.2 *Tear-Propagation Resistance*

The ASTM D1708 (9) standard is of value in rating the tear-propagation resistance of various plastic films and thin sheeting of comparable thickness. For highly extensible film or sheeting the deformation energy of the specimen legs is significantly greater than the tearing energy. The tear-propagation resistance in slightly extensible or non-extensible film or sheeting is distinguished from the tear-propagation resistance in highly extensible film or sheeting by the load-time or load-displacement data. The tear-propagation force for slightly extensible or non-extensible material is determined from the average tear force versus the initial and peak force for a highly extensible material.

3.2.3 *Oxygen Gas Transmission Rate*

The ASTM D3985-17 test method (15) is a procedure for determination of the steady state rate of transmission of oxygen gas through plastics in the form of film, sheeting, laminates, coextrusions, or plastic-coated papers or fabrics. It is useful for the determination of the (15):

1. oxygen gas transmission rate,
2. Permeance of the film to oxygen gas, and
3. Oxygen permeability coefficient in the case of homogeneous materials.

3.2.4 *Biomaterials*

The ASTM F981-04 (16) standard covers a test protocol for comparing the local tissue response evoked by biomaterials, from which medical implantable devices might ultimately be fabricated, with the local tissue response elicited by control materials currently accepted for the fabrication of surgical devices.

The materials may include metals (and metal alloys), dense aluminum oxide, and poly(ethylene) that are standardized on the basis of an acceptable, well-recognized, long-term response. The controls consistently produce cellular reaction and wound healing to a degree that has been found to be acceptable to the host.

This practice provides a series of experimental protocols for biological assays of tissue reaction to nonabsorbable biomaterials for surgical implants. It assesses the effects of the material on animal tissue in which it is implanted.

3.2.5 Eye Protectors

The ASTM F803-19 specification covers eye protectors, designed for use by players of racket sports, women's lacrosse, field hockey, basketball, baseball, and soccer that minimize or significantly reduce injury to the eye and adnexa due to impact and penetration by racket-sport rackets and balls, women's lacrosse and field hockey sticks and balls, baseballs, soccer balls, hands, elbows, and fingers.

Protective eyewear offers protection only to the eyes and does not protect other parts of the head. Protectors are divided into four types depending on their design characteristics as follows (11):

1. Type I — A protector with the lens or lenses and frame frontpiece molded as one unit. Frame temples or other devices, such as straps, to affix the lens/frontpiece may be separate pieces,
2. Type II — A protector with a single lens or lenses, either plano or prescription, mounted in a frame that was manufactured as a separate unit,
3. Type III — A protector without a lens, and
4. Type IV — A full or partial face shield.

The materials shall be tested using optical tests such as field of view, optical quality, luminous transmittance, prismatic deviation measurements, haze, refractive power measurements, surface imperfections and internal defects, and alternate optical tests; and mechanical tests such as high velocity impact resistance, and projectile simulator test. In addition, the individual grades shall conform to the general performance requirements.

The ASTM F659-10 specification (12) covers the material, design, optical, and strength requirements, and associated test procedures for goggles and faceshields used by alpine skiers, to provide a reasonable degree of protection against foreign objects that strike or lodge in the eye or surrounding soft tissue causing eye irritation or damage, as well as to minimize fogging and vision restrictions that distract or handicap the skier, thereby causing accidents. Contact lenses, sunglasses, and corrective dress eyewear are not included within the scope of this specification. When tested by the methods provided herein, these eye protective devices shall adhere to specified optical requirements in terms of field of view (temporal, nasal, superior, and inferior fields), luminous transmittance, refractive tolerances, astigmatism, refractive power imbalance, prismatic deviation and imbalance (vertical and horizontal imbalances), optical defects, and physical lens defects. The protective eyewear shall also meet light-transmitting ability requirements such as clearness, ultraviolet and infrared filtration, and resistance to fogging. Furthermore, lens strength shall be examined by means of basic impact resistance and higher impact resistance tests as well.

3.3 Eye Model with Blink Mechanism

An eye model with a physiological blink mechanism has been developed (24).

Two particularly important tests for ophthalmic biomaterials, relating to its comfort, are the deposition of tear film components (25–28) and tear break-up time (29, 30).

However, the current *in-vitro* eye models are extremely rudimentary and unable to simulate these complex physiological mechanisms (24). Most *in-vitro* studies are performed in a simple glass vial, in which the entire material is bathed in a solution of simulated tear solution (31–35).

Factors such as a low tear volume, slow tear flow and replenishment, intermittent air exposure, and the blink actuation, all of which impact tear deposition, are absent from such a simplistic vial-based model.

In the study, the designs for the eyeballs, eyelids, and acrylic chambers were designed using a 3D modeling software and a computer-aided design (CAD) program (24).

The molds for the eyelids were 3D printed using poly(ethylene terephthalate glycol) (PETG) on a commercially available 3D printer.

The printer uses fused deposition modeling to print the parts layer by layer. The print detail was set to high on a 0.35 *mm* nozzle, with a layer resolution of 75 μm. PETG was chosen due to its water-resistant properties, but other 3D printer filaments could also be used such as poly(lactic acid) or acrylonitrile-butadiene-styrene.

The eyelid design is composed of three key components: the main support structure, and a top and bottom mold.

The role of the support structure ($38.0 \times 21.4 \times 12.1$ *mm*) is to hold and secure a flexible poly(vinyl alcohol) (PVA) membrane. The two corresponding molds are used to cast a flexible polymer onto the support structure. Both the eyeball and eyelid membrane were synthesized using PVA.

All components were designed to be reusable, but the main support structure could be replaced with every experiment if necessary. A small hole, created during the molding process, is in the polymer to allow for fluid to flow into the eyelid.

Four samples of PVA with molecular weights of 89–98 *kDa*, 85–124 *kDa*, 130 *kDa*, and 146–186 *kDa* were tested at a range of concentrations between 5% and 30% weight/volume. The wettability and water content of these materials were compared with the bovine cornea and sclera.

The model was connected to a microfluidic pump, which delivers artificial tear solution to the eyelid. A corneal topographer was used to evaluate the tear break-up and tear film regeneration.

It was found that the eyelid flexes and slides across the eyeball during each blink. This ensures a direct contact between the two surfaces. When loaded with an artificial tear solution, this mechanism evenly spreads the solution over the eyeball to generate an artificial tear film.

The artificial tear film in this eye model had a tear break-up time of 5.13±0.09 *s* at a flow rate of 1.4 $\mu l\ min^{-1}$ 6 blinks per *min*, and less then 25% humidity (24).

3.4 Assessment of Cytotoxic Effects

A method for determining the cytotoxic effect of soft contact lens care solutions has been described (36). The method provides a means for the direct exposure of mammalian cells to solutions and to lenses that have been soaked in solutions.

3.4.1 Draize Eye Irritation Test

The Draize test is an acute toxicity test devised in 1944 by the US Food and Drug Administration toxicologists John H. Draize and Jacob M. Spines (37). Initially used for testing cosmetics, the procedure involves applying 0.5 *ml* or 0.5 *g* of a test substance to the eye or skin of a restrained, conscious animal, and then leaving it for a set amount of time before rinsing it out and recording its effects.

The animals are observed for up to 14 *d* for signs of erythema and edema in the skin test, and redness, swelling, discharge, ulceration, hemorrhaging, cloudiness, or blindness in the tested eye. The test subject is commonly an albino rabbit, though other species are used too, including dogs.

The animals are euthanized after testing if the test renders irreversible damage to the eye or skin. Animals may be reused for testing purposes if the product tested causes no permanent damage. Animals are typically reused after a *wash out* period during which all traces of the tested product are allowed to disperse from the test site (37).

The Draize eye test became a governmentally endorsed method to evaluate the safety of materials meant for use in or around the eyes (38). The test involves a standardized protocol for instilling agents onto the cornea and conjunctiva of laboratory animals.

A sum of ordinal-scale items of the outer eye gives an index of ocular morbidity. Advances in ocular toxicology are challenging the validity, precision, relevance, and need of the Draize eye test.

Preclinical product-safety tests with rabbits and other mammals also raise ethical concerns of animal well-being. Some use the Draize test as a rallying point for how animals are treated in science and industry. A battery of cellular systems and computer models aim to reduce and ultimately to replace whole-animal testing. Molecular measures of ocular toxicity may eventually allow comprehensive screening in humans. The Draize eye test was created and refined for humanitarian reasons and has assuredly prevented harm. Its destiny is to be progressively supplanted as *in-vitro* and clinical alternatives emerge for assessing irritancy of the ocular surface (38).

3.4.2 *Acute Eye Irritation Testing*

An acute eye irritation test has been presented by OECD (39). This method provides information on health hazards likely to arise from exposure to a test substance (liquids, solids and aerosols) applied on the eye.

The test guideline is intended preferably for use on an albino rabbit. The test substance is applied in a single dose in the conjunctival sac of one eye of each animal. The other eye, which remains untreated, serves as a control. The initial test uses an animal and the dose level depends on the test substance nature.

A confirmatory test should be made if a corrosive effect is not observed in the initial test; the irritant or negative response should be confirmed using up to two additional animals. It is recommended that it be conducted in a sequential manner in one animal at a time, rather than exposing the two additional animals simultaneously. The duration of the observation period should be sufficient to evaluate fully the magnitude and reversibility of the effects observed. The eyes should be examined at 1, 24, 48, and 72 hours after test substance application. The ocular irritation scores should be evaluated in conjunction with the nature and severity of lesions, and their reversibility or lack of reversibility (39).

3.4.3 *Benzalkonium Chlorides*

Cytotoxicity was indicated by significant increases in the number of dead cells relative to controls. The cytotoxicity of a test battery of eight compounds was determined, in particular benzalkonium chloride.

Benzalkonium chlorides are also known as alkyl dimethyl benzyl ammonium chlorides, alkyl dimethyl (phenylmethyl) quaternary ammonium chlorides, ammonium alkyl dimethyl (phenylmethyl) chlorides, or ammonium alkyl dimethyl benzyl chlorides.

They are a class of quaternary ammonium compounds. They are usually commercialized as a mixture of compounds with different lengths for the alkyl chain, ranging from C_8 to C_{18}, with higher biocide activity for C_{12} and C_{14} derivatives (40). Some of these compounds are shown in Figure 3.1.

In addition, nine commercial soft contact lens care products containing a variety of preserving/disinfecting agents were also examined.

A modification of the basic assay for assessing the kinetics of toxicity was also described (36).

The results indicate that this method is useful for identifying compounds that bind to soft contact lenses (such as benzalkonium chloride) and induce cytotoxicity; and others that should be rinsed from lenses or neutralized (such as hydrogen peroxide) to minimize the potential for irritation (36).

The binding affinity of benzalkonium chloride toward two types of contact lenses, those with the wetting agent poly(*N*-vinyl-2-pyrrolidone) (PVP) and those without wetting agent, was calculated (41). In addition, the refractive power, UV-vis transmittance, contact angle, water content, base curve, and diameter of the contact lenses after treatment with benzalkonium chloride were examined to evaluate the effects of its adsorption on the contact lens. It was found that the maximum amount of adsorbed benzalkonium chloride was 2.88 *mM* for the contact lens without PVP whereas it was 2.32 *mM* for that with PVP. In contrast, the benzalkonium chloride binding affinities were similar.

The physical properties of the contact lens changed significantly because of the adsorption of benzalkonium chloride. Although benzalkonium chloride is a widely used preservative, the results of the study suggest that use of PVP-containing contact lenses reduces the benzalkonium chloride adsorption and so the discomfort (41).

3.4.4 *Residual Monomer Content*

Poly(methyl methacrylate) is the most commonly used contact lens material due to its excellent optical properties (42). However, the presence of the residual monomer in the structure alters its transparency as well as its biocompatibility; thus, there is a need to detect any remaining methyl methacrylate.

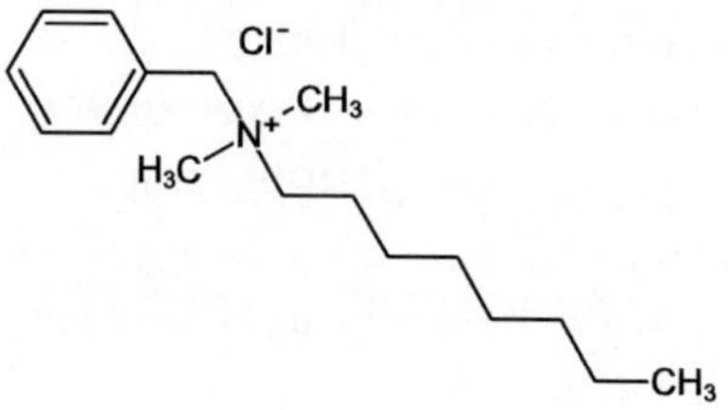

Benzyldimethyloctylammonium chloride

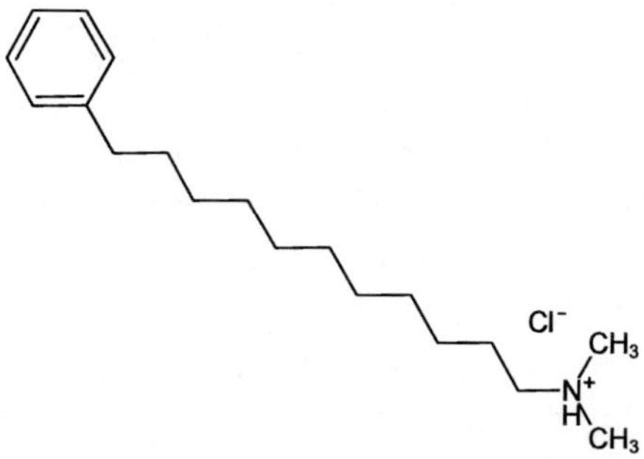

Benzyldimethyldecylammonium chloride

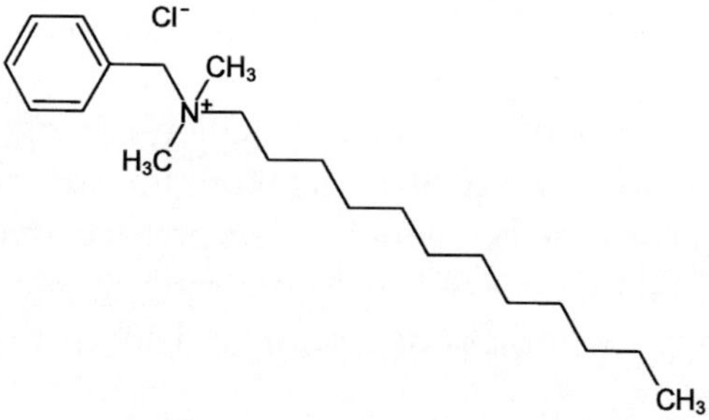

Benzyldimethyldodecylammonium chloride

Figure 3.1 Benzalkonium Chlorides.

Raman spectroscopy is a rapid, sensitive, and non-destructive method in comparison to other spectroscopic, chromatographic or polarographic methods. The spectra of some lens materials that were prepared from methyl methacrylate, 2-hydroxyethyl methacrylate, hexamethyl disiloxane, and poly(propylene glycol) with or without the addition of crosslinking agent ethylene glycol dimethylacrylate, cf. Figure 3.2, were obtained by Raman spectroscopy.

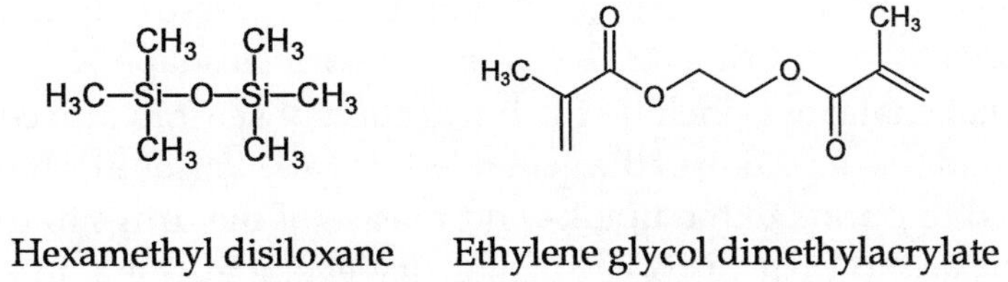

Figure 3.2 Lens materials.

It was observed that an amount of crosslinking agent present in the structure proves effective for the unpolymerized monomer content. None of the samples, except those containing hexamethyl disiloxane, demonstrated any monomer residue (42).

3.5 Special Functions

Contact lenses in the future will likely have functions other than the correction of a refractive error (43). Contact lenses as drug delivery devices and powered through advancements in nanotechnology will open up further opportunities for unique uses of contact lenses. The potential use of contact lenses aside from their role to correct refractive error has been reviewed. These issues are collected in Table 3.2.

Furthermore, new developments in contact lenses are packaging and storage cases. The use of contact lenses as devices to detect systemic disease has mostly focused on detecting changes to glucose levels in tears for monitoring diabetic control. Glucose can be detected using changes in color, fluorescence or generation of electric signals by embedded sensors such as boronic acid, Concanavalin A or glucose oxidase. Contact lenses that have gained regulatory

Table 3.2 Potential uses of contact lenses (44).

Field of Use
Detect ion in systemic and ocular surface diseases
Treatment and management of various ocular conditions
Devices that can correct presbyopia
Controlling the development of myopia
Usage for augmented vision

approval can measure changes in intraocular pressure to monitor glaucoma by measuring small changes in corneal shape (43).

Special challenges include the integration of sensors into contact lenses and the detection of the generated signals. Various techniques are used to optimize the uptake and release of the drugs to the ocular surface to treat diseases such as dry eye, glaucoma, infection and allergy. Contact lenses that either mechanically or electronically change their shape were investigated for the management of presbyopia. Contact lenses that slow the development of myopia are based upon incorporating concentric rings of plus power, peripheral optical zone(s) with add power or non-monotonic variations in power. Various forms of these lenses have shown a reduction in myopia in clinical trials and are available in various markets (43).

3.5.1 *Intraocular Pressure*

Intraocular pressure is an essential indicator of the diagnosis and treatment of glaucoma. The intraocular pressure has an apparent physiological rhythm, and it often reaches its peak value at night. To avoid missing the peak value at night and sample the entire rhythm cycle, continuous monitoring of the intraocular pressure is urgently needed. A wearable contact lens intraocular pressure sensor based on a platinum strain gauge was fabricated by the microelectromechanical process (45).

A contact lens sensor for continuous intraocular pressure monitoring using self-assembly graphene, has been developed (46). The combination of face-to-face water transfer printing and microelectromechanical systems technology can realize the batch preparation of such a sensor. The sensor has good light transmittance and temperature stability.

The continuous detection of a raised intraocular pressure could benefit the monitoring of patients with glaucoma (47). Contact lenses with embedded sensors for measuring intraocular pressure are rigid, bulky, partially block vision or are insufficiently sensitive.

The design and testing of soft and transparent contact lenses for the quantitative monitoring of the intraocular pressure in real time using a smartphone was reported (47). Such a contact lens incorporates a strain sensor, a wireless antenna, capacitors, resistors, stretchable metal interconnects and an integrated circuit for wireless communication. In human participants, the lens proved to be safe, and reliably provided accurate quantitative measurements of the intraocular pressure without inducing inflammation.

It was reported that the profiles from contact lens sensors may show significant errors (48). The intraocular pressure error from a single resonator sensor is large in a variable ocular environment. A dual-resonator sensor was developed to reduce such errors. Contact lens sensors were prototyped and tested on rubber eyes.

An intraocular pressure-signal gauge model for a dual-resonator sensor was developed that successfully removed the environmental noise. So, the error was reduced to less than 3 *mmHg*. This study showed that the new dual-resonator sensor and the intraocular pressure model reduced intraocular pressure errors to levels comparable to the errors in *ex-vivo* and *in-vivo* tonometry (48).

For continuous intraocular pressure monitoring, a pressure-measuring contact lens was developed to measure the intraocular pressure in millimeters of mercury (*mmHg*) continuously over 24 *h* (49).

The pressure-measuring contact lens is a 15 *mm* contact lens molded from medical grade silicone elastomers with surfaces treated with oxygen plasma to ensure hydrophilicity and allow overnight wear. In its center, a microelectromechanical system pressure sensor, a circular antenna and a telemetry microprocessor are embedded. The proprietary design of the lens adopts a specific geometry that holds it in place and relaxes the cornea to allow intraocular pressure measurements by individually calibrated microelectromechanical system sensor. Measurements are acquired continuously at a rate of 1 *Hz* during the entire duration of the recording, and are supplemented by intense sampling bursts at 51.2 *Hz*, for 10 *s* every 3 *min*. The readings are digitalized by the built-in microprocessor and sent wirelessly through the periorbital antenna connected to a portable recorder. Upon completion, the recording is transmitted to a computer for visualization (49).

Bland-Altman plots were used to illustrate the relationship between the pressure-measuring contact lens and pneumatonometer measurements.

A Bland-Altman plot (difference plot), in analytical chemistry or biomedicine, is a method of data plotting used in analyzing the agreement between two different assays (50–52).

3.5.1.1 Continuous Wear Contact Lens Sensor

Approaches for telemetric continuous intraocular pressure measurements have been developed and tested in animal models (53). Among these approaches, contact lens-based monitoring techniques are attractive because they are noninvasive. One contact lens system (Sensimed AG's Triggerfish) measures minute changes in corneal curvature by a contact lens equipped with an electrical strain sensor, an antenna and a microchip that are used for processing and transmitting signal wirelessly. This technology requires the patient to wear a receiver on the waist for data transmission and power transfer. Because of the thick silicone contact lens (central thickness 580 μm), it is not as comfortable as daily used contact lenses; mild to moderate adverse reactions are reported in up to 80% of patients.

The requirement of trained personnel, and the discomfort and high cost associated with this contact lens platform, precludes its usage in long-term monitoring applications and only allows tests for a single 24-hour period. For this reason, Triggerfish is found to be more suitable for determining changes in intraocular pressure on a daily scale. However, intraocular pressure change as a response to a drug is in the time scale of weeks. Similarly, the intraocular pressure change in response to certain lifestyle modifications will also be longer than a 24 h time scale.

Therefore, there is a need for a continuous wear contact lens sensor for long-term monitoring of intraocular pressure variations for determining the drug efficacy and for decreasing the number of doctor visits that a patient needs to make for routine intraocular pressure measurements (53).

A strain sensor has been presented that uses microfluidic principles integrated with a contact lens for intraocular pressure measurements. The materials used in the invention are low-cost, transparent, air permeable, and flexible. A method is provided to embed the microfluidic strain sensor in a silicone contact lens. The microfluidic contact lens sensor allows patients to measure their own intraocular pressure to better manage glaucoma.

The microfluidic contact lens sensor is capable of measuring the intraocular pressure fluctuations due to internal (i.e., metabolism, blinking and saccadic eye movements) as well as external factors (i.e., drugs, diet, lifestyle, etc.) during the lifetime of the patient. The measurements will be done at the discretion of the patient (or automatically) where a readout will be realized by a smartphone camera (or by a wearable camera for automated measurements). This allows for at-home monitoring and continuous data recording. The data then will be sent directly to a medical provider's database, which allows patients and physicians to monitor intraocular pressure variations. The aspects of this technology are as follows (53):

1. The microfluidic contact lens sensor will be built using a hybrid material system where the narrow microfluidic sensing region (as low as 0.1 *mm* wide ring at the periphery of microfluidic contact lens sensor) is embedded in a silicone or silicone/hydrogel contact lens material. The microfluidic sensing channels will be made out of transparent, soft, and oleophobic materials. The sensing material will be 6-10 orders of magnitude more air permeable compared to electronic components.
2. The microfluidic sensing technique has no actively controlled components and only works based on the principles of fluid physics. The microfluidic contact lens sensor is free of all electrical components (powerless). It is a low-cost device. In addition, it provides easier usability by eliminating the cumbersome peripheral components (e.g., antenna, microchip, etc.) for data transmission, reception and recording, which are needed in wearable electronic sensors.
3. The sensor will be sensitive to strain and responds to corneal radius of curvature changes but has low sensitivity to forces applied directly by the eyelid or due to hydration of the contact lens materials. The designed sensor has low stiffness in lateral direction (i.e., the microfluidic device is thin and

has low elastic modulus) and a high stiffness in the radial direction (i.e., the microfluidic network channels have small width), which will make it insensitive to external forces (e.g., blinking, rubbing of the eye).

4. The microfluidic contact lens sensor enables a readout with a smartphone camera and an optical adaptor. This will provide measurements at discrete time points. In one variation, a wearable camera that can track the sensor response can also be utilized for continuous and automated measurements.
5. Continuous data recorded with existing technologies show that intraocular pressure fluctuates around 5–15 *mmHg* day-to-day and hour-to-hour, and 15–40 *mmHg* second-to-second. The microfluidic network circuitry that was designed has the capability to filter out large fluctuations that occur in short time scales due to blood pressure or muscle contractions. In this case, the sensor actually acts as a fluidic low-pass filter, which only responds to changes that occur in minutes or less. In a similar manner, the fluidic components can be designed to register only the rapid intraocular pressure changes. A sensor that can measure events happening in different time scales can make better estimations of the true intraocular pressure based on the corneal radius of curvature measurements.

The microfluidic strain sensor embedded contact lens is convenient to use and has continuous measurement capability. It requires minimal training to take measurements and therefore will be used as a device for treatment at home. These measurements will enable clinical studies where recording of long-term intraocular pressure data on large patient populations is needed. Continuous recording of intraocular pressure and its analysis will improve our understanding of neurodegenerative diseases and their relation to pressure. Additionally, it will be useful for improving the efficiency and efficacy of drugs that are used for glaucoma treatment. Therefore, microfluidic contact lens sensor technology offers a promising healthcare technology for better personalized care of glaucoma patients. These advantages listed above will potentially enable the patient to use the sensor permanently and without trained personnel assistance (53).

3.5.2 *Coating Thickness*

A method for determining the thickness of coatings on the surfaces of contact lenses has been described. This method uses the steps of (54):

- Obtaining a coated contact lens in fully hydrated state, wherein the coated contact lens consists of a lens body (i.e., bulk material) and a coating thereon, wherein the lens body consists of a non-silicone hydrogel material or a silicone hydrogel material, wherein the coating consists of a coating material having negatively charged groups,
- Selectively staining the coating over the lens body of the coated contact lens by immersing the coated contact lens in an aqueous solution of a fluorescently labeled polycationic polymer for a time period of about 12 *h* or less, wherein the aqueous solution consists of buffering agents in an amount for having a pH of from about 6.5 to about 8.0
- Orthogonally cutting the selectively stained coated contact lens, and
- Determining the thickness of the coating on the coated contact lens.

Here, a polycationic polymer is a polycationic polypeptide with positively charged amino acid units. Examples of preferred positively charged amino acids include lysine, arginine, histine, or 2,3-diaminopropionic acid.

A fluorescently labeled polycationic polymer refers to a polymer which has been chemically modified to have a covalently attached moiety which is capable of emitting fluorescence upon being irradiated with a light (54).

3.6 Cleaning of Contact Lenses

Disinfecting solutions for use with contact lenses are well known in the art. The use of such lenses involves a daily disinfecting treatment (55). Flexible, or soft, contact lenses are generally made from hydrophilic polymers and the hydroxy groups of these lenses attract and retain substantial amounts of water in the plastic, which results in difficulties during cleaning and sterilization.

Hydrogen peroxide systems, containing 3% hydrogen peroxide, have emerged as the disinfectant of choice for all types of daily and extended wear hydrogel lenses (56, 57). The primary reason for hydrogen peroxide's popularity is its rapid killing of microbial contaminants and its non-residual character. After hydrogen peroxide disinfects lenses, it can be converted into innocuous and natural by-products, such as O_2 and water, which are compatible with ocular physiology (58).

In general, the hydrogen peroxide systems involve a hydrogen peroxide-containing disinfecting solution into which the contact lenses to be disinfected are placed and allowed to remain for a required period of time. The hydrogen peroxide may (55):

1. Oxidize chloride in the bacteria to hypochlorite, or
2. Decompose into nascent oxygen and hydroxyl radicals, thus providing a germicidal effect.

Following the requisite time period, a purposeful inactivation of the hydrogen peroxide is conducted, for example, with a platinum catalyst. Following inactivation, the contact lens may be reinserted into the eye.

However, harmful microorganisms, proteins, lipids, and other irritating deposits are not always sufficiently removed by a peroxide disinfection alone and the lens should be cleaned and rinsed beforehand. This is typically performed by wetting the lens with a sufficient amount of a lens cleaner and then rubbing the lens with one's fingers and rinsing the lens with saline.

The cleaning step is considered a hassle by some consumers and a peroxide disinfection system that adequately disinfects and cleans without this step (a *no rub-no rinse* regimen) would offer a great improvement in convenience to the user (55).

The addition of a surface-active agent to a peroxide disinfection solution can enhance the disinfecting properties of the solution (59). However, the surfactants disclosed are all present in amounts above 0.1% and, because of excessive foaming, are incompatible with the platinum catalyst disc typically used to deactivate hydrogen peroxide in lens disinfection systems (55).

In addition, glycerol, polyhydric alcohol, and Tween 20 will reduce the rate at which hydrogen peroxide will decompose, thus increasing its disinfecting efficacy (60). However, there are significant problems with each of these compositions that effectively preclude their use in a contact lens disinfection solution. For instance, glycerol is not stable in 3% hydrogen peroxide and both polyhydric alcohol, such as PVA, and Tween 20 will cause excessive foaming when the solution contacts the catalytic disc and decomposes (55).

Compositions and methods were reported for disinfecting and cleaning contact lenses that include a liquid medium containing hydrogen peroxide and a solid ethylene oxide/propylene oxide block copolymer surfactant having at least 70% poly(ethylene oxide) (PEO) (61). Here, the hydrogen peroxide is degraded by a catalase released into the solution and causes a reduced amount of foam. However, such compositions cause excessive foaming when a platinum catalyst is used to decompose the hydrogen peroxide (55).

Methods for treating contact lenses and compositions for the same have been developed (55). It was found that a composition for disinfecting a contact lens consisting of an effective disinfecting amount of hydrogen peroxide and a surfactant consisting of a low-foaming or non-foaming copolymer of hydrophobic and hydrophilic blocks show an outstanding disinfection efficacy, even when used without an additional rub and rinse step. The hydrophile component of the block copolymer constitutes less than 50% of the block copolymer.

The surfactant is a poly(oxyethylene) (POE) poly(oxypropylene) (POP) block copolymer having a Ross-Miles (62) foam height of less than 1 *mm* at 0.1% and 50°C.

An example of such surfactants are POE POP condensation polymers terminated with primary hydroxyl groups. They may be synthesized by first creating a hydrophobic material of desired molecular weight by the controlled addition of propylene oxide to the two hydroxyl groups of propylene glycol. In the second step of the synthesis, ethylene oxide is added to sandwich this hydrophobic material between hydrophile groups. Such block copolymers can be obtained commercially under the trademark Pluronic®.

Specific examples of Pluronic surfactants that are satisfactory are listed in Table 3.3.

The Pluronic letter-number combinations (as shown in Table 3.3) are used to identify the various products of the series. The alphabetical designation explains the physical form of the product: *L* for liquids, *P* for pastes, *F* for solid forms (all at 20°C). The first digit

Table 3.3 Pluronic® surfactants (55).

Liquid compounds	Compounds with reverse structure	
Pluronic® L42	Pluronic® 12R3	Pluronic® 17R1
Pluronic® L43	Pluronic® 25R1	Pluronic® 17R2
Pluronic® L61	Pluronic® 31R1	Pluronic® 17R4
	Pluronic® 31R2	

(two digits in a three-digit number) in the numerical designation, multiplied by 300, indicates the approximate molecular weight of the hydrophobe (polypropylene oxide). The last digit, when multiplied by 10, indicates the approximate PEO content in the molecule in percent.

The letter *R* found in the middle of the designation of the Pluronic R series signifies that this product has a reverse structure compared to the Pluronic products, i.e., the hydrophile (ethylene oxide) is sandwiched between the propylene oxide blocks. The numeric designation preceding the *R*, when multiplied by 100, indicates the approximate molecular weight of the propylene oxide block. The number following the *R*, when multiplied by 10, indicates the approximate weight percent of ethylene oxide in that product (55).

Several other properties of these compounds, such as molecular weight, content of PEO, melting pour point, Brookfield viscosity, surface tension, cloud point, and others, have been shown in a review article (63).

Particularly good results are obtained with the Pluronic 17R4 surfactant (55).

It was suspected that the block copolymer surfactants provide a defoaming or antifoaming action by forming an insoluble monolayer at the air-water interface of the foam. For this reason, the defoaming/antifoaming activity of a block copolymer is a function of both the cloud point of the copolymer and the use temperature. To select an effective defoamer/antifoamer, one should choose a block copolymer whose cloud point is lower than the intended use temperature. Block copolymers with a low ethylene oxide content are the most effective defoamers. Within each series of block copolymer products, defoaming performance increases as the ethylene oxide content decreases and the molecular weight increases.

Also, the compositions preferably contain a hydrogen peroxide stabilizer. The stabilizer can be a diphosphonic acid alkanol (56). The most preferred phosphonic acid-containing stabilizer is diethylenetriamine penta(methylenephosphonic acid) or a physiologically compatible salt thereof (57). Diethylenetriamine penta(methylenephosphonic acid) is shown in Figure 3.3.

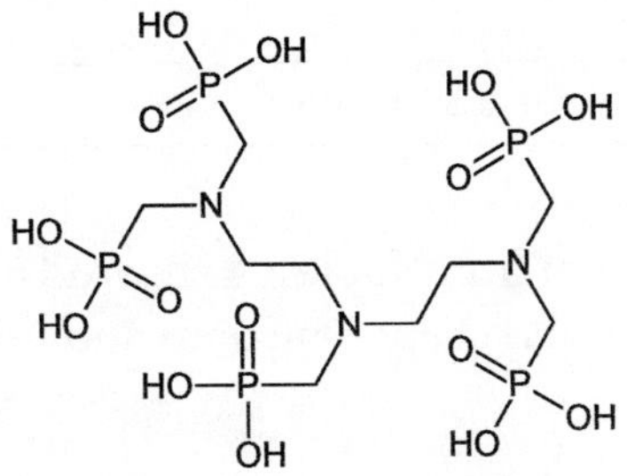

Figure 3.3 Diethylenetriamine penta(methylenephosphonic acid).

This compound is manufactured by Solutia under the name Dequest® 2060. This stabilizer is preferably present in the solution in an amount between about 0.006% and 0.0120%.

Furthermore, the cleaning composition contains a buffer. The buffer maintains the pH preferably in the desired range, so, in a physiologically acceptable range of 5.5 to about 8. Such a buffer is selected from inorganic or organic bases, preferably basic phosphates, borates, citrates, tartrates, carbonates, bicarbonates and mixtures thereof. The buffer component may include sodium dibasic phosphate (Na_2HPO_4), sodium monobasic phosphate (NaH_2PO_4), and potassium monobasic phosphate (KH_2PO_4).

A liquid composition has been prepared by blending together the ingredients shown in Table 3.4.

The solution prepared according to Table 3.4 was evaluated using ISO 14729 (21). Three lots of product were each challenged with 5 panel organisms: *Fusarium solani, Candida albicans, Serratia marcescens, Staphylococcus aureus,* and *Pseudomonas aeruginosa.* The prepared solution achieved a total kill against all five panel organisms.

Also, the protein cleaning efficacy of a solution and others were compared. The protein removal effectiveness shown by the solu-

Table 3.4 Cleaning composition for contact lenses (55).

Compound	Amount/[g]
Hydrogen peroxide	35.0
Sodium Phosphate, monobasic (monohydrate)	0.772
Sodium Phosphate, dibasic (anhydrous)	1.555
Dequest® 2060	0.120
Sodium Chloride	7.900
Pluronic® 17R4	0.500
USP Purified Water QS to 1 liter	

tions of the composition from Table 3.4 showed a significantly better cleaning efficacy than EasySept One Step and OxySept 1 Step.

3.7 Biofouling

The issue of biofouling has been described in a monograph (64).

3.8 Wettability

The maintenance of contact lens surface wettability is important because surface properties such as wettability can change during wear, affecting the wearer's comfort (44, 65, 66).

Several factors, including individual tear composition, blinking and related tear evaporation, ocular temperature, types of lens materials worn, duration of lens wear and lens replacement schedule may affect wettability of worn contact lenses (44).

Wettability is one of the most crucial properties determining a material's solid surface and material applications (67).

For contact lenses, the wettability indicates how easily liquids spread over the lens surface. this can be observed through the interaction between the lens surface and tears and can be defined by the contact angle (68).

Lenses that exhibit and sustain complete water wetting allow thick tear film deposition, minimize film rupture, and permit smooth tear recovery upon lid closure (69). The water contact angles determined using an air bubble captive on a lens are the best gauge of the *in-vivo* wetting state.

To achieve highly water wetting lenses demands that contact angle hysteresis be eliminated and that the advancing and receding angles both approach zero. Since lens wear exposes the anterior surface to tear proteins, lens wettability should be measured in the presence of tear film components.

A method has been proposed to improve the lubricity of contact lenses by polymerizing a thin film of a hydrophilic polymer made from *N,N*-dimethylacrylamide (DMA) on the contact lens (70).

This approach involves soaking the lens in a solution of 2,2′-azobisisobutyronitrile (AIBN) in methanol to load the hydrophobic thermal initiator into the lens. The AIBN-loaded lens is then placed in a DMA solution at elevated temperature to initiate the thermal polymerization of the monomer to polymerize a film on the surface of the lens. Though AIBN is hydrophobic, it is released into the solution at high temperatures due to the high solubility of the free radicals generated by decomposition of the initiator, which results in polymerization of the bulk solution as well.

The processing parameters must be optimized to achieve a surface DMA film of desired thickness without causing the bulk solution to gel and without significant changes to the lens shape. Acuvue® Advance® lenses were successfully modified using 3.4% AIBN solution to load the initiator and then placing that in a 4% DMA solution at 70°C for 12 *h* (70).

Fourier transform infrared spectroscopy spectra confirmed a surface DMA film and the results were further substantiated by measuring the weight of the surface film as well as wettability (contact angle) and lubricity (coefficient of friction). The optimized poly-DMA film had a hydrated weight of about 10 *mg* with a water content of about 400%. The film reduces the contact angle from 105.9±0.1° to 45.3±0.12° for Acuvue Advance lenses, and reduces the coefficient of friction in contact with excised cornea significantly from 0.0385±0.010 to 0.0063±0.0017 (70).

This method is effective only in lenses in which the release duration of the AIBN is sufficiently long to initiate the DMA film within the release duration. The release duration is about 30 *min* in Acuvue Advance and Air Optix® contact lenses. For other lens types, a modified approach can be developed by first loading Vitamin E, which is an effective diffusion barrier, into the lens to slow the AIBN release from the lens. This method can be successfully used with other lenses, such as Acuvue Oasys (70).

3.8.1 *Blister Pack Solutions*

An approach to increase the wettability of lenses is to reduce the surface tension of the liquid in which the contact lenses are stored (44). This can result in a reduction of interfacial tension between the blister pack solution and the lens surface, thus promoting the adhesion of the solution to the contact lens surface. Traditionally, buffered saline is used as the blister pack solution for contact lenses (71).

The wettability and the physical properties of blister pack solutions of hydrogel contact lenses have been discussed (72, 73).

The advancing and receding contact angles were measured directly out of the blister pack for five daily disposable lenses. These are listed in Table 3.5.

Table 3.5 Daily disposable lenses (73).

Designation	Manufacturer	Main materials
Omafilcon A	CooperVision	HEMA, PC
Nelfilcon A	CIBA Vision	HPMC, PEG, PVA
Modified Nelfilcon A	CIBA Vision	
Etafilcon A	Johnson & Johnson	HEMA, MAA
Narafilcon A	Johnson & Johnson	SIH

Abbreviations	
HEMA	2-Hydroxyethyl methacrylate
PC	Poly(carbonate)
HPMC	Hydroxypropyl methylcellulose
PEG	Poly(ethylene glycol)
CPVA	Crosslinked poly(vinyl alcohol)
MA	Methacrylic acid
SIH	Silicone hydrogel

Advancing contact angles were measured using the sessile drop method and the Wilhelmy balance method. Receding contact angles were measured using the Wilhelmy balance method (73).

The sessile drop method is a method used for the characterization of solid surface energies, and in some cases, aspects of liquid surface energies (74). The main premise of the method is that by placing a droplet of liquid with a known surface energy, the shape of the drop, specifically the contact angle, and the known surface energy of the liquid are the parameters which can be used to calculate the surface energy of the solid sample. The liquid used for such experiments is referred to as the probe liquid, and the use of several different probe liquids is required (74).

The Wilhelmy balance method, invented in 1863, uses a plate to measure the interfacial tension (75). In particular, a Wilhelmy plate is a thin plate that is used to measure equilibrium surface or interfacial tension at an air-liquid or liquid-liquid interface. In this method, the plate is oriented perpendicular to the interface, and the force exerted on it is measured (76).

Surface tension, pH, and osmolality were measured for each blister pack solution from all the daily disposable lenses (73). Osmolality is a variation of molality that takes into account only solutes that contribute to a solution's osmotic pressure (77).

The advancing contact angles for the Nelfilcon A lenses were statistically lower ($P<0.05$) than the advancing contact angles of the other three lenses. The receding contact angles for Etafilcon A were statistically lower ($P<0.05$) than the receding contact angles for the other four lenses. The pH of all the blister pack solutions was relatively neutral (7.01–7.43). The surface tension of the blister pack solution for the modified Nelfilcon A was significantly lower ($P<0.05$) than the surface tension of all other blister pack solutions. The osmolality of the blister pack solutions for the Etafilcon A and Narafilcon A lenses were significantly higher ($P<0.05$) than the other blister pack solutions (73).

3.8.2 *Captive Bubble Method*

The captive bubble method is a method for measuring contact angle between a liquid and a solid, by using drop shape analysis (78, 79). In this method, a bubble of air is injected beneath a solid, the surface of which is located in the liquid, instead of placing a drop on the solid as in the case of the sessile drop technique.

The method is particularly suitable for solids with high surface free energy on which liquids spread out. Hydrogels, such as soft contact lenses for example, are likewise inaccessible for the standard arrangement; the captive bubble method is also used in such cases (80).

A contact angle is formed on a smooth, periodically heterogeneous solid surface. Above the solid surface, a liquid drop is submerged in a fluid. The measurement of contact angles usually contributes to the measurement of the surface energy of solids in the industry. Different from other methods of measuring the contact angle, such as the sessile drop method, the system utilized in the captive bubble method has the fluid bubble attached from below to the solid surface, in which both the liquid bubble and the solid interact with a fluid (79).

For contact lenses, an air bubble immersed in aqueous solution is brought into contact with the contact lens. The contact angle through water during bubble expansion yields the receding angle. Bubble contraction gives the water advancing angle. Contact angle hysteresis is the difference between the advancing and receding angles.

3.8.2.1 *Exemplary Tests*

A captive bubble method has been applied to measure the advancing and receding contact angles of two commercial silicone hydrogel lenses: PureVision and Focus Night & Day and a standard 2-hydroxyethyl methacrylate (HEMA) hydrogel lens, i.e., Acuvue.

In an isotonic solution, all three lenses display considerable contact angle hysteresis with advancing angles of almost 90°. When lysozyme and/or mucin were added to the aqueous solution, hysteresis was eliminated, and equivalent and high water wetting was achieved for the three lenses. Only the advancing angle in isotonic solution provided discriminating evidence for differences in surface chemistry. Covalent attachment of poly(ethylene glycol) (PEG) to the PureVision lens surface achieved a complete water wetting independent of the presence of a tear protein in the solution.

The captive bubble technique provides contact angles that are relevant to on-eye lens wear. Both advancing and receding contact angles are important to lens wettability performance. When lysozyme and/or mucin are present in the solution, PureVision, Focus Night & Day, and Acuvue lenses display low advancing and receding contact angles indicative of equivalent wettability performance. This result is due to molecular adsorption of the proteins onto the lens external surface. Covalently attached PEG on the PureVision lens not only provides complete water wetting but also minimizes or even eliminates protein adsorption (69).

3.8.3 Tethered Hyaluronic Acid-Based Coatings

The wettability of contact lenses can be improved and the protein adsorption can be reduced by a surface functionalization.

A simple *click chemistry* approach has been described to functionalize the surface of poly(2-hydroxyethyl methacrylate) (PHEMA)-based contact lenses with hyaluronic acid (HA), a carbohydrate naturally contributing to the wettability of the native tear film (81, 82). HA is shown in Figure 4.41

A two-step preparation technique consisting of a laccase/TEMPO-mediated oxidation followed by covalent grafting of hydrazide-functionalized HA via simple immersion resulted in a model lens surface that is significantly more wettable, more water retentive, and less protein binding than unmodified PHEMA while maintaining the favorable transparency, refractive, and mechanical properties of a native lens.

The dipping/coating method that was developed to covalently tether the HA wetting agent is simple, readily scalable, and a highly efficient route for contact lens modification (81).

The uptake of a fluorescently labeled HA and a low-molecular-weight HA derivative in four types of contact lenses was investigated using fluorescent microscopy and confocal laser scanning microscopy (83).

The four lens types were used to compare efficacy in improving hydrophilicity, as well as maintenance of contact angle measurements, in commercially available multipurpose solutions that contained either HA, the low-molecular-weight HA derivative, or an alternative wetting agent.

The low-molecular-weight HA derivative was found to sorb more readily to silicone hydrogel lenses and exhibited a greater accumulation over time than conventional HA (83). Multipurpose solutions containing the low-molecular-weight HA derivative showed an increase in lens hydrophilicity through decreases in contact angle measurements when compared with those obtained from lenses treated with multipurpose solutions containing conventional HA or alternative wetting agents.

This increase in the hydrophilicity of the lens is associated with the low-molecular-weight HA derivative. This property was also maintained over multiple cycles in phosphate buffered saline, while alternative solutions with conventional HA did not show this effect (83).

3.9 Material Properties and Antimicrobial Efficacy

Two series of silicone hydrogel materials were investigated for their characterization, water content, surface wettability, transmittance, mechanical property, oxygen permeability, and bacterial attachment as potential contact lens materials (84). The relationships between water affinity and optical, mechanical, oxygen permeable and biological properties were discussed (84).

One of the series of silicone hydrogels was fabricated on the basis of 3-(methacryloyloxy)propyltris(trimethylsiloxy)silane (TRIS), 3-(3-methacryloxy-2-hydroxypropoxy)propylbis(trimethylsiloxy) methylsilane (BIS), and HEMA with different silicone monomers/HEMA ratios.

The other series of silicone hydrogels was fabricated on the basis of TRIS, BIS, HEMA, and DMA with different ratios of DMA and HEMA.

The results showed that the water affinity could be modulated by the hydrophilic methacrylate. The equilibrium water content increased and the water static contact angle value decreased with the increase of hydrophilic monomers. The equilibrium water content versus monomer content is shown in Figure 3.4.

Overall, the results demonstrated that visible light transmittance tends to increase and tensile mechanical properties presented in declining trend depending on the increasing equilibrium water content (84).

The transparency versus monomer content is shown in Figure 3.5.

The oxygen permeability value decreased first and then increased when the equilibrium water content increased from 20% to 60%. The reversion point of equilibrium water content was about 42.5% The

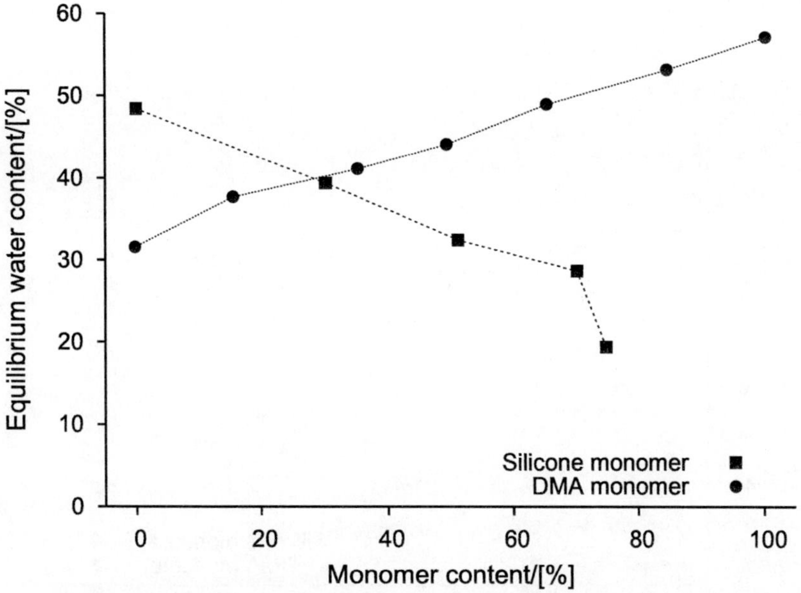

Figure 3.4 Equilibrium water content vs. monomer content (84).

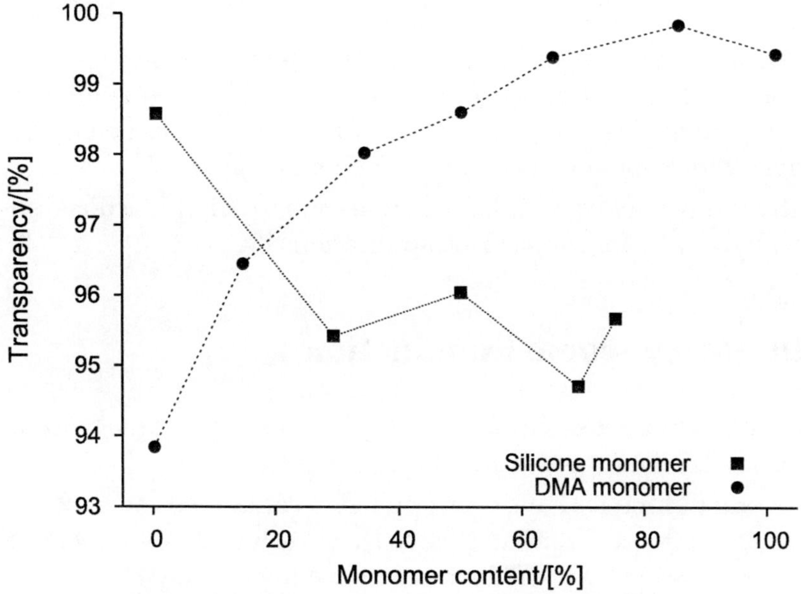

Figure 3.5 Transparency vs. monomer content (84).

oxygen permeability versus monomer content is shown in Figure 3.6.

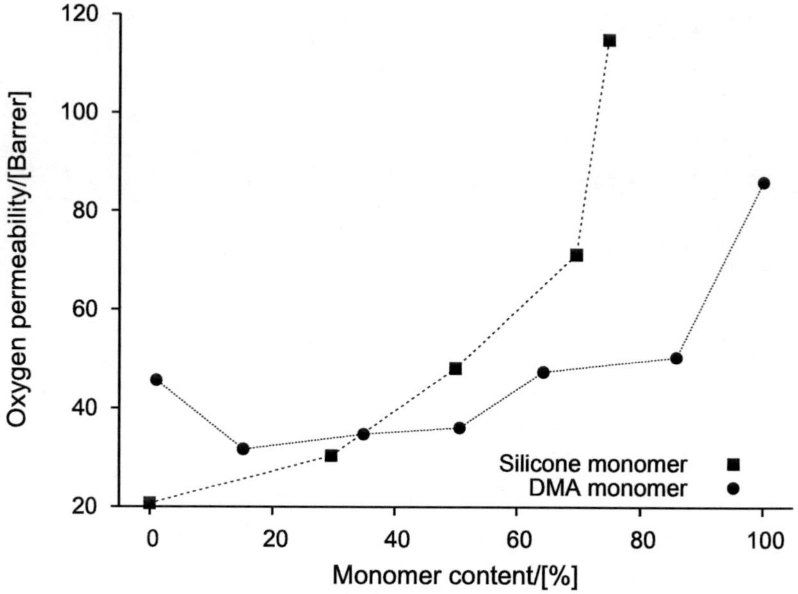

Figure 3.6 Oxygen permeability vs. monomer content (84).

The amount of *Staphylococcus aureus* attached on the surface of the silicone hydrogels dropped from 104 to 103 while the equilibrium water content was at 55°. The amount of *S. aureus* attached on the surface versus monomer content is shown in Figure 3.7.

This study may provide information for preparing functional silicone hydrogels for contact lens applications (84).

3.10 Microscopic Examination

A smooth surface is essential for the optical quality and the biocompatibility of contact lenses and the ocular surface.

Several techniques have been applied to contact lens microscopic examination for different purposes. These include X-ray photoelectron spectroscopy (XPS) (85), atomic force microscopy (AFM) (86), scanning electron microscopy (SEM) (87), and time-of-flight secondary ion mass spectrometry (88).

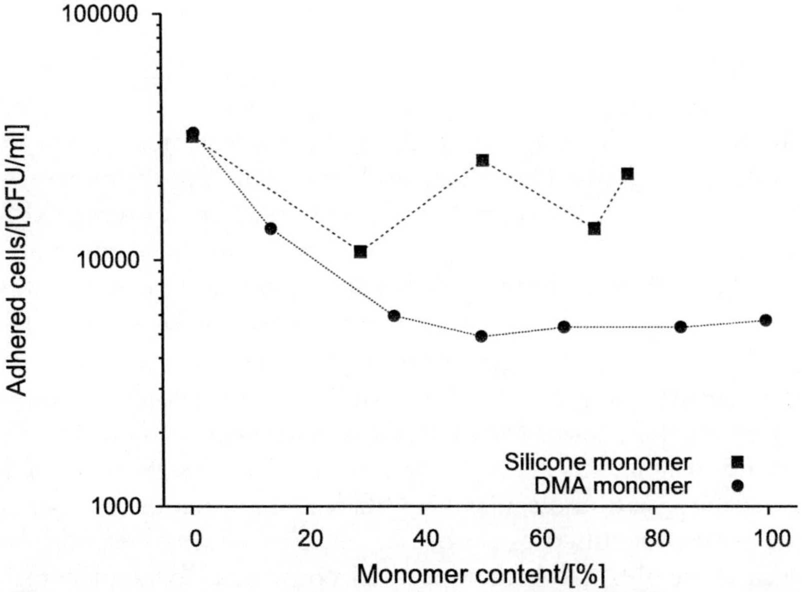

Figure 3.7 Amount of *Staphylococcus aureus* on the surface vs. monomer content (84).

3.10.1 X-Ray Photoelectron Spectroscopy

X-Ray photoelectron spectroscopy (XPS) is a surface-sensitive quantitative spectroscopic technique that measures the elemental composition at the parts per thousand range, empirical formula, chemical state and electronic state of the elements that exist within a material (89). XPS is a useful measurement technique because it not only shows what elements are within a film but also what other elements they are bonded to.

The practical concepts of XPS have been presented in a monograph (90). This book first introduces the reader to the concepts used in this field and then demonstrates how these concepts are applied. Including how the spectra are produced, and factors that can influence the spectra with respect to initial and final state effects are discussed.

3.10.1.1 *Exemplary Tests*

X-Ray photoelectron spectroscopy (XPS) and matrix-assisted laser desorption/ionization time-of-flight mass spectrometry (MALDI-TOF) were used to analyze initial adsorption events in the fouling of HEMA-based contact lenses (85). All of the lenses tested accumulated tear film deposits within 10 *min* of wear. XPS indicated the presence of mainly proteinaceous deposits, with indications of some contributions by mucins or lipids on some lenses and the nature of the deposit being influenced by the lens chemistry.

MALDI-TOF detected the presence of surface-adsorbed species with molecular weights <15 *kDa*. While lysozyme could be identified by comparison of MALDI-TOF signals with known protein mass and assignments are suggested for some other signals, several other species, with molecular weights less than that of lysozyme, could not be identified as no ocular proteins with corresponding molecular weights had been reported in previous biochemical tear film analysis experiments. These species, and others, were also detected in MALDI-TOF analysis of reflex tear film, suggesting that the adsorbed unidentified species were not simply products of surface-induced dissociation of adsorbing higher molecular weight proteins (85).

This short-term wear study detected rapid interface conversion and demonstrated the utility and surface sensitivity of XPS and MALDI-TOF in characterizing contact lens deposits at the initial stages when sub-monolayer adsorbed amounts are present on lenses (85).

3.10.2 *Atomic Force Spectroscopy*

In atomic force microscopy (AFM), a sharp tip stylus attached to a small cantilever scans the sample surface within a sub-nanometer range or resolution. Several studies have revealed that AFM is a proper technique to study hydrogel contact lens surface because it can explore the contact lens surface in aqueous environments and can provide microscopic information with a spatial resolution relevant to the size of polymeric functional groups proteins and cells. Because the sample for AFM does not need to be electrically conductive, no metallic coating is required as it is in SEM. Therefore, some of the surface irregularities such as ondulations or wrinkles observed under conventional SEM that are artifacts of the critical point dehydration and subsequent metallic coating process, are not seen in the AFM samples.

3.10.2.1 *Exemplary Tests*

Samples of Lotrafilcon A, Balafilcon A, and Galyfilcon A contact lenses were observed by AFM in tapping mode at areas ranging from 0.25 μm^2 to 400 μm^2.

The mean roughness, root-mean-square roughness and maximum roughness in nanometers were obtained for the three lens materials at different magnifications. The three contact lenses showed significantly different surface topography.

However, roughness values were dependent on the surface area to be analyzed. For a 1 μm^2 area, statistics revealed significantly more irregular surface of Balafilcon A compared with Lotrafilcon A and Galyfilcon A. The parameters are collected in Table 3.6.

Table 3.6 Roughness values (91).

Lens material	Mean	Root-mean-square roughness/[nm]	Maximum
Balafilcon A	6.44	8.30	96.82
Lotrafilcon A	2.40	3.19	40.89
Galyfilcon A	1.40	1.79	15.33

The mean roughness and the root-mean-square roughness were the most consistent parameters, with maximum roughness presenting more variability for larger surface areas. The higher roughness of Balafilcon A is attributed to the plasma oxidation treatment used to improve wettability. Conversely, Galyfilcon A displays a smoother surface. These observations could have implications in clinical aspects of siloxane-hydrogel contact lens wear such as lens spoliation, resistance to bacterial adhesion, or mechanical interaction with the ocular surface (91).

3.10.3 *Electrochemical Impedance Spectroscopy*

Plasma polymerization techniques are very useful for tailoring unique surface properties for specific applications such as for biomaterials. The systematic selection of monomer gases and plasma discharge conditions can provide characteristic surface state properties that behave virtually independent from the substrate for a wide range of materials (92, 93).

It is believed that a good wettability insures the stability of the tear film over and under a lens, providing good on-eye mobility and comfort. Plasma polymerization coatings can modify the surface wettability easily.

The influence of ultrathin (i.e., 5 *nm* to 50 *nm*) plasma polymer coatings on siloxane-based hydrogel contact lenses was investigated by electrochemical impedance spectroscopy (EIS) (94).

The rather unconventional EIS method is used for evaluating free-standing polymeric films. However, some EIS studies have illustrated the effects of surface and interfacial factors introduced by plasma polymers on water and ion permeability of free-standing films (95–97).

Impedance measurements as a function of frequency (Bode plots) were taken at regular intervals until steady impedance was obtained, indicating that the lenses were saturated. Appropriate equivalent circuit models were constructed to describe the salt intrusion characteristics of the plasma polymer-coated contact lenses. This provided information pertaining to the resistance and capacitance of interfacial and bulk layers in the plasma polymer-coated lenses. Resistance relates to ion permeability and capacitance for water uptake.

The study showed that some of an ultrathin layer of plasma polymer applied onto a dry hydrogel remains a contiguous film after the substrate hydrogel swells upon hydration. In some cases, however, the overall impedance of the coated lens is so low that the state of the plasma polymer layer after the hydration of the substrate hydrogel could not be judged by EIS (94).

3.10.4 *Scanning Electron Microscopy*

A scanning electron microscope is a type of electron microscope that produces images of a sample by scanning the surface with a focused beam of electrons (98).

The electrons interact with atoms in the sample, producing various signals that contain information about the surface topography and composition of the sample. The electron-beam is scanned in a raster scan pattern, and the position of the beam is combined with the intensity of the detected signal to produce an image. In the most common SEM mode, secondary electrons emitted by atoms excited by the electron-beam are detected using a secondary electron detector (Everhart-Thornley detector) (98).

The Everhart-Thornley detector is a secondary electron and backscattered electron detector used in SEM (99). It is named after its designers, Thomas E. Everhart and Richard F. M. Thornley, who published their design in 1960 to increase the efficiency of existing secondary electron detectors by adding a light pipe to carry the photon signal from the scintillator inside the evacuated specimen chamber of the SEM machine to the photomultiplier outside the chamber (100). The Everhart-Thornley detector with its light-guide and highly efficient photomultiplier is the most frequently used detector for SEM.

The number of secondary electrons that can be detected, and thus the signal intensity, depends, among other things, on specimen topography. SEM can achieve a resolution better than 1 *nm* (98).

3.10.4.1 *Exemplary Tests*

The surface and bulk structures of hydrogel contact lenses that contain siloxane moieties, PureVision™ (Balafilcon A) and Focus Night & Day™ (Lotrafilcon A) were investigated (87). Standard hydrogel lenses of low (Seequence®), medium (Acuvue®), and high water content (Precision UV®) were used as controls.

All the lenses were dehydrated in a series of ethanol solutions of increased concentration, critical point dried in CO_2, and sputter coated with gold/palladium before they were examined by SEM.

Of all the lenses examined, only the Balafilcon lenses presented, in addition to the polymer network porosity characteristic of all hydrogels, a macroporous structure that was observed on the front and back surfaces, and in their bulk. The average diameter of the macropores appears to be much larger, from one to several orders of magnitude, than the network porosity of standard hydrogel lenses. The macropores might contribute to the gas and water permeability of these lenses, as well as to their mobility on the cornea (87).

3.11 Schirmer Tear Test

The Schirmer tear test was invented by Otto Schirmer, a German ophthalmologist. The test was already published in 1903 (101).

The Schirmer tear test determines whether the eye produces enough tears to keep it moist (102). This test is used when a person experiences very dry eyes or excessive watering of the eyes. It poses no risk to the subject.

The Schirmer tear test uses paper strips inserted into the eye for several minutes to measure the production of tears. Both eyes are tested at the same time. Most often, this test consists of placing a small strip of filter paper inside the lower eyelid (inferior fornix). The eyes are closed for 5 *min*. Then, the paper is removed and the amount of moisture is measured. Sometimes a topical anesthetic is placed into the eye before the filter paper to prevent tearing due to the irritation from the paper. The use of an anesthetic ensures that only basal tear secretion is being measured.

A young person normally moistens 15 *mm* of each paper strip. Because hypolacrimation occurs with aging, 33% of normal elderly persons may wet only 10 *mm* in 5 *min*. Persons with Sjögren's syndrome moisten less than 5 *mm* in 5 *min*.

A negative test result with more than 10 *mm* of moisture on the filter paper in 5 *min* is normal. Both eyes normally secrete the same amount of tears.

3.12 Ocular Surface Disease Index Test

Individuals treated for dry eye disease, increasing tear production, or improving ocular discomfort can provide important information used to diagnose their condition and determine the severity of dry eye symptoms through questionnaires. A well-designed questionnaire can be validated for reproducibility and should consist of relevant questions that elicit responsive answers.

One example of a dry eye questionnaire is the Ocular Surface Disease Index (OSDi), a 12-question survey for dry eye patients that has been shown to be a reliable and valid instrument for directly assessing symptom frequency.

The ocular symptoms that are evaluated include burning/stinging, itching, foreign body sensation, eye discomfort, eye dryness, photophobia, and pain. Most people are familiar with questionnaires and understand that they are an efficient way for a health provider to gather information. Questionnaires also reduce bias, as there are no verbal or visual cues to inadvertently influence the respondent.

The OSDi score can be used to evaluate the severity of the ocular symptom, and the effectiveness of a particular treatment of an individual. Higher numbers indicate a higher severity of dry eye disease. Reduction in OSDi scores over time is evidence of a reduction in or alleviation of the ocular symptoms and generally indicates an improvement in the individual's condition. A decrease in the OSDi score is also evidence that the treatment is effective in treating dry eye disease, increasing tear production, or improving ocular discomfort.

3.13 Corneal Fluorescein Staining Test

Corneal surface changes are associated with insufficient tear flow and excessive dryness, as well as dry eye disease and ocular discomfort. Corneal surface changes may include disruption of the mucin coating protecting the surface epithelial cells, and/or damage to the epithelial cell walls.

The corneal fluorescein staining test is a diagnostic test for determining corneal surface health and can indicate areas of damage on the corneal surface (103). The normal corneal surface does not take up water-soluble dyes instilled in the tear film. However, damaged epithelial cells allow water-soluble dyes to diffuse into the surface cells. Fluorescein, which stains damaged epithelial cells, may be visualized on the corneal surface, indicating damage as a result of desiccation on the corneal surface.

To administer the corneal fluorescein staining test, fluorescein is applied to one or both eyes. Fluorescein is allowed to penetrate and stain the area between surface cells.

Devitalized cells and strands of devitalized surface tissue (filaments) can be visualized with this stain. A test administrator then uses a corneal surface scoring system that has been developed to rate the severity of damage observed. This scoring system is useful for monitoring dry eye treatment over time.

The test may be administered multiple times to monitor any change in the severity of the individual's ocular surface over a period of time. In general, higher numbers indicate more damage to the corneal surface compared to lower numbers, which indicate lower levels of damage to the corneal surface (103).

The reduction in corneal scores over time is evidence of a reduction in the damage to corneal surface. The decrease in corneal scores generally indicates an improvement in the individual's condition. The decrease in corneal scores over time is also evidence that the treatment is effective in treating a dry eye disease, increasing tear production, or improving ocular discomfort.

As reported, a corneal fluorescein staining test was performed as follows (104, 105):

The ocular surface was examined with a biomicroscope and the ×10 objective under blue-light illumination 2 *min* after fluorescein instillation into the tear film. The density of the corneal fluorescein staining was assessed in each of 4 quadrants on the cornea (temporal, nasal, superior, and inferior) using a standardized 4-point scale. Here, 0 = none, 1 = mild, 2 = moderate, and 3 = severe. So, the staining scores could range from 0 to 12.

3.14 Ion Permeability

3.14.1 *Ionoflux Technique*

The ionoflux technique is a preferred method for determining the ion permeability of a lens (6). This technique may be used to determine the likelihood of adequate on-eye movement.

The ionoflux technique involves the use of a conductometer (LF 2000/C, catalog no. 35 300105, Wissenschaftlich-Technische Werkstätten GmbH (WTW), Germany), an electrode equipped with a temperature sensor (LR 01/T, catalog no. 302 520, WTW), a donor chamber containing a salt solution, a receiving chamber containing about 60 *ml* of deionized water, a stir bar and a thermostat.

The donor chamber is specially designed for sealing a contact lens thereto, so that the donor solution does not pass around the lens (i.e., ions may only pass through the lens). The donor chamber is composed of a glass tube which is threaded at the end which is immersed in the receiving solution. The glass tube includes a centrally located hole of about 9 *mm* in diameter. A lid, which is threaded to mate with the glass tube, holds a lens-retaining member which includes a centrally located hole of about 8 *mm* in diameter. The lens-retaining member includes a male portion adapted to mate with and seal the edges of the inner (concave) surface of a lens and a female portion adapted to mate with and seal the edges of the outer (convex) surface of a lens.

The lens to be measured is placed in the lens-retaining member, between the male and female portions. The male and female portions include flexible sealing rings which are positioned between the lens and the respective male or female portion. After positioning the lens in the lens-retaining member, the lens-retaining member is placed in the threaded lid. The lid is screwed onto the glass tube to define the donor chamber. The donor chamber is filled with 16 *ml* of 0.1 *M* NaCl solution. The receiving chamber is filled with 60 *ml* of deionized water. The leads of the conductivity meter are immersed in the deionized water of the receiving chamber and a stir bar is added to the receiving chamber. The receiving chamber is placed in a thermostat and the temperature is held at about 35°C. Finally, the donor chamber is immersed in the receiving chamber.

Measurements of conductivity are taken every 20 *min* for about 3 *h*, starting 10 *min* after immersion of the donor chamber into the receiving chamber. The ionoflux diffusion coefficient, D, is determined by applying Fick's law as follows:

$$D = -\frac{n'}{A \times dc/dx} \tag{3.1}$$

Here, n' is the rate of ion transport ($mol\ min^{-1}$), A is the area of the lens exposed (mm^2), D is ionoflux diffusion coefficient ($mm^2\,min^{-1}$), dc is the concentration difference ($mol\,l^{-1}$), and dx is the thickness of the lens (mm).

An ionoflux diffusion coefficient of greater than about 1.5×10^{-6} $mm^2\,min^{-1}$ is preferred for achieving sufficient on-eye movement. Most preferably, the ionoflux diffusion coefficient is greater than about 6.4×10^{-6} $mm^2\,min^{-1}$. It must be emphasized that the ionoflux diffusion coefficient correlates with ion permeability through the lens, and thereby is a predictor of on-eye movement (6).

3.14.2 *Ionoton Measurement Technique*

The ionoton technique is a preferred method for determining the relative ion permeability of a lens (6). The technique is based on measurement of the diffusion of sodium chloride through a lens.

The ionoton technique involves the use of a pH meter (Beckman, VWR catalog no. BK123142), a VSC-1 diffusion cell drive console (CrownBio, Somerville, NJ), a DCB-100B diffusion cell (CrownBio), and a 6 *cm* sodium ion-specific electrode (Microelectronics, Londonderry, NH, catalog no. MI-414P).

First, a contact lens is mounted onto an orifice of the DCB-100B cell chamber, the donor chamber. Next, the connecting cell chamber (receptor chamber) is placed against the cell chamber containing the contact lens and tightly clamped on the clamp holder supplied with the VSC-1 drive console. Then, a phosphate-buffered saline (PBS, MediaTech catalog no. 21-031-LV) is placed into the receptor side of the cell chamber. Stir bars are added to each cell chamber. The 6 *cm* electrode is placed into the PBS saline receptor side. After the electrode has equilibrated in the PBS saline, the pH meter is placed in the mV function to establish the 0 mV point. PBS which has been saturated with sodium chloride is added to the donor chamber.

The millivolt signal is recorded at 5, 10, 15, 30, 60, 120, and 180 *min* intervals. The millivolt signal is converted to a sodium ion concentration by a standard curve of sodium ion concentration vs. millivolt signal. The ionoton ion permeability coefficient, P, is then determined in accordance with the following equation:

$$\ln \frac{1 - 2C(t)}{C(0)} = \frac{2APt}{Vd} \tag{3.2}$$

Here, $C(t)$ is the concentration of sodium ions at time t in the receiving cell, $C(0)$ is initial concentration of sodium ions in donor cell, A is membrane area, i.e., lens area exposed to cells, V is volume of cell compartment (3.0 *ml*), d is average lens thickness in the area exposed, and P is permeability coefficient.

The average thickness of the lens in the exposed test area may be determined by averaging a number of readings, e.g., 10 readings, with a low-pressure thickness-measuring instrument, such as a Mitutoyo VL-50 micrometer, or equivalents thereof.

An ionoton ion permeability coefficient, P, greater than 0.4×10^{-6} $cm^2 sec^{-1}$ is most preferred. It must be emphasized that the ionoton ion permeability coefficient correlates with the ion permeability through the lens, and thereby is a predictor of on-eye movement (6).

3.15 Hydrodell Water Permeability Technique

The Hydrodell technique can be used for determining the water permeability of a lens (6). This technique may be used to determine the likelihood of adequate on-eye movement.

The Hydrodell technique involves the measurement of the rate of transfer of the radiolabeled solutes THO (3H-HO or tritiated water) and ^{14}C-glucose across the contact lens using a two-chamber apparatus. ^{14}C-Glucose is used in this measurement technique to reveal any leak in the system during testing.

The lens is mounted between chambers, which are stirred at a controllable rate. Chamber I contains a solution with a high concentration of labeled solute. Chamber II, the receiving chamber, contains an identical solution but without the labeled solute. Samples of the solution in Chambers I and II are taken at intervals over the test period. The radioactivity in the samples is measured. The permeability of the lens is calculated from the measured radioactivity, the sample times, the chamber volumes and the lens area exposed to the solutions (6).

3.16 Oxygen Permeability and Transmissibility

The oxygen permeability is the rate at which oxygen will pass through a material (6). The oxygen permeability is conventionally expressed in units of barrers. The oxygen permeability of a lens and oxygen transmissibility of a lens material may be determined by the following technique:

Oxygen fluxes (J) are measured at 34°C in a wet cell (i.e., gas streams are maintained at about 100% relative humidity) using a Dk1000 instrument (available from Applied Design and Development Co., Norcross, Ga.) or a similar analytical instrument. An air stream, having a known percentage of oxygen (e.g., 21%), is passed across one side of the lens at a rate of about 10 $cm^3\ min^{-1}$ to 20 $cm^3\ min^{-1}$, while a nitrogen stream is passed on the opposite side of the lens at a rate of about 10 $cm^3\ min^{-1}$ to 20 $cm^3\ min^{-1}$. The barometric pressure surrounding the system, P, is measured. The thickness (t) of the lens in the area being exposed for testing is determined by measuring about 10 locations with a Mitotoya VL-50 micrometer, or similar instrument, and averaging the measurements. The oxygen concentration in the nitrogen stream (i.e., oxygen which diffuses through the lens) is measured using the Dk1000 instrument. The oxygen permeability of the lens material, D_k, is determined from the following formula (6):

$$D_k = \frac{Jt}{P_{oxygen}} \tag{3.3}$$

Here, J is the oxygen flux $\mu lcm^{-2}min^{-1}$, P_{oxygen} is the partial pressure of oxygen in the air stream, t is the average thickness of the lens over the exposed test area in mm, and D_k is expressed in units of barrers.

The oxygen transmissibility (D_k/t) of the material may be calculated by dividing the oxygen permeability (D_k) by the average thickness (t) of the lens (6).

3.16.1 Contact Lens Solutions

Chitosan (CS) is a nontoxic biopolymer with a weak antimicrobial activity. However, the use of CS to preserve pharmaceutical compositions has been hampered by its insolubility at pH above 6 (106).

The water solubility at near neutral pH can be improved by derivatization with hydrophilic functional groups, such as carboxymethyl or glycol substituents, or by selective *N*-acetylation.

The acetylation can be done in aqueous acidic solution by the reaction with an acetylating agent in the presence of a phase transfer reagent. Phase transfer reagents include quaternary ammonium salts, quaternary phosphonium salts, crown ethers, and pyridinium salts. Several procedures of the preparation have been described in detail (106).

The CS derivatives with borate or phosphate buffers have higher antimicrobial activity in comparison to citrate, tris buffers, and in water. Surfactant additives may help in the cleaning of the lenses. PEO polymers are suitable surfactants.

A series of compositions based on glycol CS have been prepared and tested with respect to their antimicrobial activity, biocompatibility, and other required properties (106).

3.17 Optical Biometer

3.17.1 Ophthalmologic Apparatus

A lot of ophthalmologic apparatus engines have been described in the recent patent literature (107–116).

In the conventional ophthalmologic apparatus, when the eye to be examined is examined, the focal aim of the light radiated to the eye to be examined is adjusted to match the axis of vision of the eye (112). However, a normal direction of the crystalline lens typically shifts from the axis of vision of the eye to be examined.

For this reason, even when the focal aim of the light radiated to the eye is adjusted so as to match the axis of vision thereof, the light is radiated obliquely to the crystalline lens and light scattering occurs on the surface of the crystalline lens. As a result, in some patients, the light with a sufficient intensity is not reflected from the crystalline lens, and the position of the crystalline lens cannot be determined with good accuracy.

So, an ophthalmologic apparatus for examining an interior, for example, crystalline lens and retina of an eye, has been developed (112). The ophthalmologic apparatus of this type is an optical measurement system that radiates light from a light source to inside the eye to be examined and guides the reflected light therefrom, and an optical reference system that radiates light from the light source to a reference surface and guides the reflected light therefrom.

A position of a measuring portion (for example, the crystalline lens and retina) inside the eye to be examined is determined from the interfering light between the reflected light guided by the optical measurement system and the reflected light guided by the optical reference system. The ophthalmologic apparatus includes (112):

1. A light source,
2. An optical measurement system that radiates light from the light source to inside an eye to be examined and guides reflected light from the eye,
3. An optical reference system that radiates light from the light source to a reference surface and guides reflected light from the reference surface,
4. A photodetector that detects interfering light between the reflected light from the optical measurement system and the reflected light from the optical reference system, and
5. A processor that determines a position of a measuring portion inside the eye based on the interfering light detected by the photodetector.

A schematic view of the system is shown in Figure 3.8.

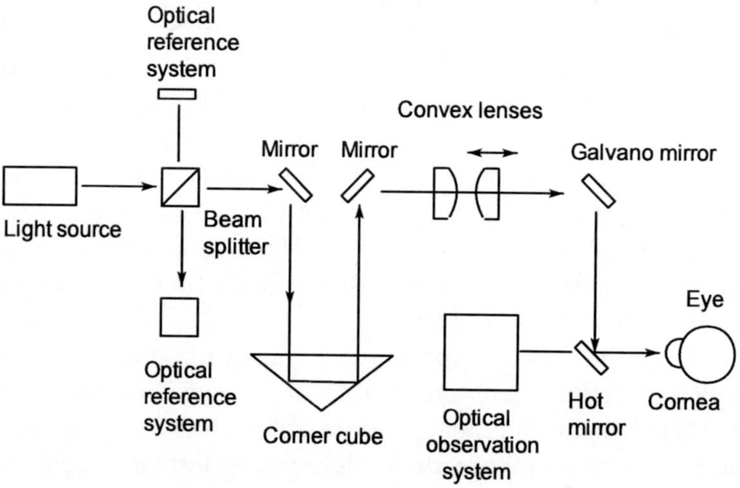

Figure 3.8 Optical measurement system (112).

The optical measurement system has an incident angle changing member that changes an incident angle of the light radiated to the eye within a predetermined angular range relative to an axis of vision of the eye (112).

The ophthalmologic apparatus contains a measurement unit for examining an eye.

The measurement unit contains an optical interference system that causes an interference of a reflected light that is reflected from the eye and a reference light, an optical observation system that observes an anterior part of the eye, and an optical alignment system for aligning the measurement unit with respect to the eye in a predetermined positional relationship.

The optical system is configured by a light source, an optical measurement system that radiates light from the light source to inside the eye and guides reflected light thereof, an optical reference system that radiates light from the light source to a reference surface and guides the reflected light thereof, and a photodetector that detects interfering light between the reflected light guided by the optical measurement system and the reflected light guided by the optical reference system.

The light source is of a wavelength sweep type, and a wavelength of the emitted light changes with a predetermined period. Where the wavelength of the light emitted from the light source changes, the reflection position of the reflected light that causes interference with the reference light changes correspondingly to the wavelength of the emitted light. This change in the reflection position takes place in the depth direction of the eye.

Therefore, the position of each portion, i.e., the crystalline lens and retina, inside the eye can be determined by measuring the interfering light, while changing the wavelength of the emitted light.

The optical measurement system is constituted by a beam splitter, a mirror, a 0 point adjustment mechanism, a mirror, a focal point adjustment mechanism, an incident angle adjustment mechanism, and a hot mirror. The light emitted from the light source irradiates the eye via the beam splitter, mirror, 0 point adjustment mechanism, mirror, focal point adjustment mechanism, incident angle adjustment mechanism, and hot mirror. The reflected light from the eye is guided to the photodetector via the hot mirror, incident angle adjustment mechanism, focal point adjustment mechanism, mirror, 0 point adjustment mechanism, mirror, and beam splitter.

The optical reference system is constituted by the beam splitter and a reference mirror. Part of the light emitted from the light source is reflected by the beam splitter, radiated to the reference mirror, and reflected by the reference mirror. The light reflected by the reference mirror is guided to the photodetector via the beam splitter. The reference mirror, beam splitter, and photodetector are disposed inside an interferometer, and the positions thereof are fixed. Therefore, in this ophthalmologic apparatus the reference optical path length of the optical reference system is constant and does not change.

The photodetector detects the interfering light between the light guided by the optical reference system and the light guided by the optical measurement system. For example, a photodiode can be used as the photodetector.

The incident angle adjustment mechanism 46 is provided with a galvano mirror and a fourth driver that drives the galvano mirror. The galvano mirror is disposed on the focal aim and can be tilted within a predetermined angular range with respect to the focal aim. Where the fourth driver moves the galvano mirror within the predetermined angular range, the incident position and incident angle of the light radiated to the eye change. Thus, the incident position and incident angle of the light on the cornea change according to the displacement angle of the galvano mirror (112).

The tilting direction of the galvano mirror is set so that the incident position of the light radiated to the eye changes in the transverse direction (i.e., direction connecting the left and right eyes). Therefore, the occurrence of the event in which the eye is not irradiated with the light from the light source because of eyelids or eyelashes is prevented.

The ophthalmologic apparatus is controlled by a processor. The processor may be part of a microcomputer.

The light source, the drivers, and the optical observation system are connected with the processor. The processor performs ON/OFF control of the light source and controls the drivers. The processor also controls the optical observation system and displays the anterior eye part image picked up by the optical observation system on the monitor. The photodetector is also connected with the processor, and the interference signal corresponding to the intensity of the interfering light detected by the photodetector is introduced to the processor (112).

3.17.2 *Ophthalmologic Information Processing*

In conventional techniques, for a plurality of eyes having various axial lengths, it is necessary to calculate in advance the correction amount of the scanning angle corresponding to all the pixels in the scannable range of the scanning means (117). Therefore, when the angle of view is large, it is difficult to accurately correct the distortion of the tomographic image for each subject's eyes having various eyeball optical systems.

An ophthalmologic information processing apparatus has been described that consists of (117):

1. An image forming unit configured to form a tomographic image of a subject's eye based on data acquired using optical coherence tomography; the optical coherence tomography uses an optical scanner disposed at an optically substantially conjugate position with a first site of the subject's eye,
2. An intraocular distance calculator configured to obtain an intraocular distance between predetermined sites of the subject's eye based on the data, and
3. An image correcting unit configured to correct the tomographic image formed by the image forming unit, based on the intraocular distance obtained by the intraocular distance calculator.

3.17.3 *Swept-Source Optical Coherence Tomography*

A method and apparatus for a swept source optical coherence tomography system has been developed (107).

The system uses a fast scanning mechanism in the sample arm and a slowly swept light source. The position data are collected rapidly while the wavelength of the source is swept slowly.

The system reduces the sweep speed requirements of the light source enabling higher power, greater imaging range, and linear sweeps of the source frequency. The optical coherence tomography components (or most of them) may be implemented within a handheld imaging probe. In operation, a triangulation scan may be used to orient the imaging probe with respect to a fixed coordinate system; preferably, optical coherence tomography data captured by the device is then transformed to that same orientation with respect to the fixed coordinate system to improve the scanning results (107).

A schematic view of the system is shown in Figure 3.9.

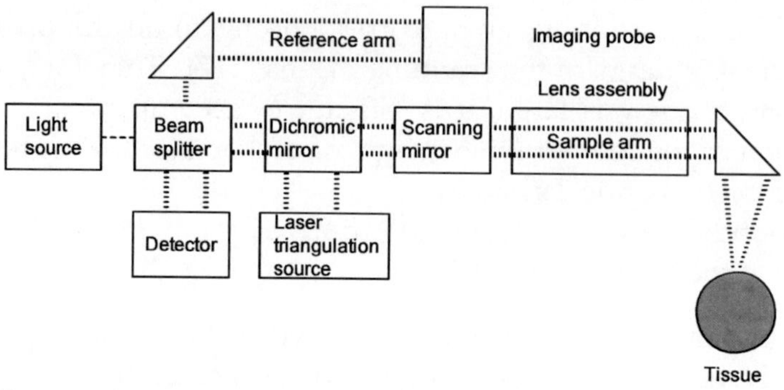

Figure 3.9 Swept source optical coherence tomography system (107).

A handheld imaging probe is connectable to an optical coherence tomography light source through an optical fiber, and the imaging probe is used to capture the optical coherence tomography data. In this approach, preferably the sample, reference, and detection arms of the optical coherence tomography interferometer are incorporated into the imaging probe using free space optics. Preferably, a triangulation scan is used to orient the imaging probe device with respect to a fixed coordinate system, and the optical coherence tomography data collected by that device are transformed to that same orientation with respect to the fixed coordinate system (107).

References

1. J.S. Wolffsohn, The visual experience with contact lens wear, *Contact Lens Spectrum*, Vol. 35, p. 29, November 2020.
2. D. Troilo, E.L. Smith III, D.L. Nickla, R. Ashby, A.V. Tkatchenko, L.A. Ostrin, T.J. Gawne, M.T. Pardue, J.A. Summers, C.-s. Kee, F. Schroedl, S. Wahl, and L. Jones, IMI — Report on Experimental Models of Emmetropization and Myopia, *Investigative Ophthalmology & Visual Science*, Vol. 60, p. M31, 02 2019.

3. V. Naël, K. Pérès, I. Carrière, V. Daien, A.-C. Scherlen, A. Arleo, J.-F. Korobelnik, C. Delcourt, and C. Helmer, Visual Impairment, Undercorrected Refractive Errors, and Activity Limitations in Older Adults: Findings from the Three-City Alienor Study, *Investigative Ophthalmology & Visual Science*, Vol. 58, p. 2359, 04 2017.
4. M.K. Margolis, K. Coyne, T. Kennedy-Martin, T. Baker, O. Schein, and D.A. Revicki, Vision-specific instruments for the assessment of health-related quality of life and visual functioning, *PharmacoEconomics*, Vol. 20, p. 791, 2002.
5. O.A. Hunt, J.S. Wolffsohn, and C. García-Resúa, Ocular motor triad with single vision contact lenses compared to spectacle lenses, *Contact Lens and Anterior Eye*, Vol. 29, p. 239, 2006.
6. P.C. Nicolson, R.C. Baron, P. Chabrecek, J. Court, A. Domschke, H.J. Griesser, A. Ho, J. Hopken, B.G. Laycock, Q. Liu, D. Lohmann, G.F. Meijs, E. Papaspiliotopoulos, J.S. Riffle, K. Schindhelm, D. Sweeney, W.L. Terry, Jr., J. Vogt, and L.C. Winterton, Extended wear ophthalmic lens, US Patent 6 951 894, assigned to Ciba Vision Corporation (Duluth, GA), October 4, 2005.
7. ISO Standards concerning Contact Lenses, ISO Standards, International Organization for Standardization, Geneva, Switzerland, 2020. https://www.iso.org/search.html?q=contact%20lens&hPP=10&idx=all_en&p=0.
8. Standard test method for tensile properties of plastics by use of microtensile specimens, ASTM Standard D1708-18, ASTM International, West Conshohocken, PA, 2018. https://www.astm.org/Standards/D1708.htm.
9. Standard test method for tear-propagation resistance (trouser tear) of plastic film and thin sheeting by a single-tear method, ASTM Standard D1938-19, ASTM International, West Conshohocken, PA, 2019. https://www.astm.org/Standards/D1938.htm.
10. Standard guide for choosing a method for determining the index of refraction and dispersion of glass, ASTM Standard C1648-12, ASTM International, West Conshohocken, PA, 2018. https://www.astm.org/Standards/C1648.htm.
11. Standard specification for eye protectors for selected sports, ASTM Standard F803-19, ASTM International, West Conshohocken, PA, 2019. https://www.astm.org/Standards/F803.htm.
12. Standard specification for ski and snowboard goggles, ASTM Standard F659-10, ASTM International, West Conshohocken, PA, 2018. https://www.astm.org/Standards/F659.htm.
13. Standard specification for eye protective devices for airsoft sports, ASTM Standard F2879-19, ASTM International, West Conshohocken, PA, 2019. https://www.astm.org/Standards/F2879.htm.

14. Standard specification for eye protective devices for paintball sports, ASTM Standard F1776-19, ASTM International, West Conshohocken, PA, 2019. https://www.astm.org/Standards/F1776.htm.
15. Standard test method for oxygen gas transmission rate through plastic film and sheeting using a coulometric sensor, ASTM Standard D3985-17, ASTM International, West Conshohocken, PA, 2017. https://www.astm.org/Standards/D3985.htm.
16. Standard practice for assessment of compatibility of biomaterials for surgical implants with respect to effect of materials on muscle and insertion into bone, ASTM Standard F981-04, ASTM International, West Conshohocken, PA, 2016. https://www.astm.org/Standards/F981.htm.
17. Ophthalmic optics — Contact lenses and contact lens care products — Labelling, ISO Standard 11978, International Organization for Standardization, Geneva, Switzerland, 2017. https://www.iso.org/standard/72603.html.
18. Air quality — Particle size fraction definitions for health-related sampling, ISO Standard 7708, International Organization for Standardization, Geneva, Switzerland, 1995. https://www.iso.org/standard/14534.html.
19. Contact lenses — Determination of back vertex power — Part 1: Method using focimeter with manual focusing, ISO Standard 9337-1, International Organization for Standardization, Geneva, Switzerland, 1999. https://www.iso.org/standard/17021.html.
20. Ophthalmic optics — Contact lens care products — Method for evaluating Acanthamoeba encystment by contact lens care products, ISO Standard 19045, International Organization for Standardization, Geneva, Switzerland, 2015. https://www.iso.org/contents/data/standard/06/38/63807.html.
21. Ophthalmic optics — Contact lens care products — Microbiological requirements and test methods for products and regimens for hygienic management of contact lenses, ISO Standard 14729, International Organization for Standardization, Geneva, Switzerland, 2001. https://www.iso.org/standard/25382.html.
22. Ophthalmic optics — Contact lens care products — Antimicrobial preservative efficacy testing and guidance on determining discard date, ISO Standard 14730, International Organization for Standardization, Geneva, Switzerland, 2014. https://www.iso.org/contents/data/standard/06/51/65165.html.
23. Ophthalmic optics — Contact lens care products — Method to assess contact lens care products with contact lenses in a lens case, challenged with bacterial and fungal organisms, ISO Standard 18259, International Organization for Standardization, Geneva,

Switzerland, 2014. https://www.iso.org/contents/data/standard/06/19/61901.html.

24. C.-M. Phan, H. Walther, H. Qiao, R. Shinde, and L. Jones, Development of an eye model with a physiological blink mechanism, *Translational Vision Science & Technology*, Vol. 8, p. 1, 09 2019.
25. D. Fonn and K. Dumbleton, Dryness and discomfort with silicone hydrogel contact lenses, *Eye & Contact Lens*, Vol. 29, p. S101, 2003.
26. L. Jones, M. Senchyna, M.-A. Glasier, J. Schickler, I. Forbes, D. Louie, and C. May, Lysozyme and lipid deposition on silicone hydrogel contact lens materials, *Eye & Contact Lens*, Vol. 29, p. S75, 2003.
27. H. Lorentz and L. Jones, Lipid deposition on hydrogel contact lenses: How history can help us today, *Optometry and Vision Science*, Vol. 84, p. 286, 2007.
28. H. Lorentz, M. Heynen, D. Trieu, S.J. Hagedorn, and L. Jones, The impact of tear film components on in vitro lipid uptake, *Optometry and Vision Science*, Vol. 89, p. 856, 2012.
29. N. Keir and L. Jones, Wettability and silicone hydrogel lenses: A review, *Eye & Contact Lens*, Vol. 39, p. 100, 2013.
30. H. Walther, L.N. Subbaraman, and L. Jones, Novel in vitro method to determine pre-lens tear break-up time of hydrogel and silicone hydrogel contact lenses, *Contact Lens and Anterior Eye*, Vol. 42, p. 178, 2019.
31. H. Lorentz, M. Heynen, L.M.M. Kay, C.Y. Dominici, W. Khan, W.W.S. Ng, and L. Jones, Contact lens physical properties and lipid deposition in a novel characterized artificial tear solution, *Molecular Vision*, Vol. 17, p. 3392, 2011.
32. H. Lorentz, M. Heynen, W. Khan, D. Trieu, and L. Jones, The impact of intermittent air exposure on lipid deposition, *Optometry and Vision Science*, Vol. 89, p. 1574, 2012.
33. A. Ng, M. Heynen, D. Luensmann, and L. Jones, Impact of tear film components on lysozyme deposition to contact lenses, *Optometry and Vision Science*, Vol. 89, p. 392, 2012.
34. H. Walther, H. Lorentz, M. Heynen, L. Kay, and L.W. Jones, Factors that influence in vitro cholesterol deposition on contact lenses, *Optometry and Vision Science*, Vol. 90, p. 1057, 2013.
35. H. Walther, L. Subbaraman, and L.W. Jones, In vitro cholesterol deposition on daily disposable contact lens materials, *Optometry and Vision Science*, Vol. 93, p. 36, 2016.
36. J.S. Vaughan and D.A. Porter, A new in vitro method for assessing the potential toxicity of soft contact lens care solutions, *The CLAO Journal: Official publication of the Contact Lens Association of Ophthalmologists, Inc*, Vol. 19, p. 54, 1993.

37. Wikipedia contributors, Draize test — Wikipedia, the free encyclopedia, https://en.wikipedia.org/w/index.php?title=Draize_test&oldid=950709774, 2020. [Online; accessed 26-May-2020].
38. K.R. Wilhelmus, The Draize eye test, *Survey of Ophthalmology*, Vol. 45, p. 493, 2001.
39. OECD, Acute eye irritation/corrosion, OECD Test 405, OECD, Paris, 2017.
40. EU Reference Laboratory, Analysis of quaternary ammonium compounds (QACs) in fruits and vegetables using QuEChERS and LC-MS/MS, EURL-SRM SRM-08, Reference Laboratory for Single Residue Methods, Fellbach, Germany, 2012.
41. J. Ahn and M. Choi, Binding affinity of benzalkonium chloride on contact lens surfaces and the effects on their physical properties, *Colloids and Surfaces B: Biointerfaces*, Vol. 203, p. 111744, 2021.
42. Z. Kantarci, S. Aksoy, and N. Hasirci, Estimation of monomer content in polymethyl methacrylate contact lens materials by raman spectroscopy, *The International Journal of Artificial Organs*, Vol. 20, p. 407, 1997.
43. L. Jones, A. Hui, C.-M. Phan, M.L. Read, D. Azar, J. Buch, J.B. Ciolino, S.A. Naroo, B. Pall, K. Romond, P. Sankaridurg, C.M. Schnider, L. Terry, and M. Willcox, CLEAR - contact lens technologies of the future, *Contact Lens and Anterior Eye*, Vol. 44, p. 398, 2021.
44. M. Willcox, N. Keir, V. Maseedupally, S. Masoudi, A. McDermott, R. Mobeen, C. Purslow, J. Santodomingo-Rubido, S. Tavazzi, F. Zeri, and L. Jones, CLEAR - contact lens wettability, cleaning, disinfection and interactions with tears, *Contact Lens and Anterior Eye*, Vol. 44, p. 157, 2021.
45. Z. Dou, J. Tang, Z. Liu, Q. Sun, Y. Wang, Y. Li, M. Yuan, H. Wu, Y. Wang, W. Pei, and H. Chen, Wearable contact lens sensor for non-invasive continuous monitoring of intraocular pressure, *Micromachines*, Vol. 12, 2021.
46. Z. Liu, G. Wang, C. Ye, H. Sun, W. Pei, C. Wei, W. Dai, Z. Dou, Q. Sun, C.-T. Lin, Y. Wang, H. Chen, and G. Shen, An ultrasensitive contact lens sensor based on self-assembly graphene for continuous intraocular pressure monitoring, *Advanced Functional Materials*, Vol. n/a, p. 2010991, 2021.
47. J. Kim, J. Park, Y.-G. Park, E. Cha, M. Ku, H.S. An, K.-P. Lee, M.-I. Huh, J. Kim, T.-S. Kim, D.W. Kim, H.K. Kim, and J.-U. Park, A soft and transparent contact lens for the wireless quantitative monitoring of intraocular pressure, *Nature Biomedical Engineering*, Vol. 5, p. 772, 2021.
48. I. Karunaratne, C.H.C. Lee, P.W. Or, Y. Wei, I.T. Chong, Y. Yang, M. Yu, and D. Lam, Wearable dual-element intraocular pressure contact lens sensor, *Sensors and Actuators A: Physical*, Vol. 321, p. 112580, 2021.

49. K. Gillmann, R. Wasilewicz, K. Hoskens, S. Simon-Zoula, and K. Mansouri, Continuous 24-hour measurement of intraocular pressure in millimeters of mercury (mmHg) using a novel contact lens sensor: Comparison with pneumatonometry, *PloS one*, Vol. 16, p. e0248211, 2021.
50. D.G. Altman and J.M. Bland, Measurement in medicine: The analysis of method comparison studies, Vol. 32, p. 307, 1983.
51. J.M. Bland and D.G. Altman, Measuring agreement in method comparison studies, *Statistical Methods in Medical Research*, Vol. 8, p. 135, 1999.
52. Wikipedia contributors, Bland-Altman plot — Wikipedia, the free encyclopedia, https://en.wikipedia.org/w/index.php?title=Bland%E2%80%93Altman_plot&oldid=1021311044, 2021. [Online; accessed 29-May-2021].
53. I.E. Araci, S. Agaoglu, M. Baday, and P. Diep, Closed microfluidic network for strain sensing embedded in a contact lens to monitor intraocular pressure, US Patent 10 898 074, assigned to Smartlens Inc., January 26, 2021.
54. Y. Chang, Y. Zheng, J. Ge, S.Y. Zhang, K.B. Sentell, and J. Dou, Method for determining coating thickness on coated contact lenses, US Patent Application 20 210 131 923, assigned to Alcon Inc., May 06, 2021.
55. F.-P. Tsao, Compositions and methods for cleaning contact lenses, US Patent 7 022 654, assigned to Novartis AG, April 04, 2006.
56. F.-P. Tsao and M.A. Sills, Stabilized hydrogen peroxide contact lens disinfecting solution, US Patent 4 812 173, assigned to Novartis Corp, March 14, 1989.
57. F. Tsao, Method of disinfecting a soft contact lens with a diethylene triamine penta(methylenephosphonic acid) stabilized hydrogen peroxide solution, US Patent 4 889 689, assigned to Novartis Corp., December 26, 1989.
58. J.Z. Krezanoski and R.D. Houlsby, A comparison of new hydrogen peroxide disinfection systems, *Journal of the American Optometric Association*, Vol. 59, p. 193, 1988.
59. L.C. Winterton and K.C. Su, Hydrogen peroxide disinfection solutions, US Patent 5 523 012, assigned to Novartis Corp., June 04, 1996.
60. J. Holloway, Contact lens solution, EP Patent 0 855 188, assigned to Waverley Pharmaceutical Ltd, November 25, 1998.
61. J.Y. Park, L.K. Thomas, L. Peng, and D.P. Cafaro, Compositions and methods for disinfecting and cleaning contact lenses, US Patent 5 746 972, assigned to Allergan Inc., May 05, 1998.
62. J. Ross and G.D. Miles, Method and apparatus for foam determination, US Patent 2 315 983, assigned to Colgato Palmolive Peet Co., April 06, 1943.

63. P. Alexandridis and T.A. Hatton, Poly(ethylene oxide)-poly(propylene oxide)-poly(ethylene oxide) block copolymer surfactants in aqueous solutions and at interfaces: Thermodynamics, structure, dynamics, and modeling, *Colloids and Surfaces A: Physicochemical and Engineering Aspects*, Vol. 96, p. 1, 1995.
64. S. Dürr and J.C. Thomason, *Biofouling*, Wiley, 2009.
65. M. Guillon, K.A. Dumbleton, P. Theodoratos, S. Wong, K. Patel, G. Banks, and T. Patel, Association between contact lens discomfort and pre-lens tear film kinetics, *Optometry and Vision Science*, Vol. 93, p. 881, 2016.
66. M. Vidal-Rohr, J.S. Wolffsohn, L.N. Davies, and A. Cerviño, Effect of contact lens surface properties on comfort, tear stability and ocular physiology, *Contact Lens and Anterior Eye*, Vol. 41, p. 117, 2018.
67. B. Samuel, H. Zhao, and K.-Y. Law, Study of wetting and adhesion interactions between water and various polymer and superhydrophobic surfaces, *The Journal of Physical Chemistry C*, Vol. 115, p. 14852, 2011.
68. S. Wong, A review of contact angle technique, *Contact Lens Update Clinical Insights Based in Current Research*, 2017.
69. L. Cheng, S.J. Muller, and C.J. Radke, Wettability of silicone-hydrogel contact lenses in the presence of tear-film components, *Current Eye Research*, Vol. 28, p. 93, 2004.
70. Y. Yu, R. Macoon, and A. Chauhan, Improving wettability and lubricity of commercial contact lenses by polymerizing a thin film of dimethylacryamide, *Colloids and Surfaces A: Physicochemical and Engineering Aspects*, Vol. 583, p. 123974, 2019.
71. E. Lum, I. Perera, and A. Ho, Osmolality and buffering agents in soft contact lens packaging solutions, *Contact Lens and Anterior Eye*, Vol. 27, p. 21, 2004.
72. K.L. Menzies, *In Vitro Analysis of Wettability and Physical Properties of Blister Pack Solutions of Hydrogel Contact Lenses*, University of Waterloo, 2010.
73. K.L. Menzies, R. Rogers, and L. Jones, In vitro contact angle analysis and physical properties of blister pack solutions of daily disposable contact lenses, *Eye & Contact Lens*, Vol. 36, p. 10, 2010.
74. Wikipedia contributors, Sessile drop technique — Wikipedia, the free encyclopedia, https://en.wikipedia.org/w/index.php?title=Sessile_drop_technique&oldid=966871708, 2020. [Online; accessed 29-November-2020].
75. L. Wilhelmy, Ueber die Abhängigkeit der Capillaritäts-Constanten des Alkohols von Substanz und Gestalt des benetzten festen Körpers, *Annalen der Physik*, Vol. 195, p. 177, 1863.

76. Wikipedia contributors, Wilhelmy plate — Wikipedia, the free encyclopedia, https://en.wikipedia.org/w/index.php?title=Wilhelmy_plate&oldid=989575010, 2020. [Online; accessed 29-November-2020].
77. Wikipedia contributors, Molality — Wikipedia, the free encyclopedia, https://en.wikipedia.org/w/index.php?title=Molality&oldid=1024920264, 2021. [Online; accessed 27-May-2021].
78. A. Marmur, Contact-angle hysteresis on heterogeneous smooth surfaces: Theoretical comparison of the captive bubble and drop methods, *Colloids and Surfaces A: Physicochemical and Engineering Aspects*, Vol. 136, p. 209, 1998.
79. Wikipedia contributors, Captive bubble method — Wikipedia, the free encyclopedia, https://en.wikipedia.org/w/index.php?title=Captive_bubble_method&oldid=958689737, 2020. [Online; accessed 25-May-2020].
80. Y. Baek, J. Kang, P. Theato, and J. Yoon, Measuring hydrophilicity of RO membranes by contact angles via sessile drop and captive bubble method: A comparative study, *Desalination*, Vol. 303, p. 23, 2012.
81. X. Deng, M. Korogiannaki, B. Rastegari, J. Zhang, M. Chen, Q. Fu, H. Sheardown, C.D.M. Filipe, and T. Hoare, Click chemistry-tethered hyaluronic acid-based contact lens coatings improve lens wettability and lower protein adsorption, *ACS Applied Materials & Interfaces*, Vol. 8, p. 22064, 2016.
82. M. Korogiannaki, J. Zhang, and H. Sheardown, Surface modification of model hydrogel contact lenses with hyaluronic acid via thiol-ene click chemistry for enhancing surface characteristics, *Journal of Biomaterials Applications*, Vol. 32, p. 446, 2017.
83. K. Yamasaki, E. Drolle, H. Nakagawa, R. Hisamura, W. Ngo, and L. Jones, Impact of a low molecular weight hyaluronic acid derivative on contact lens wettability, *Contact Lens and Anterior Eye*, Vol. 44, p. 101334, 2021.
84. H.-W. Chien and C.-J. Kuo, Preparation, material properties and antimicrobial efficacy of silicone hydrogel by modulating silicone and hydrophilic monomer, *Journal of Biomaterials Science, Polymer Edition*, Vol. 30, p. 1050, 2019.
85. S.L. McArthur, K.M. McLean, H.A.W. St. John, and H.J. Griesser, XPS and surface-MALDI-MS characterisation of worn HEMA-based contact lenses, *Biomaterials*, Vol. 22, p. 3295, 2001. Opthalmic Special Issue.
86. S.H. Kim, A. Opdahl, C. Marmo, and G.A. Somorjai, AFM and SFG studies of pHEMA-based hydrogel contact lens surfaces in saline solution: Adhesion, friction, and the presence of non-crosslinked polymer chains at the surface, *Biomaterials*, Vol. 23, p. 1657, 2002.

87. A. López-Alemany, V. Compañ, and M.F. Refojo, Porous structure of PureVision™ versus Focus® Night&Day™ and conventional hydrogel contact lenses, *Journal of Biomedical Materials Research*, Vol. 63, p. 319, 2002.
88. C. Maldonado-Codina, P.B. Morgan, N. Efron, and J.-C. Canry, Characterization of the surface of conventional hydrogel and silicone hydrogel contact lenses by time-of-flight secondary ion mass spectrometry, *Optometry and Vision Science*, Vol. 81, 2004.
89. Wikipedia contributors, X-ray photoelectron spectroscopy — Wikipedia, the free encyclopedia, https://en.wikipedia.org/w/index.php?title=X-ray_photoelectron_spectroscopy&oldid=950986388, 2020. [Online; accessed 25-May-2020].
90. P. van der Heide, *X-ray Photoelectron Spectroscopy: An Introduction to Principles and Practices*, Wiley, 2011.
91. J.M. González-Méijome, A. López-Alemany, J.B. Almeida, M.A. Parafita, and M.F. Refojo, Microscopic observation of unworn siloxane-hydrogel soft contact lenses by atomic force microscopy, *Journal of Biomedical Materials Research Part B: Applied Biomaterials*, Vol. 76B, p. 412, 2006.
92. C.M. Weikart, M. Miyama, and H.K. Yasuda, Surface modification of conventional polymers by depositing plasma polymers of trimethylsilane and of trimethylsilane + o2: I. static wetting properties, *Journal of Colloid and Interface Science*, Vol. 211, p. 18, 1999.
93. C.M. Weikart, M. Miyama, and H.K. Yasuda, Surface modification of conventional polymers by depositing plasma polymers of trimethylsilane and of trimethylsilane + o2: Ii. dynamic wetting properties, *Journal of Colloid and Interface Science*, Vol. 211, p. 28, 1999.
94. C.M. Weikart, Y. Matsuzawa, L. Winterton, and H.K. Yasuda, Evaluation of plasma polymer-coated contact lenses by electrochemical impedance spectroscopy, *Journal of Biomedical Materials Research*, Vol. 54, p. 597, 2001.
95. M. Chen, Q.S. Yu, C.M. Reddy, and H.K. Yasuda, Model study investigating the role of interfacial factors in electrochemical impedance spectroscopy measurements, *Corrosion*, Vol. 56, p. 709, 2000.
96. H. Yasuda, Q. Yu, and M. Chen, Interfacial factors in corrosion protection: an EIS study of model systems, *Progress in Organic Coatings*, Vol. 41, p. 273, 2001. Keystone Special issue.
97. L. Jianguo, G. Gaoping, and Y. Chuanwei, EIS study of corrosion behaviour of organic coating/dacromet composite systems, *Electrochimica Acta*, Vol. 50, p. 3320, 2005.
98. Wikipedia contributors, Scanning electron microscope — Wikipedia, the free encyclopedia, https://en.wikipedia.org/w/index.php?title=Scanning_electron_microscope&oldid=956693769, 2020. [Online; accessed 25-May-2020].

99. Wikipedia contributors, Everhart-Thornley detector — Wikipedia, the free encyclopedia, https://en.wikipedia.org/w/index.php?title=Everhart-Thornley_detector&oldid=933653368, 2020. [Online; accessed 25-May-2020].
100. T.E. Everhart and R.F.M. Thornley, Wide-band detector for micro-microampere low-energy electron currents, *Journal of Scientific Instruments*, Vol. 37, p. 246, July 1960.
101. O. Schirmer, Studien zur physiologie und pathologie der tränenabsonderung und tränenabfuhr, *Albrecht von Graefes Archiv für Ophthalmologie*, Vol. 56, p. 197, 1903.
102. Wikipedia contributors, Schirmer's test — Wikipedia, the free encyclopedia, https://en.wikipedia.org/w/index.php?title=Schirmer%27s_test&oldid=924587267, 2019. [Online; accessed 4-June-2020].
103. J.A. Nau and J. Ackermann, Douglas Michael, Methods of treating ocular conditions, WO Patent 2 020 014 217, assigned to Oyster Point Pharma, Inc., January 16, 2020.
104. A.A. Afonso, D. Monroy, M.E. Stern, W.J. Feuer, S.C.G. Tseng, and S.C. Pflugfelder, Correlation of tear fluorescein clearance and Schirmer test scores with ocular irritation symptoms, *Ophthalmology*, Vol. 106, p. 803, 1999.
105. A. Macri and S. Pflugfelder, Correlation of the Schirmer 1 and Fluorescein Clearance Tests with the Severity of Corneal Epithelial and Eyelid Disease, *Archives of Ophthalmology*, Vol. 118, p. 1632, 12 2000.
106. W.M. Hung, K.L. Bergbauer, K.C. Su, and G. Wang, Water soluble, randomly substituted partial *N*-, partial *O*-acetylated chitosan, preserving compositions containing chitosan, and processes for making thereof, US Patent 7 683 039, assigned to Adjuvant Pharmaceuticals, LLC (Alpharetta, GA), March 23, 2010.
107. G.T. Bonnema, H.S. Quadling, and M.S. Quadling, Swept source optical coherence tomography (OCT) method and system, US Patent 8 928 888, assigned to D4D Technologies LP, January 06, 2015.
108. H. Ogura, Ophthalmologic apparatus, control method, US Patent 9 314 158, assigned to Canon Inc., April 19, 2016.
109. K. Watanabe, S. Yamaguchi, N. Sekine, and W. Kaku, Ophthalmologic measurement apparatus, method and program of controlling the same, US Patent 9 427 145, assigned to Canon Inc, August 30, 2016.
110. K. Watanabe, H. Matsumoto, and T. Sekine, Ophthalmologic apparatus, US Patent 9 662 007, assigned to Canon Inc., May 30, 2017.
111. H. Okada, T. Kogawa, T. Fujimura, and K. Fujii, Ophthalmologic apparatus, US Patent 9 706 920, assigned to Topcon Corp., July 18, 2017.

112. C. Kato, T. Ohmori, and Y. Nozawa, Ophthalmologic apparatus, US Patent Application 20 180 279 873, assigned to Tomey Corp., October 04, 2018.
113. Z. Wang, Z. Mao, H. Suzuki, K. Oomori, and M. Fujino, Ophthalmologic apparatus, US Patent Application 20 200 337 552, assigned to Topcon Corp., October 29, 2020.
114. M. Kobayashi, Ophthalmologic apparatus, US Patent 10 702 145, assigned to Topcon Corp., July 07, 2020.
115. Y. Fukuma, H. Suzuki, Z. Wang, K. Oomori, and M. Fujino, Ophthalmologic apparatus, US Patent Application 20 200 163 545, assigned to Topcon Corp., May 28, 2020.
116. T. Yamaguchi, M. Nakanishi, and T. Yuasa, Ophthalmologic apparatus, US Patent Application 20 200 138 283, assigned to Topcon Corp., May 07, 2020.
117. T. Yamaguchi, R. Hirose, and M. Nakanishi, Ophthalmologic apparatus, and ophthalmologic information processing apparatus, US Patent Application 20 200 288 966, assigned to Topcon Corp., September 17, 2020.

4

Drug Delivery

Contact lens materials are developing alongside the advances made in related biomaterials for applications such as drug delivery (1–4).

The introductory literature on ocular delivery using contact lenses, their classification and manufacturing process, and the recent advances on drug delivery techniques using such lenses have been described (5).

With the prevalence of electronic devices and an aging population, the number of people affected with eye disease is increasing year by year (6). In spite of the large number of eye drops on the market, most of them do not perform sufficiently, due to rapid clearance mechanisms and ocular barriers. To enhance drug delivery to the eye, a number of novel formulations for ocular diseases have been investigated over recent decades, aiming to increase drug retention and permeation while also allowing for sustained drug release over prolonged periods. The contact lens, initially used to correct visual acuity and beautify female eyes, is one such novel formulation with outstanding potential.

Recently, contact lenses have been extensively used for ocular drug delivery to enhance the ocular bioavailability and reduce side effects, and are particularly suitable for the treatment of chronic diseases, and thus are of interest to ophthalmic scientists. The current state of ocular drug therapy has been reviewed (6).

The issues of therapeutic contact lenses for ocular drug delivery have been reviewed (4, 7).

The *in-vivo* efficacy of different contact lens drug-delivery systems has been reviewed (8). Here, 126 studies were identified following a literature search adhering to the preferred reporting items for systematic reviews and meta-analysis guidelines. After full-text evaluation, 19 studies about contact lens drug-delivery systems were included. The following drug-delivery systems have been investigated *in vivo* (8):

- Drug-soaked contact lenses,
- Contact lenses with physical barriers, e.g.,vitamin E,
- Molecularly imprinted contact lenses,
- Contact lenses with implants, and
- Nanoparticle-loaded contact lenses.

Nanoparticle-loaded contact lenses and contact lenses with implants seem the most promising drug-delivery systems, although initial burst drug release and patient acceptance may limit their widespread use in current practice. Also, clinical trials are warranted to understand the role of contact lenses as a drug-delivery system in improving glaucomatous patient care (8).

4.1 Basic Issues

Eye drop solutions are widely used to treat the anterior segment eye diseases. However, eye drop solutions have many limitations, including low bioavailability, high-dose requirements, and poor patient compliance (9).

Contact lenses can be used to deliver the ocular drugs with high ocular bioavailability due to their immediate location to the cornea. To attend controlled and prolonged drug release from the contact lenses, various systems are explored, including polymeric nanoparticles, molecular imprinting, microemulsion, micelles, liposomes, implantation, supercritical fluids, and use of Vitamin E (9).

A great challenge in using contact lenses for drug delivery is to achieve a prolonged drug release profile within the therapeutic range for various eye-related problems and diseases (10). In general, the desired release kinetics to avoid the initial burst release is the zero-order kinetics within the therapeutic range. New technologies developed to achieve efficient and extended drug delivery have been reviewed. Also, the materials and methods for fabrication of contact lenses and their mechanical and optical properties have been detailed (10).

However, the changes in the critical lens properties like swelling, optical transparency, ion permeability, tensile strength, oxygen permeability, high burst release, issues during monomer extraction, sterilization and storage are still not completely solved (9).

The commercial challenges with different methodologies to develop therapeutic contact lenses for the commercial market have been reviewed. Many animal and clinical studies are in the pipeline and it is likely that therapeutic contact lenses will be commercialized in the next few years (9).

4.2 Methodologies for the Design of Therapeutic Contact Lenses

Several methodologies to design therapeutic contact lenses have been analyzed (7, 11). The basic issues of this analysis is given subsequently.

4.2.1 *Soaking Method*

The soaking method is the most simple, cost-effective and conventional way to load drugs into the contact lenses. This method involves soaking the preformed contact lenses in the drug solution, followed by drug uptake and release in pre- and post-lens tear film.

The so-prepared contact lenses are available as a solid or may have a cavity for receiving the drug solution. Their drug reservoir ability strongly depends on the water content, thickness of lenses, the molecular weight of the drug, soaking time period and concentration of drug in soaking solution.

As an alternative, it is possible to insert contact lenses into the eyes and then apply eye drops. By this means, the drugs can be absorbed and released by the contact lens.

4.2.2 *pH-Sensitive Lenses*

The characteristics of human tears such as pH and composition can vary significantly depending on physical and environmental factors

(12). Contact lenses directly contact with human tears and therefore can swell or de-swell depending on the pH of the solution due to the nature of the hydrogel. For example, when the pH of the solution is low, anionic hydrogels can shrink due to the electric attraction force within the hydrogel network. The opposite phenomenon may appear when the solution is basic.

pH-sensitive hydrogels have developed greatly over the past few years (13). This has been possible due to the synthesis of new hydrogel systems with an increased sensitivity; a sensitivity of up to 10^{-5} pH units has already been established. Recently, pH-sensitive hydrogels have shown to be very useful in biomedical applications. The synthesis of pH-sensitive hydrogels is also quick and cost-effective. The properties of pH-sensitive hydrogels have been reviewed (13). Also, a range of synthesis processes have been reported along with the fabrication of different structures such as microcantilevers and contact lenses.

Contact lenses have been evaluated as drug delivery media (14). The effect of tear physiological pH on the drug release behavior was tested. Anionic or cationic 2-hydroxyethyl methacrylate (HEMA) lenses were polymerized with either *N*-vinyl-2-pyrrolidone (NVP) or *N*-isopropylacrylamide (NIPAAm). The pH of artificial tears was prepared as between 5.8 and 8.35. In one common treatment, hydroxypropyl methylcellulose (HPMC) was used as a test drug for dry eye disease.

As a result, drug releases from an anionic 100% poly(2-hydroxyethyl methacrylate) (PHEMA) and PHEMA-NVP lens were both increased with increasing tear pH. However, released drug amounts from cationic PHEMA-NIPAAm lens were decreased with increasing pH. With a weak basicity of pH 8.03, the PHEMA-NVP (20%) lens swelled, resulting in drugs being released 3.5 times more compared to in weak acidity at a pH of 5.80. On the other hand, the PHEMA-NIPAAm (20 wt%) lens de-swelled in a basic solution, resulting in a decreased drug release as compared to in an acidic solution.

The hydrogel contact lenses showed various physical properties and drug-releasing properties, including diffusion coefficients in response to ionization reactions between ionic groups in the lens and pH of solution. This suggests that a hydrogel contact lens has potential as selective drug delivery media (14).

4.2.3 *Magnetic Micropump*

A thin magnetic micropump has been described that is embedded in a contact lens, which is capable of on-demand one-directional drug delivery (15).

This micropump has great potential to be inserted into a soft or rigid contact lens and fixed with an adhesive, or the simple structure of the micropump can be realized in a rigid contact lens through a photolithography-based master mold.

Such a micropump can be actuated by an external magnetic field whenever needed without the need of a battery.

A micro check valve was integrated with the micropump for one-directional drug delivery from the micropump to the post-lens tear film. With actuation of the external magnetic field, the micro check valve is opened, and on-demand drug release can be realized.

In contrast, without an external magnetic field, the micro check valve is closed, and the undesired drug diffusion can be prevented. Through the control of the strength and the frequency of the magnetic field pulse, on-demand drug release and controlled dose can be realized (15).

The fabrication process of the magnetic micropump runs as follows (15):

1. Fabricating a poly(dimethyl siloxane) (PDMS) master mold using the standard photolithographic method,
2. Casting the main body of the micropump, which is composed of Ostemer 322, using the PDMS master mold, and
3. The total assembly of the magnetic micropump through oxygen plasma treatment.

The apertures on the PDMS membrane and Ostemer layer were punched by using biopsy punches (15).

4.2.4 *Molecular Imprinting*

The use of the molecular imprinting technique is believed to be important progress in this line of work. The spatial arrangement of monomers becomes permanent when the polymerization process is completed. Molecular imprinting is one of the advanced methodologies using hydrogel contact lenses for high drug loading and controlled drug delivery.

The procedure consists of synthesizing the contact lens in the presence of the drug molecules which act as a mold, causing monomers to arrange themselves according to their affinity.

4.2.5 *Colloidal Nanoparticles*

This technique is based on the ability of colloidal nanoparticles to entrap or encapsulate drug and control its release rate from contact lenses. Such a formulated nanoparticulate system (10 to 100 *nm*) is dispersed in HEMA monomers and polymerized using ethylene glycol dimethacrylate (EGDMA) and a photoinitiator to fabricate therapeutic materials.

Drug-laden nanoparticles prevent the interaction of drug with polymerization mixture and also offer additional resistance to drug release. Thus, the nanoparticles-loaded contact lenses can deliver drugs at a controlled rate for an extended period of time. Drug-loaded nanoparticles or globules (microemulsion) also bypass, to some extent, drug metabolism from the enzymes like lysosomes, present in the tear/corneal epithelial surface.

This technique is successful in developing therapeutic contact lenses for extended drug delivery, while at the same time the transparency (optical), oxygen permeability, ion permeability, mechanical properties, and swelling behavior of contact lenses was altered for comfort wear.

4.2.6 *Polymeric Nanoparticles*

A lot of research has been done with regard to polymeric nanoparticles using biodegradable and non-biodegradable polymers to formulate therapeutic contact lenses to treat ocular diseases. These polymeric nanoparticles have been developed to treat glaucoma by dispersing timolol-loaded propoxylated glyceryl triacrylate nanoparticles in contact lenses.

This system showed a sustained release as a result of the incorporation of nanoparticle in the silicone hydrogel contact lenses, which caused reduction in both ion and oxygen permeability, and an increase in storage modulus, suggesting the limitation of the technique.

4.2.7 *Cyclodextrins*

Polymers like cyclodextrins and their derivatives were used to achieve sustained drug delivery of hydrophobic drugs. α-Cyclodextrin is shown in Figure 4.1. Cyclodextrins can accommodate many different hydrophobic molecules in their hydrophobic interior (ring-shaped structure) to achieve controlled drug delivery. The incorporation of cyclodextrins in the hydrogels results in an increased swelling and tensile strength. The cyclodextrins-loaded contact lenses are effective in treating glaucoma. *In-vitro* studies, reported an increase in the drug solubility in poly(cyclodextrin), an increase of its concentration in the cornea and an extended release over several weeks.

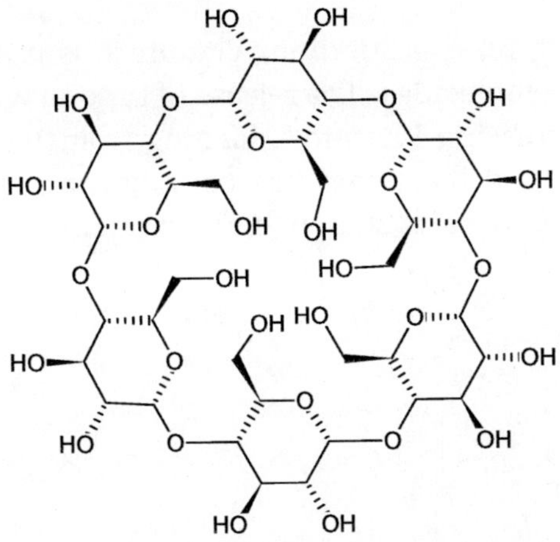

Figure 4.1 α-Cyclodextrin.

4.2.8 *Liposomes*

Due to their biological membrane-like structure, liposomes are biocompatible and biodegradable, and can be used in numerous drug delivery applications, including ophthalmic drug delivery through contact lenses.

4.2.9 *Microemulsion and Micelles*

Drug-loaded microemulsion and micelle-loaded therapeutic contact lenses showed promising results, due to their thermodynamic stability, easy preparation, high drug-loading capacity, increased wettability (low protein adherence) and easy tailoring of drug release pattern. Due to their nano size (5100 *nm*), the optical property of hydrogels remains unaltered, e.g., timolol-contact lenses with o/w type.

The microemulsion showed controlled release of timolol, due to the presence of a tightly packed surfactant at the oil-water interface. This system involves the use of surfactant. The presence of surfactant did not alter the optical property of the contact lenses, and also had the advantage of increase in wettability, i.e., reduction in protein absorption on contact lens surface.

4.2.10 *Vitamin E*

To improve drug release duration, Vitamin E is used as transport barriers for drug molecules. The release of timolol was significantly extended by increasing Vitamin E loading from 10 to 40% in contact lenses, while at the same time complicating oxygen and ion permeability. Vitamin E is shown in Figure 4.2.

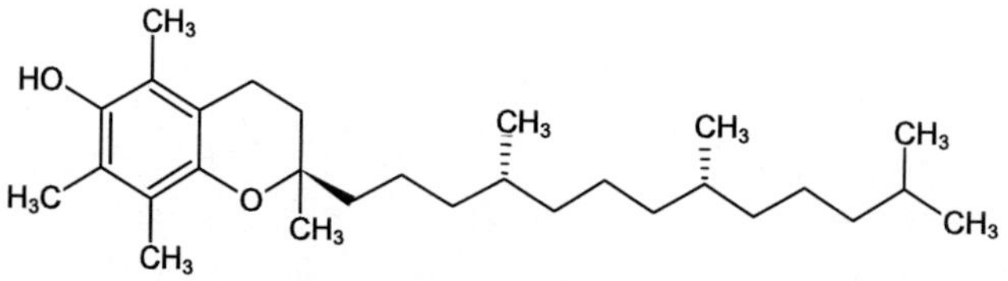

Figure 4.2 Vitamin E.

4.2.11 *Supercritical Fluid Technology*

Supercritical fluid technology is one of the most effective technologies to load/impregnate both hydrophilic and hydrophobic drug in contact lenses using supercritical solvent like CO_2. The impregnation process involves the dissolution of drug in supercritical solvent like CO_2 (at subcritical or supercritical conditions), followed by interaction with hydrogel contact lenses. The drug loading amount and its release kinetics are controlled by tailoring operational parameters like pressure, temperature, processing time and depressurization rate.

4.2.12 *Hydrophobic Drug Loading*

A cholesterol-hyaluronate micelle-embedded contact lens was developed for efficient hydrophobic drug loading and long-term controlled drug delivery (16).

The contact lens was fabricated via the photopolymerization of HEMA using EGDMA as crosslinking agent. The C-HA micelle-loaded contact lens showed statistically significant improvement in wettability and mechanical strength, maintaining the optical transmittance. *In-vitro* drug release tests revealed the controlled delivery of cyclosporine (cf. Figure 4.9) for more than 12 *d*.

Furthermore, the Schirmer tear test, a corneal fluorescein staining test, and MMP-9 fluorescein analysis confirmed its therapeutic effect on dry eye syndrome in disease model rabbits (16).

4.2.13 *Cationic Drugs*

The use of surface-active anionic unsaturated fatty acids in commercial contact lenses to extend drug release duration and regulate delivery dosage has been described (17).

The effect of oleic acid on the *in-vitro* release kinetics of three cationic drugs, and two anionic drugs from silicone hydrogel contact lenses, was investigated. Oleic acid is shown in Figure 4.3.

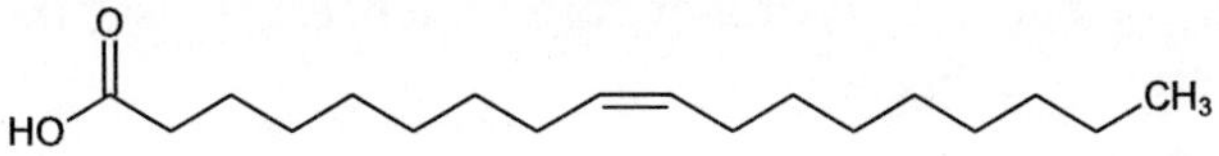

Figure 4.3 Oleic acid.

The release duration of the cationic drugs tetracaine hydrochloride, bupivacaine hydrochloride, cf. Figure 4.4, and ketotifen fumarate, cf. Figure 4.23, was found to be significantly extended from less than a day to more than a month due to the presence of oleic acid in the contact lenses.

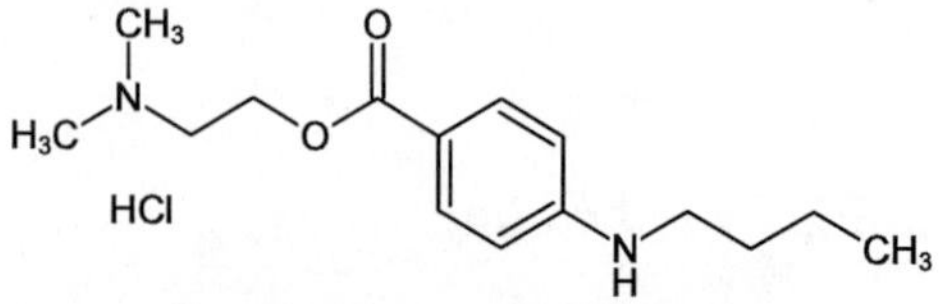

Tetracaine hydrochloride

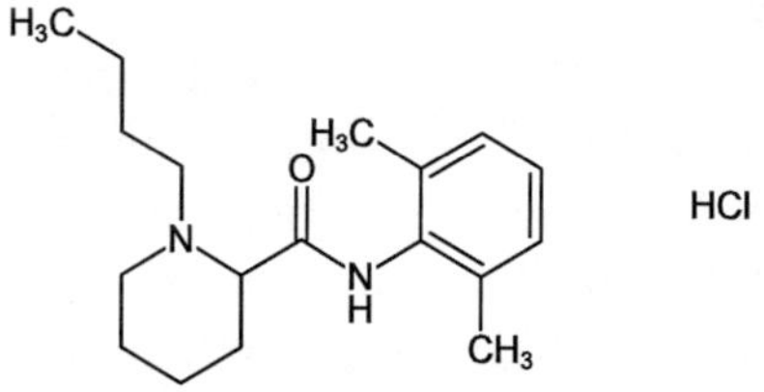

Bupivacaine hydrochloride

Figure 4.4 Cationic drugs.

With a simple change in the fatty acid loading media, a similar efficacy could be duplicated by loading oleic acid in conventional non-silicone hydrogel contact lenses. The fitted effective diffusivity values of the three cationic drugs significantly decrease when the amount of oleic acid in the lenses was increased.

By using two other unsaturated fatty acids, linoleic and α-linolenic acid ((9Z,12Z,15Z)-9,12,15-octadecatrienoic acid), the release duration of ketotifen fumarate was also significantly extended in the silicone hydrogel contact lenses. Unsaturated fatty acids are shown in Figure 4.5.

In contrast, the release of two anionic drugs, diclofenac sodium, cf. Figure 4.46, and flurbiprofen sodium, cf. Figure 4.18, was accelerated for oleic acid-modified lenses. These results show the dominating impact of coupling charge interactions between the drug and the fatty acid carrier molecules to precisely adjust delivery rate and dosage from a contact lens (17).

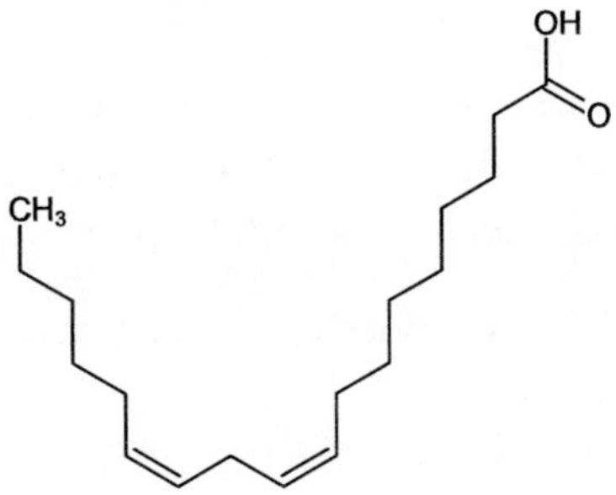

Linoleic acid

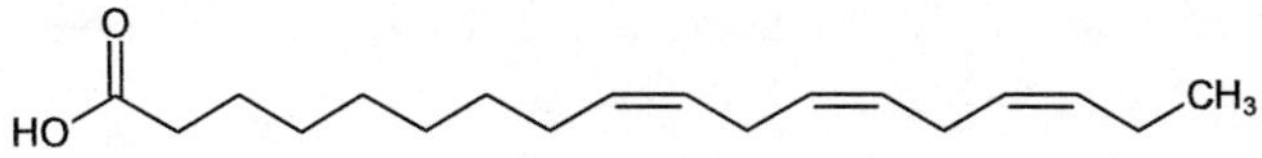

α-Linolenic acid

Figure 4.5 Unsaturated fatty acids.

4.3 Hydrogels

Various types of hydrogels for contact lens-based ophthalmic drug delivery systems, their advantages and drawbacks were critically analyzed in a review (18).

The term hydrogel refers to a network or matrix of polymer chains, some or all of which may be water soluble, and which may contain high percentages of water (19). Hydrogels refer to polymeric materials, including contact lenses, that are water swellable or water swelled. Thus, a hydrogel may be unhydrated and be water swellable, or may be partially hydrated and swollen with water, or may be fully hydrated and swollen with water. The term silicone hydrogel refers to a hydrogel that includes a silicon component or a silicone component.

The different methods of drug loading used throughout a polymer hydrogel have been detailed (20).

Soft contact lenses can improve the bioavailability and prolong the residence time of drugs and, therefore, are ideal drug carriers for ophthalmic drug delivery. Hydrogels are the leading materials of soft contact lenses because of their biocompatibility and transparent characteristic (21). In order to increase the amount of drugs loaded and control their release at the expected intervals, many strategies are developed to modify the conventional contact lens as well as the novel hydrogel contact lenses, including (21):

1. Polymeric hydrogels with controlled hydrophilic/hydrophobic copolymer ratio,
2. Hydrogels for inclusion of drugs in a colloidal structure dispersed in the contact lenses,
3. Ligand-containing hydrogels,
4. Molecularly imprinted polymeric hydrogels, and
5. Hydrogels with the surface containing multilayer structure for drug loading and releasing.

The advantages and disadvantages of the abovementioned strategies in modifying or designing hydrogel contact lenses for extended ophthalmic drug delivery have been analyzed (21).

Conventional hydrogel soft contact lenses have the ability to absorb some drugs and release them into the post-lens lacrimal fluid, minimizing clearance and sorption through the conjunctiva (22).

Their ability to be a drug reservoir strongly depends on the water content and thickness of the lens, the molecular weight of the drug, the concentration of the drug loading solution and the time the lens remains in it. However, the ability of contact lenses to load drugs and to control their release is generally inadequate, and the following approaches, based on modifications of the polymer network, have been under evaluation (22):

1. Covalent binding of the drug to the lens network via labile bonds,
2. Inclusion of the drug in colloidal structures that are dispersed in the lens and are responsible for controlling drug release,
3. Functionalization of the network with chemical groups that work as ion exchange resins, and
4. Creating a structure of imprinted pockets in the lens that memorize the spatial features and bonding preferences of the drug and provide the lens with a high affinity and selectivity for a given drug.

The possibilities and the advantages and drawbacks of these types of contact lenses as drug delivery systems have been critically analyzed in a review (22).

In order to evaluate the state of recent research, the latest hydrogel formulations and their associated chemistries for use in ocular therapies, spanning from external anterior to internal posterior regions of the eye, have been reviewed (23). The utility of hydrogels have been discussed concerning soft contact lenses, intraocular lenses, vitreous drug release hydrogels, and other issues.

4.3.1 *Salt-Induced Modulation*

Low drug loading efficiency is one of the main obstacles hindering the application of contact lenses as the carrier for extended ocular drug delivery. A simple and effective drug loading method based on salt-induced modulation was proposed and demonstrated with mechanism elucidation (24).

In this study, poly-*HEMA* was used as the contact lens material. Betaxolol hydrochloride, diclofenac sodium and betaxolol base were used as model drugs with a different solubility. As salts, sodium salts of sulfate, chloride, and sulfocyanate were used. Betaxolol hydrochloride (1-4-[2-(Cyclopropylmethoxy)ethyl]phenoxy-3-(isopropylamino)-2-propanol hydrochloride) is shown in Figure 4.6.

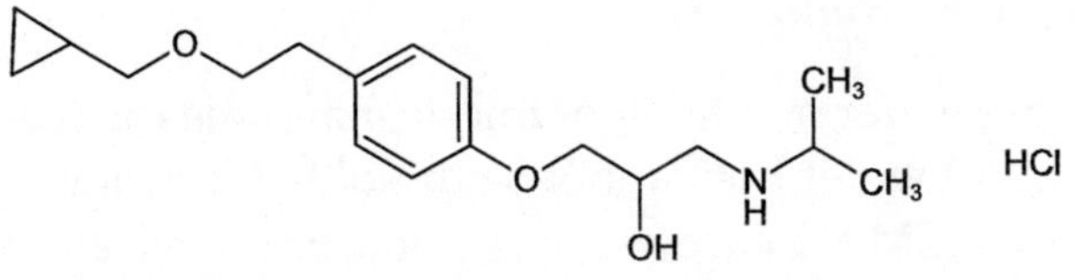

Figure 4.6 Betaxolol hydrochloride.

The mechanism of enhanced drug loading in the contact lens was explored via studying the influence of salt on the absorption isotherm, drug solubility and water content of contact lenses. It could be demonstrated that adjusting the ionic strength of loading solutions resulted in a significant increase of the drug loading in the contact lenses.

The empirical Setschenow equation with little modification was used to describe the influence of salts on drug solubility, as follows:

$$log\frac{S_0}{S_{app}} = K_s I \tag{4.1}$$

Here, where S_0 is the drug solubility in water, S_{app} is its solubility in salt solutions, K_s is the Setschenow constant, I is the ionic strength of the solution. The Setschenow constants are shown in Table 4.1.

Table 4.1 Setschenow constants.

Salt type	Diclofenac Sodium	Betaxolol Base
NaCl	1.37±0.13	0.19±0.02
Na_2SO_4	1.03±0.08	0.25±0.01
NaSCN	1.14±0.12	-0.12±0.02

The type and the concentration of the salts and the solubility of the drug were the main factors influencing the ratio of drug loading. The mechanism for the improved drug loading was related to the reduced drug solubility in the loading solutions and the reduced bound water content in contact lenses (24).

The modulation of the drug loading by adjusting the ionic strength was also applicable to other contact lenses and here the light transmittance was not affected. This method was more suitable for salt-form drugs with high solubility (24).

4.3.2 *Polymeric Hydrogels*

Hydrogels are water-swollen polymeric materials that can absorb a large amount of water but cannot be dissolved in water (25).

After poly-HEMA hydrogels were first prepared as soft contact lenses in the 1960s, the hydrogel contact lenses have been used to deliver ophthalmic drugs. However, the conventional contact lenses have some limitations in the application of long-time therapy due to the fast release rate of drugs and low loaded drug amount (26–28).

In order to enhance the potential capacity of hydrogel to load drugs and prolong the sustained release time of drugs, hydrophobic monomers, such as 4-vinylpyridine, or ionic monomers, such as *N*-(3-aminopropyl)methacrylamide, were incorporated into poly-HEMA hydrogels (29).

The incorporation of a ionic or hydrophobic monomer could increase the interaction between hydrogel and drugs so that the drugs have more difficulties diffusing from the hydrogel.

In order to increase the oxygen permeability, silicone polymers replace the conventional contact lenses monomers (30–32). It was found that the sustained drug release process of silicone hydrogels varied from 20 *d* up to more than three months depending on the compositions of hydrophobic and hydrophilic components of silicone hydrogels.

4.3.3 *Colloid-Laden Hydrogels*

Colloidal carriers have been investigated to achieve ophthalmic drug delivery (33). These colloidal systems consist of microparticles or nanoparticles, microemulsions or nanoemulsions, nanosuspensions, and liposomes.

It was reported that drug carriers via nanotechnology are favorable in enhancing the permeation of drugs, controlling the release of drug and targeting drug (34).

The encapsulation of drugs into these colloidal carriers can also significantly prevent degradation from the ocular enzymes (35, 36).

In addition, the size of these nanocarriers is small enough so as to not affect the vision of the patient. Therefore, colloid carriers can be incorporated into hydrogel contact lenses in order to prolong sustained release time of drugs and further increase their bioavailability (37–40).

Furthermore, it has also been proposed to create colloid-laden hydrogel *in situ* in one step. Surfactant-laden hydrogels can be prepared by the addition of surfactants to the polymerizing mixture. During the process of fabrication, the surfactants interact with the polymer chains and form micelles that create hydrophobic cores. In these cores, the hydrophobic drugs will preferentially enter (21).

4.3.4 *Ligand-Containing Hydrogels*

Weak interactions between drugs and ligands in a polymer matrix, including hydrogen bond, electrostatic interactions, and host-guest interactions, can induce the loading of a drug and control its release by ions in solution (27, 41–47).

Hydrogels containing cationic functional groups were synthesized for the delivery of anionic drugs and hydrogels containing anionic functional groups were synthesized for delivery of cationic drugs (41, 42). The resulting hydrogels were capable of storing the anionic drugs or cationic drugs depending on the charge of functional groups based on ion exchange reaction. The incorporated drugs could be released into tear fluid by ion exchange. Study results also show that these hydrogels are suitable for soft contact lenses as ophthalmic drug delivery. However, the sustained release time of these ion ligand-containing hydrogels is only several hours, which make these hydrogels unsuitable for extended delivery of ophthalmic drugs

4.3.5 *Amphiphilic Polymers*

An amphiphilic HEMA-chitosan polymer has been developed which can be used as a contact lens material (48).

The manufacturing method of such a polymer includes the following steps (48):

1. HEMA-NH_2 is provided. HEMA is dissolved in dichloromethane, and then, 4-toluenesulfonyl chloride is added and uniformly stirred in a reaction flask to cause a reaction. As the catalyst, 4-dimethylaminopyridine is added. After the reaction, the pH value of an obtained mixture is adjusted to a neutral value with hydrochloric acid and deionized water, and then the mixture is extracted to obtain a crude product of HEMA-4-toluenesulfonyl-grafted. The product is purified by column chromatography to obtain the pure compound. Then, ethylene diamine and potassium carbonate are added into tetrahydrofuran, and HEMA-4-toluenesulfonyl-grafted is dissolved, and the solution is heated and refluxed. After the reaction, the solution is naturally cooled to room temperature, and is subjected to vacuum drying to get the crude product HEMA-NH_2.
2. Then, amphiphilic chitosan is provided. Amphiphilic chitosan powder having a carboxyl modified hydrophilic end (carboxyl group) and a long carbon chain modified hydrophobic end (hexanoyl group) is dissolved in water to form an amphiphilic chitosan solution.

3. Next, the $HEMA\text{-}NH_2$ is bonded to the amphiphilic chitosan. In this step *N*-hydroxysuccinimide is added to the amphiphilic chitosan solution while stirring, and the compound $HEMA\text{-}NH_2$ is added to the amphiphilic chitosan solution while stirring to ensure that the mixture is uniformly distributed. Then, 1-ethyl-3-(3-dimethylaminopropyl)carbodiimide is added to the solution and stirred for reaction.
4. Finally, the product is purified by a dialysis membrane and subjected to vacuum drying to obtain the final product, the HEMA-amphiphilic chitosan polymer.

Some of the abovementioned chemicals are shown in Figure 4.7.

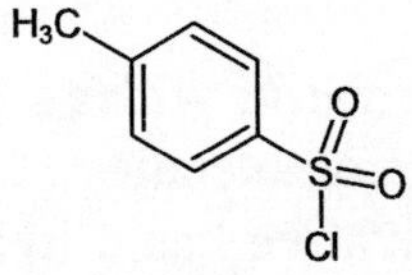

4-Toluenesulfonyl chloride

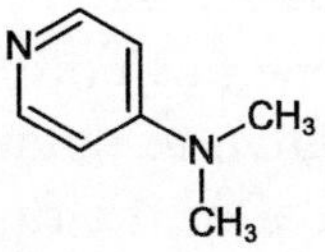

4-Dimethylaminopyridine

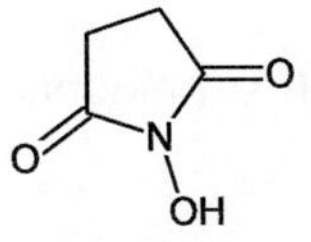

N-Hydroxysuccinimide

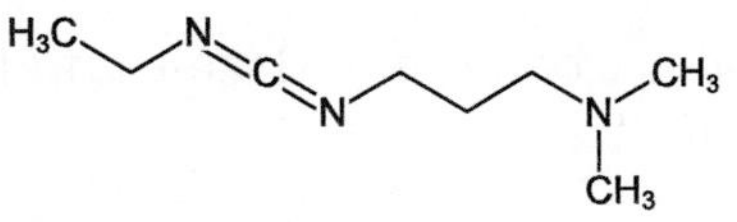

1-Ethyl-3-(3-dimethylaminopropyl) carbodiimide

Figure 4.7 Chemicals for the synthesis of a HEMA-chitosan polymer.

The amphiphilic polymer was tested as a contact lens material. Various amounts of the HEMA-amphiphilic chitosan polymer were added to a HEMA hydrogel. It was shown that the addition of a small amount of the HEMA-amphiphilic chitosan polymer can effectively increase the mechanical properties of HEMA hydrogel, which can increase the comfort of use and structural integrity (48).

It was shown that the amphiphilic polymer has good mechanical properties, penetration, extensibility, water content, water retention and cell compatibility as a contact lens material. Also, it improves the problem that occurs when silicone components are added to commercially available contact lenses in order to increase the oxygen permeability, thereby causing the phenomena of reduced transparency and insolubility.

On the other hand, these lenses are able to be loaded with a drug and are capable of releasing the drug. These drugs are not limited to glaucoma drugs, and may include, for example, an allergy drug, a pinkeye drug, and others (48).

A manufacturing method of amphiphilic macromolecules has been described. This method is carried out by (49):

- First reacting a acrylic acid derivative, i.e., hydroxyethyl methacrylate or hydroxymethyl methacrylate, with *N,N′*-carbonyldiimidazole to obtain a modified acrylic acid derivative, and
- Reacting the modified acrylic acid derivative with a siloxane derivative to obtain amphiphilic macromolecules. Here, a terminal of the first acrylic acid derivative has a hydroxyl group. The siloxane derivative is a hydroxyl-terminated, acrylamide-terminated, epoxy-terminated, or amine-terminated poly(siloxane) molecule.

N,N′-Carbonyldiimidazole and the reaction products are shown in Figure 4.8.

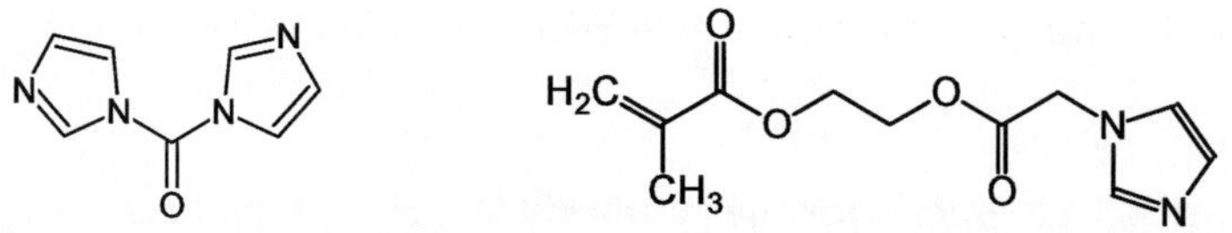

N,N′-carbonyldiimidazole Methacrylic acid derivative

Figure 4.8 *N,N′*-Carbonyldiimidazole and its methacrylic acid derivative.

The amphiphilic macromolecules have a good miscibility with the hydrophilic monomers in the contact lens, thus achieving the purpose of reducing phase separation. Because the amphiphilic macromolecules include siloaxane, the oxygen permeability and Young's modulus of the contact lens may increase. Therefore, a contact lens that contains amphiphilic macromolecules has excellent oxygen permeability while maintaining its high transmittance (49).

4.3.6 *Silicone Hydrogel Contact Lenses*

Cyclosporine A is effective in treating chronic dry eyes and contact lens-mediated dry eyes (50). Cyclosporine A is shown in Figure 4.9.

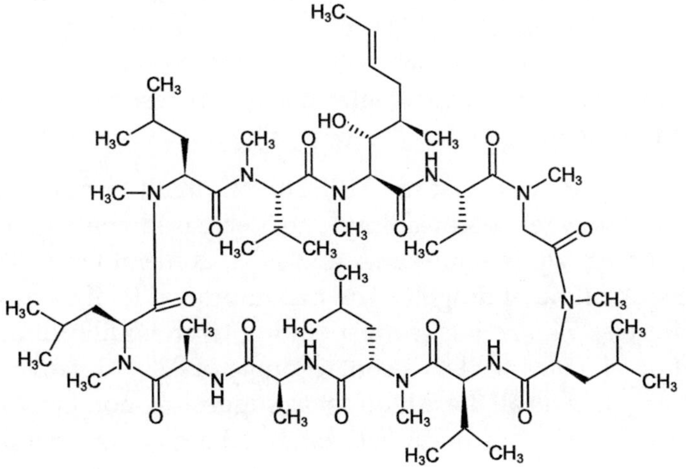

Figure 4.9 Cyclosporine A.

Cyclosporine A is delivered through oil-in-water emulsion eye drops, which has a small residence time in the eyes, leading to low bioavailability.

The delivery of cyclosporine A from contact lenses was tested to provide a controlled and extended drug delivery with an increased bioavailability due to enhanced ocular residence time. Loading and release profiles of cyclosporine A from commercial contact lenses are presented to show that 1-Day Acuvue® releases cyclosporine A for about a day and extended wear silicone hydrogel (SiH) lenses release cyclosporine A for about 2 weeks. The longer duration from SiH lenses compared to the 1-Day Acuvue lens is due to larger partition coefficients in the gel.

A novel approach could be presented for increasing release duration from the Si–H lenses to the desired 1-month through incorporation of Vitamin E. The results show that Vitamin E-loaded lenses can provide cyclosporine A release within the therapeutic window for a period of about a month. So, this study demonstrated the promising potential of delivering cyclosporine A from a contact lens for the treatment of chromic dry eyes and contact lens-mediated dry eyes (50).

Silicone-based hydrogel contact lenses were prepared by the polymerization of 3-(methacryloyloxy)propyltris(trimethylsiloxy)silane (TRIS), *N,N*-dimethylacrylamide (DMA), NVP, and HEMA (51). The properties of silicone hydrogel lenses were analyzed based on methods such as equilibrium water content, oxygen permeability, optical transparency, contact angle, mechanical test, protein adsorption, and cell toxicity.

The results showed that the TRIS content in all formulations increased the oxygen permeability and decreased the equilibrium water content, while both DMA and NVP contributed to the hydrophilicity of the hydrogels. The maximum value of oxygen permeability was 74.9 *barrers*, corresponding to an equilibrium water content of 44.5% as well as a contact angle of 82°. Moreover, L929 fibroblasts grew on all these hydrogels, suggesting non-cytotoxicity. In general, the silicone hydrogels exhibited a good oxygen permeability, stiffness, and optical transparency, as well, as anti-protein adsorption. Hence, these silicone hydrogel polymers would be feasible for making contact lenses (51).

4.3.7 *Zwitterionic Hydrogels*

It has been found that a zwitterionic material is stable in ophthalmic solutions (52). In the study, a material with a zwitterionic hydrogel was developed using an ion-exchange reaction. A monomer with a quaternary ammonium salt group and a carboxyl group as ionic monomer was used.

Then, the compounds were evaluated as a drug delivery system. Disodium cromoglycate was used as a model drug (52). This drug prevents the release of inflammatory chemicals such as histamine from mast cells (53). Disodium cromoglycate is shown in Figure 4.10.

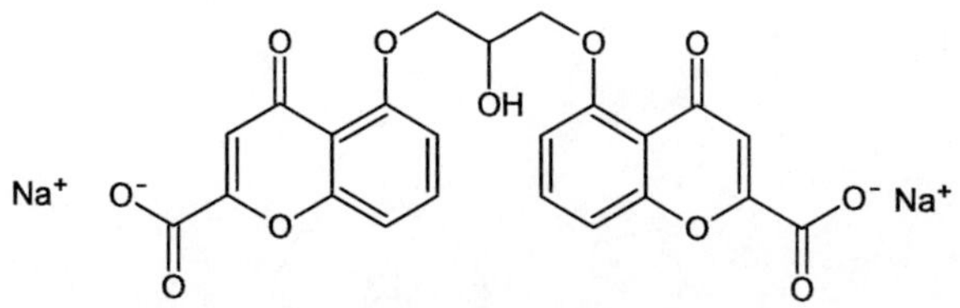

Figure 4.10 Disodium cromoglycate.

4.3.8 Surface-Modified Hydrogels

Some efforts have been made to modify the surface of commercial contact lenses for ophthalmic drug delivery. Drugs were encapsulated into liposomes and then subsequently bound these intact lipid vesicles onto both the anterior and posterior surfaces of commercial contact lenses (54). The process of immobilizing liposomes includes three steps (21):

1. Poly(ethylene imine) was grafted onto the surface of a commercial contact lens (Hioxifilcon B) via amidation under the catalyzation of disuccinimidyl carbonate, cf. Figure 4.11. Next, NHS-PEG-biotin molecules were covalently bounded onto the surface by carbodiimide chemistry.
2. NeutrAvidin was immobilized on the PEG-biotin layer via biotin-avidin affinity. Liposomes containing PEG-biotinylated lipids were then docked onto the surface-immobilized NeutrAvidin.
3. Multilayers of liposomes were fabricated by consecutive addition of further NeutrAvidin and liposome layers or by exposing contact lenses coated with NeutrAvidin to liposome aggregates produced by the addition of free biotin in solution. Biotin is shown in Figure 4.12.

Avidin is a tetrameric biotin-binding protein, which is produced in the oviducts of birds, reptiles and amphibians and deposited in the whites of their eggs (55).

In chicken egg white, avidin makes up approximately 0.05% of the total protein. The tetrameric protein contains four identical subunits, i.e., homotetramers. Each of these subunits can bind to biotin (Vitamin B7, Vitamin H) with a high degree of affinity and specificity (55).

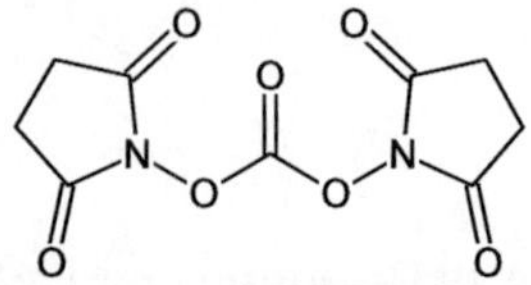

Figure 4.11 Disuccinimidyl carbonate.

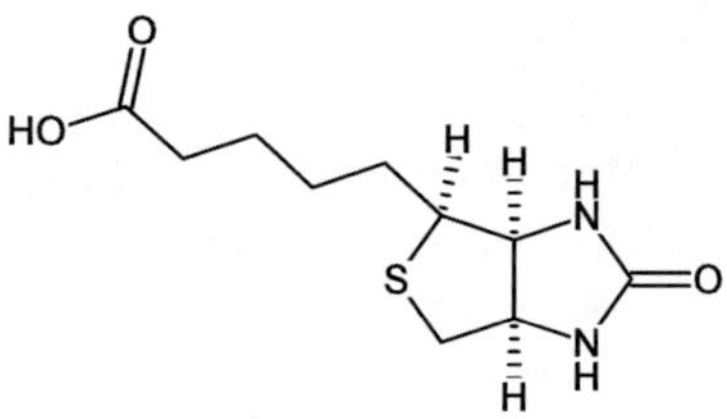

Figure 4.12 Biotin.

The results showed that the surface-immobilized, drug-filled liposome multilayers provide a promising avenue for site-specific delivery (21). However, no actual drug was investigated in this research (54).

Also, layer-by-layer platforms have been applied for drug delivery due to their simple, mild aqueous manufacturing conditions at room temperature (56–58)

Yet, layer-by-layer platforms cannot deliver small molecule drug with highly controlled release kinetics, and the release time scales delivered by layer-by-layer platforms is short. Some efforts have been made to modify the conventional layer-by-layer technique for small molecule drug delivery such as by incorporating the cyclodextrin into layer-by-layer platform. Layer-by-layer platforms were designed to deliver small molecule therapeutics from virtually any surface, regardless of geometry or surface chemistry, with programmable zero-order release kinetics through hydrolytic top-down degradation (56).

4.3.9 *Cyclodextrin-Hyaluronan Hydrogels*

A series of poly-HEMA hydrogels containing crosslinked β-cyclodextrin-hyaluronan, with a tear protein adsorption resistance and sustained drug delivery, were developed as contact lens materials for eye diseases (59).

β-Cyclodextrin-hyaluronan was synthesized from aminated β-cyclodextrin and hyaluronan and then crosslinked within poly-*HEMA* hydrogel using poly(ethylenimine) as a crosslinking agent.

The incorporation of β-cyclodextrin-hyaluronan significantly improved the surface hydrophilicity, water uptake ability, oxygen permeability, and flexibility of poly-*HEMA* hydrogel, but did not compromise light transmission.

Poly-*HEMA*/β-cyclodextrin-hyaluronan hydrogels not only decreased the tear protein adsorption because of the electrostatically mutual repulsion and the improved hydrophilicity, leading to the reduced adhesion of *Staphylococcus aureus* on the hydrogel surface, but also enhanced the encapsulation capacity and the sustainable delivery of diclofenac due to the formation of inclusion complexes between β-cyclodextrin and drugs (59).

Among these hydrogels with different β-cyclodextrin-hyaluronan contents, the poly-*HEMA*/β-cyclodextrin-hyaluronan$_1$0 hydrogel showed the lowest water contact angle of 52°, the highest water content of 65%, the largest *Dk* value of 36.4 *barrer*, and the optimal modulus of 1.8 *MPa*, as well as a good light transmission of more than 90%.

An *in-vivo* conjunctivitis treatment of rabbits for 72 *h* indicated that drug-loaded pHEMA/β-cyclodextrin-hyaluronan$_1$0 hydrogel presented a better therapeutic effect than both one dose administration of drug solution per day and drug-loaded poly-*HEMA* hydrogel (59).

So, the poly-*HEMA*/β-cyclodextrin-hyaluronan$_1$0 hydrogel is a promising contact lens material for ophthalmic diseases (59).

4.3.10 *Bioinspired Hydrogels*

Efficient ocular drug delivery that can overcome the challenges of topical application has been greatly pursued (60). Contact lenses may act as light-transparent cornea/sclera bandages for prolonged drug release towards the post-lens tear fluid, if their composition and inner architecture are fitted to the features of the drug molecules.

The foundations and advantages of using contact lenses as ocular drug depots were reviewed. Also, the pros and cons of common strategies to prepare drug-loaded contact lenses were analyzed on the basis of recent examples, and bioinspired strategies that can overcome some limitations of current designs are highlighted.

Most bioinspired strategies resemble a reverse engineering process to create artificial receptors for the drug inside the contact lens network by mimicking the natural binding site of the drug in humans. Related bioinspired strategies were also tested for designing contact lenses that elute comfort ingredients mimicking the blinking-associated renewal of eye mucins. Other bioinspired approaches exploit the natural eye variables as stimuli to trigger drug release or take advantage of bio-glues to specifically bind active components to the contact lens surface.

Overall, biomimicking approaches are being revealed as valuable tools to fit the amounts loaded and the release profiles to the therapeutic demands of each pathology. Biomimetic and bioinspired strategies are remarkable tools for the optimization of drug delivery systems. Translation of the knowledge about how drugs interact with the natural pharmacological receptor and about components and dynamics of the anterior eye segment may shed light on the design criteria for obtaining efficient drug-eluting contact lenses. Current strategies for endowing contact lenses with controlled drug release performance still require optimization regarding the amount loaded and drug retained in the contact lens structure during storage, regulation of drug release once applied onto the eye, and maintenance of contact lens physical properties. All these limitations may be addressed through a variety of recently growing bioinspired approaches, which are expected to pave the way towards the use of medicated contact lenses in clinics (60).

4.3.11 Tobramycin Release

Tobramycin is an aminoglycoside antibiotic derived from *Streptomyces tenebrarius* that is used to treat various types of bacterial infections, particularly Gram-negative infections (61). It is especially effective against species of *Pseudomonas*. It was patented in 1965 and approved for medical use in 1974 (61, 62). Tobramycin is shown in Figure 4.13.

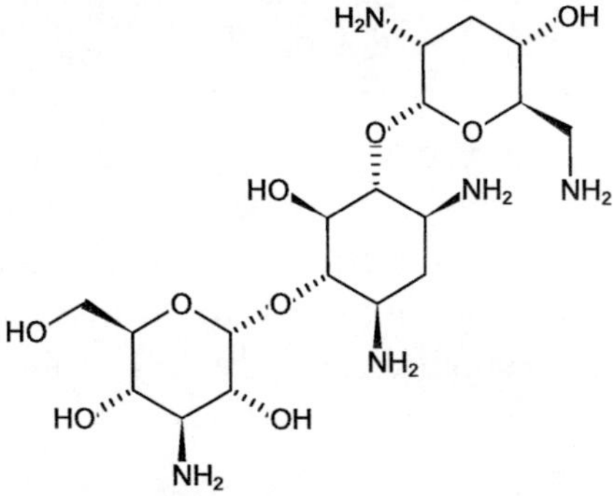

Figure 4.13 Tobramycin.

The controlled delivery of hydrophilic drugs can be difficult to achieve due to the burst release of drug that is associated with materials of high water content, such as hydrogels.

Silicone hydrogels have significant potential for drug delivery due to their increased hydrophobicity and the tortuous nature of the pores, overcoming some of the limitations associated with conventional hydrogel materials (63).

The potential of model poly(ethylene glycol) (PEG)-containing silicone hydrogels was examined for the delivery of hydrophilic aminoglycoside antibiotics. It was hypothesized that PEG, a polymer that has seen extensive use in biomedical applications, in addition to providing hydrophilicity and protein repulsion, will also provide a mechanism for controlling the delivery of this hydrophilic antibiotic. PEG was combined with the macromer TRIS to create model silicone hydrogel materials.

The optical and physical properties of the TRIS-*co*-PEG silicone hydrogels exhibited excellent transparency, appropriate refractive index and high transmittance, indicating minimal phase separation. Desirable properties such as wettability and protein repulsion were maintained across a wide range of formulations. The water content was found to be highly correlated with the ethylene oxide content.

Drug release could be influenced through the PEG content and was found to fit Higuchi-like kinetics (63).

The study could demonstrate that the incorporation of PEG into a model silicone hydrogel could be used to control the release of a hydrophilic compound. The data suggest this is related to the unique structure and properties of PEG, which alter the types of water found in each formulation and the water content (63).

In another study, the use of an interpenetrating network of hydrogel was tested as a vehicle for the delivery of ocular topical antibiotics (64). The drug release of two commonly use topical antibiotics, vancomycin and tobramycin, from a hydrogel was measured. Vancomycin is shown in Figure 4.14. Tobramycin is shown in Figure 4.13.

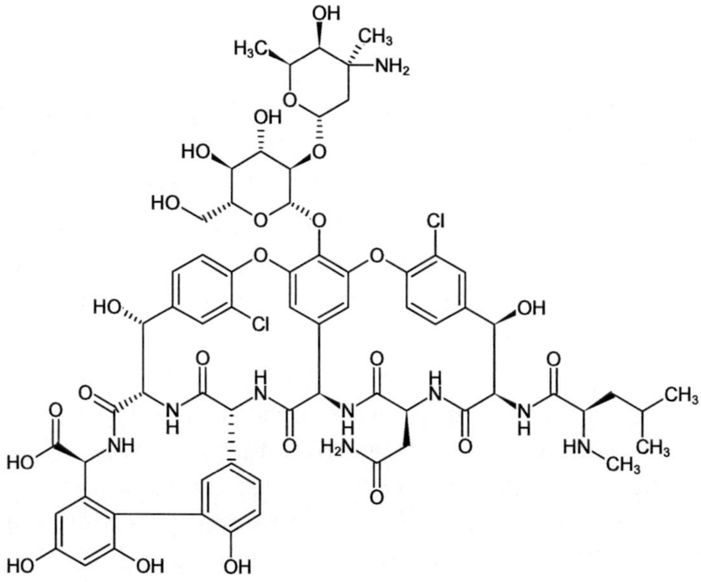

Figure 4.14 Vancomycin.

Hydrogels composed of a PEG/poly(acrylic acid) double network with high strength and high water content were synthesized and cut into 1 *cm* diameter discs. The hydrogel discs were then dried overnight in a dessicator. They were then loaded with vancyomycin 50 $mg\,ml^{-1}$ or tobramycin 40 $mg\,ml^{-1}$, by soaking for 48 *h*. The antibiotic release was monitored by measuring the percentage transmittance at 201 *nm* for vancomycin and 198 *nm* for tobramycin using UV/VIS spectrophotometry (64).

The amount of drug release versus time is shown in Figure 4.15.

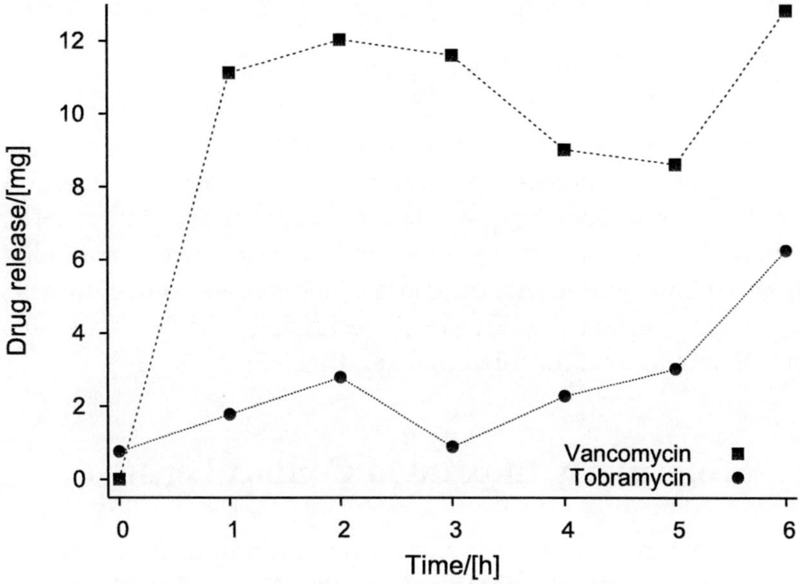

Figure 4.15 Amount of drug release vs. time (64).

4.4 Contact Lens Gels

Microbial keratitis is a serious sight-threatening infection affecting approximately two million individuals worldwide annually (65).

A nitric oxide releasing contact lens gel displaying broad spectrum antimicrobial activity against two of the most common causative pathogens of microbial keratitis was assessed (65).

The contact lens gel is composed of poly(ε-lysine) functionalized with nitric oxide releasing diazeniumdiolate moieties, cf. Figure 4.16, which enables the controlled and sustained release of bactericidal concentrations of nitric oxide at a physiological pH over a period of 15 *h*. Diazeniumdiolate functionalization was confirmed by Fourier transform infrared spectroscopy, and the concentration of nitric oxide released from the gels was determined by chemiluminescence.

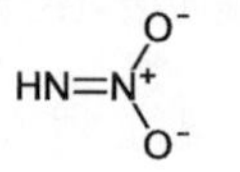

Figure 4.16 Diazeniumdiolate.

The bactericidal efficacy of the gels against *Pseudomonas aeruginosa* and *Staphylococcus aureus* was ascertained, and between 1 and 4 log reductions in bacterial populations were observed over 24 *h*. Additional cell cytotoxicity studies with human corneal epithelial cells also demonstrated that the contact lens gels were not cytotoxic, thus suggesting that the developed technology could be a viable alternative treatment for microbial keratitis (65).

4.5 Molecularly Imprinted Contact Lenses

The manufacture of substrate-selective polymers by host-guest polymerization was initially described in 1982 (66). Also, the issues of molecularly imprinted polymers as drug delivery vehicles have been reviewed (67–69).

4.5.1 *Molecular Imprinting Technology*

Molecular imprinting is used in a wide variety of applications, such as polymer electrochemical sensors, biosensors, and drug delivery (70).

Molecular imprinting can function as biomimetic way of natural antibody-antigen systems (71). Their mechanism can be understood from a lock and key mechanism, thus indicating that molecular imprinted polymers selectively bind the molecule with which they were templated during synthesis. Among many beneficial applications of molecular imprinted polymers, drug delivery is considered an excellent and promising method of sustained release of drug to achieve desired therapeutic results.

The issues of molecular imprinted polymers as drug delivery systems and their progress over the last three years have been reviewed (71).

In the preparation of molecular imprinted polymers, a complex is formed between a target analyte and a functional monomer followed by polymerization in the presence of excess of crosslinking monomer and appropriate solvent. The polymerization can be carried out via thermal polymerization, electricity, UV, etc. In different cases, other constituents may also be required such as an initiator. Once the polymerization is stopped, the trapped template molecules are extracted from the polymer with the help of organic solvents, leaving behind a 3D polymer. This polymer possesses recognition sites with the exact shape, size and chemical functionality as the template molecule.

Usually, non-covalent and covalent bonding drive the molecular recognition phenomena between the template analytes and functional monomer groups. The non-covalent bonding interaction is commonly preferred owing to convenient binding and rebinding phenomenon (72–77).

4.5.2 *Molecularly Imprinted Contact Lenses*

Contact lens-based opthalmic drug delivery systems with significant potential for use in ocular therapeutics have been reviewed (78, 79).

The ocular delivery route is a widely used method for drug delivery systems. However, serious obstacles arise, including high lachrymal turnover and dynamics that cause quick precorneal removal of the drug, subsequently reducing bioavailability and therapeutic response of the drug. Furthermore, high frequency of drugs or excessive dosage of drugs may pose potential risks to the patients. Due to obstacles, such as low bioavailability and loading capacity of various ophthalmic solutions, ointments and gels, applications in drug delivery systems involving the treatment of ocular diseases is the most active research area involving molecularly imprinted polymers, as they offer solutions for many problems in this area (69).

Molecular imprinting has been used to produce therapeutic contact lenses with enhanced loading and delayed release. The progress in the field has mostly included low-molecular-weight therapeutics such as antiglaucoma, antihistamine, antibiotic and anti-inflammatory therapeutics used to treat anterior eye disorders (78).

The preparation of molecularly imprinted polymers involves the self-assembly of functional monomers and target molecules, followed by polymerization with crosslinking agent in the presence of an inert solvent as a porogen (28). Upon removal of the target molecules, cavities that can recognize the spatial features and bonding preferences of the target molecules are created, providing the contact lens with a high affinity and selectivity for a given drug. Although the polymerization is usually performed in an organic solvent to give a macroporous structure that allows the target molecules access to the imprinted sites, one can avoid the use of any solvent by taking advantage of the liquid state of the monomers in preparation of molecular imprinted polymer hydrogels.

Molecularly imprinted polymer hydrogels have been prepared by dissolution of EGDMA as crosslinking agent in HEMA with methacrylic acid (MA) as functional monomer or methyl methacrylate as functional monomer (28).

The application of molecular imprinting technology during soft contact lens manufacturing enables the creation of imprinted pockets in the lens structure that memorize the spatial features and bonding preferences of the drug and provide the lens with a high affinity for a given drug (80). Imprinted soft contact lenses could prolong the permanence of the drug in the precorneal area and provide sustained drug levels, increasing ocular bioavailability and avoiding systemic side effects. The potential and advantages and drawbacks of drug-imprinted soft contact lenses were reviewed and examples of the application of the molecular imprinting technology were shown (80).

In a review of the patent literature it was stated that among all noninvasive alternatives, contact lenses offer the highest bioavailability to the cornea due to the location of the lens in the immediate vicinity of the cornea (81). Several approaches have been patented to improve contact lens design for an extended release duration of drugs. Many technologies have successfully integrated suitable drug release profiles into contact lenses, but drug-eluting contacts are not yet commercialized, which is likely due to regulatory challenges, including the high cost of clinical trials.

Furthermore, the technique of imprinting has been criticized as follows: The imprinting leads to an increase in the partition coefficients and slower release of drugs, but the increase is not very substantial, and these lenses typically have an initial burst release (82).

In the following sections, several substances that are used for drug delivery in molecularly imprinted contact lenses are described. These materials are listed in Table 4.2. Also, the characterization of some imprinted hydrogels have been given in a review (68). Parts of these issues are also summarized in Table 4.2.

Table 4.2 Drugs for molecularly imprinted contact lenses (68).

Compound	References
Acetazolamide	(83)
Ciprofloxacin	(84, 85)
Dexamethasone	(86)
Diclofenac	(87)
Dorzolamide	(88)
Ethoxzolamide	(83, 89)
Flurbiprofen	(86)
Hyaluronic acid	(90)
Hydroxypropyl methylcellulose	(91)
Ibuprofen	(92)
Ketotifen fumarate	(93–97)
Norfloxacin	(98)
Bimatoprost	(99, 100)
Polymyxin B	(101)
Prednisolone	(28, 92, 102)
Timolol	(103–109)
Trehalose	(92)
Vancomycin	(101)

Acetazolamide is shown in Figure 4.17. Other drugs are detailed subsequently.

4.5.3 *Hydrogels*

Molecularly imprinted polymers were investigated for drug delivery due to their active sites of specific recognition (110–113).

The general imprinting process includes five steps (21):

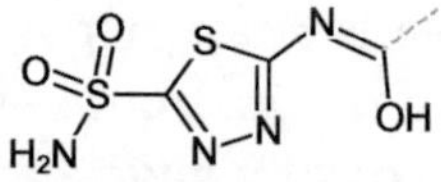

Figure 4.17 Acetazolamide.

1. A template, functional monomer, crosslinking monomer, and initiator in solution were self-assembled into the pre-polymerization complex via covalent or non-covalent chemistry.
2. The complex was initiated via UV light or heat to form crosslinked network.
3. The original template was removed via a washing step, the crosslinked polymer network with cavities was formed.
4. A new template (potential drug) was rebonded into the crosslinked polymer.
5. The new template diffuses into solution via stimulation, such as swelling.

During this imprinting process, the bioactivity of drugs can also be preserved (110).

4.5.4 Supercritical Fluid-Assisted Preparation

An innovative supercritical fluid-assisted molecular imprinting method was developed to endow commercial soft contact lenses with the ability to load specific drugs and to control their release (86). This approach seeks to overcome the limitation of the common loading of preformed soft contact lenses by immersion in concentrated drug solutions (only valid for highly water-soluble drugs) and of the molecular imprinting methods that require choice of the drug before polymerization and thus create drug-tailored networks.

In particular, the study focused on improving the flurbiprofen load/release capacity of daily wear Hilafilcon B commercial soft contact lenses by the use of sequential supercritical fluid flurbiprofen impregnation and extraction steps. Flurbiprofen was approved for medical use in 1987 by BASF (114). Flurbiprofen

((2R)-2-(2-Fluoro-4-biphenylyl)propanoic acid) is shown in Figure 4.18.

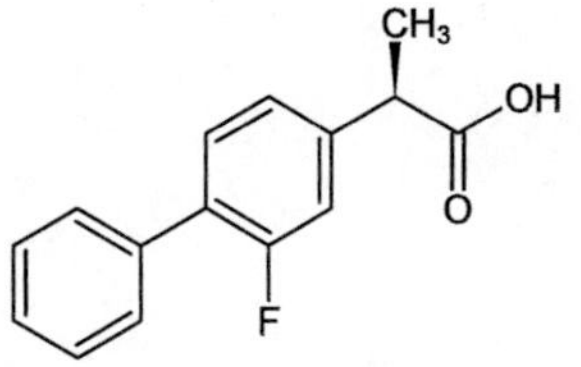

Figure 4.18 Flurbiprofen.

Supercritical carbon dioxide impregnation assays were performed at 12.0 *MPa* and 40°C, while supercritical carbon dioxide extractions were performed at 20.0 *MPa* and 40°C (86).

Conventional flurbiprofen sorption and drug removal experiments in aqueous solutions were carried out for comparison purposes. Supercritical fluid-processed soft contact lenses showed a recognition ability and a higher affinity for flurbiprofen in aqueous solution than for the structurally related ibuprofen and dexamethasone, which suggests the creation of molecularly imprinted cavities driven by both physical (swelling/plasticization) and chemical (carbonyl groups in the network with the C–F group in the drug) interactions.

Processing with supercritical carbon dioxide did not alter some of the critical functional properties of soft contact lenses (glass transition temperature, transmittance, oxygen permeability, contact angle), enabled the control of drug-loaded/released amounts (by the application of several consecutive processing cycles) and permitted the preparation of hydrophobic drug-based therapeutic soft contact lenses in much shorter process times than those using conventional aqueous-based molecular imprinting methods (86).

4.6 Special Drugs

4.6.1 *Timolol*

The usefulness of molecular imprinting technology was evaluated in order to obtain therapeutic soft contact lenses capable of prolonging the permanence of timolol in the precorneal area, compared to conventional contact lenses and eye drops (103, 104, 115). Timolol is shown in Figure 4.19.

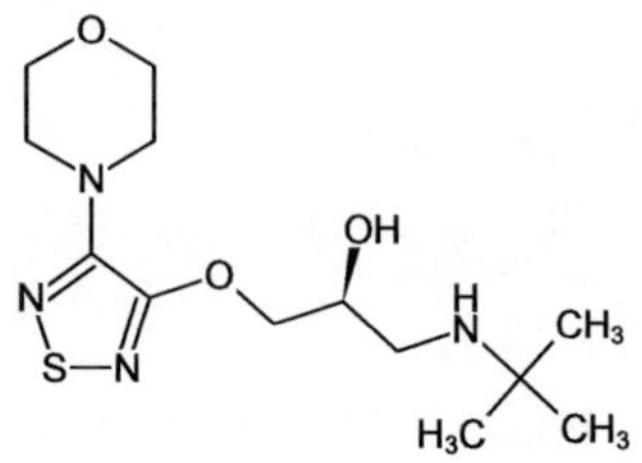

Figure 4.19 Timolol.

Timolol is used to treat increased pressure inside the eye such as in ocular hypertension and glaucoma (116).

4.6.1.1 Ocular Release of Timolol

The influence of the composition of soft contact lenses on the achievement of a significant increase in drug loading and control release capability was evaluated (117). Four types of timolol imprinted lenses were prepared by UV irradiation of *N,N*-diethyl acrylamide, HEMA, tris(trimethylsiloxy)silyl propyl methacrylate, and DMA (50:50 v/v), or methyl methacrylate and *N,N*-diethyl acrylamide (50:50 v/v) solutions. To these solutions, a functional monomer, methacrylic acid, ethylene glycol dimethacrylate as crosslinking agent, and timolol maleate were previously added. Non-imprinted systems were synthesized in the same way but with the omission of timolol.

Timolol did not interfere in the polymerization process. All lenses were optically clear and, once wet, showed adequate mechanical properties. Nevertheless, the lenses significantly differed in temperature of glass transition, as estimated by differential scanning calorimetry and oscillatory rheometry, equilibrium water content and drug loading and release properties (117).

In addition, soft contact lenses with a diameter of 14 *mm* and a center thickness of 0.08 *mm* were assessed (104). The lenses were prepared from *N,N*-diethyl acrylamide as a main component of the matrix, MA as functional monomer and EGDMA as crosslinking agent.

These materials were prepared by a conventional methodology or by applying a molecular imprinting technique using timolol as the template.

After washing and reloading, timolol release studies that were carried out in rabbits showed that the soft contact lenses made by the molecular imprinting method with a 34 μg dose provided measurable timolol concentrations in the tear fluid for 2.0-fold and 3.0-fold longer than the non-imprinted contact lenses with a 21 μg dose and eye drops with doses of 34 μg and 125 μg, respectively (104).

Furthermore, the area under the timolol concentration-time curve was 3.3- and 8.7-fold greater for imprinted contact lenses than non-imprinted contact lenses and eye drops, respectively.

The timolol concentration of the eye drops did not affect the precorneal residence time of drug significantly. On the other hand, the timolol loading capacity of the contact lenses was improved by the molecular imprinting method. The sustained drug levels in the tear fluid were proportional to the loading capacity of the contact lenses. These results indicate that imprinted soft contact lenses are promising drug devices able to provide greater and more sustained drug concentrations in tear fluid with lower doses than conventional eye drops (104).

4.6.1.2 Sustained Timolol Release

A molecular imprinted structural color contact lens for sustained timolol release has been fabricated, which could self-report the release process by a color change (118).

The specific recognition of target timolol by molecular imprinted sites can not only increase the loading amount and the residence time of the drug but also endow the structure color of lens remarkable blue shift with the accumulative release of timolol. This contact lens type can be further used for controlling the release of a large number of other ophthalmic drugs and has a high potential to be a new generation of functional contact lenses (118).

4.6.1.3 *Optimal Timolol to Functional Monomer Ratio*

Isothermal titration calorimetry was used to assess the optimal timolol:functional monomer ratio for preparing soft contact lenses able to sustain drug release (119). The isothermal titration calorimetry profiles revealed that each timolol molecule required six to eight acrylic acid (AA) monomers to saturate the binding and that these ratios could be the most suitable for creating imprinted cavities. Various poly(HEMA-*co*-AA) hydrogels 0.2 *mm* and 0.9 *mm* thick were prepared with timolol:AA molar ratios ranging from 1:6 to 1:32, and also in the absence of timolol.

The hydrogels were reloaded with timolol by immersion in 0.04, 0.06, 0.08, and 0.10 *mM* drug solutions. Both imprinted and non-imprinted hydrogels showed a high affinity for the drug because of the presence of AA. Nevertheless, the 1:6 and 1:8 imprinted hydrogels loaded less timolol but sustained the release better than the other hydrogels. These differences were explained in terms of the different arrangement of the functional monomers along the network (119).

The imprinting effect was more noticeable in the case of the thinnest hydrogels, where the contribution of the diffusion path to the release rate was smaller. The results obtained prove the interest of isothermal titration calorimetry for the rational design of drug-imprinted networks to be used as medicated soft contact lenses (119).

4.6.1.4 *Glaucoma Therapy*

Glaucoma is a leading cause of irreversible blindness in the world (120). Glaucoma is asymptomatic, which means that it is difficult to diagnose until a permanent vision loss occurs (121). Tonometric screenings for high intraocular pressure in eye exams can reduce vision losses. However, some early studies showed that the intraocular pressure screening is only effective for approximately 50% of the glaucomatous cases (122, 123).

Laboratory-based timolol release studies and *in-vivo* pharmacodynamics studies in beagle dogs were combined to evaluate the efficacy of glaucoma therapy through extended wear contact lenses (107). Commercial contact lenses cannot provide an extended delivery of ophthalmic drugs and so the studies here focused on increasing the release duration of timolol from Acuvue® TruEye™ contact lenses by incorporating Vitamin E diffusion barriers.

The efficacy of timolol delivered via extended wear contact lenses was then compared to eye drops in beagle dogs that suffer from spontaneous glaucoma. The lenses were either replaced every 24 *h* or continuously worn for 4 *d*, and the pharmacodynamics effect of changes in the intraocular pressure of timolol from the Acuvue TruEye contact lenses can be significantly increased by incorporation of Vitamin E. The changes of the rate of drug release versus Vitamin E concentration is shown in Figure 4.20.

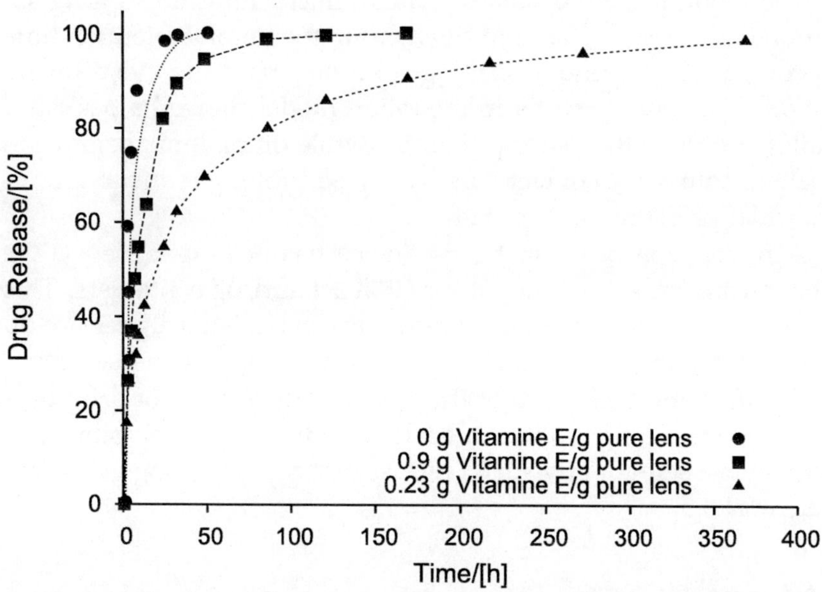

Figure 4.20 Change of drug release rate vs. Vitamin E concentration (107).

The *in-vivo* studies showed that intraocular pressure reduction from baseline by pure contact lens on a daily basis was comparable with that by eye drops but with only 20% of drug dose, which suggested higher drug bioavailability for contact lenses. In addition, by including Vitamin E in the lenses, the intraocular pressure was reduced significantly during the 4 *d* treatment with continuous wear of lens (107).

In another study, the influence of a microemulsion on timolol loading from the soaking solution and its ability to control the drug release kinetics was investigated (124). The contact lenses were soaked in the timolol-microemulsion soaking solution and compared with the timolol soaking solution without microemulsion.

The loading of a timolol-laden microemulsion in the contact lenses did not alter the swelling and transmittance properties. The two-fold improvement in the timolol loading was noted from the timolol-microemulsion soaking solution in comparison to timolol soaking solution. The flux report showed improvement in the release rate profiles of timolol-microemulsion soaking solution lenses (up to 48–96 *h*) in comparison to timolol soaking solution lenses (up to 24 – 36 *h*) (124).

The rabbit tear fluid data of timolol-microemulsion soaking solution lenses showed an improvement in the timolol retention time in comparison to timolol soaking solution lenses and eye drop solution. The efficacy study in the rabbit model showed a peak and valley profile with eye drop therapy, while timolol-microemulsion soaking solution-2 contact lenses showed prolong reduction in intraocular pressure for 96 *h* (124).

A novel type of contact lens device has been designed (125). Therein are embedded microtubes that act as drug containers. This device can provide a simple, noninvasive, extended drug release up to 45 *d* with higher bioavailability and lower risk for adverse effects.

Another unique feature of the device is the release of drug triggered by stretching of the contact lens, indicating the possibility of achieving a self-adaptive drug release device for treating glaucoma patients (125).

4.6.2 *Dexamethasone*

The release duration of dexamethasone from commercial contact lenses by loading Vitamin E into the lenses has been investigated (126). Dexamethasone with the systematic name: (11-β,16-α)-9-fluoro-11,17,21-trihydroxy-16-methylpregna-1,4-diene-3,20-dione is shown in Figure 4.21.

The Vitamin E was loaded into the lenses by soaking the lenses in a Vitamin E-ethanol solution followed by ethanol removal through evaporation.

The results showed that with about 30% of Vitamin E loading in the contact lens, the dexamethasone release time can be increased

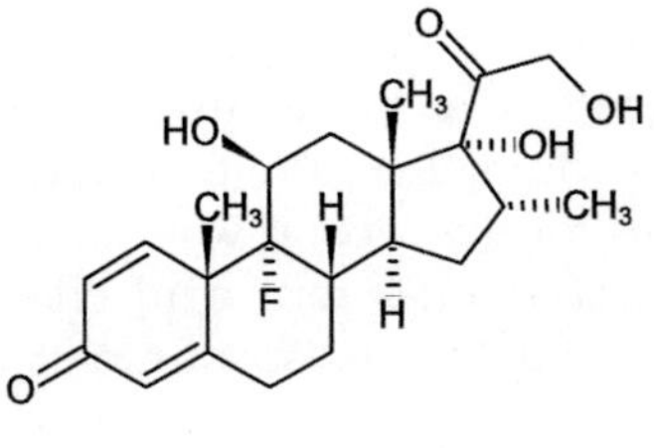

Figure 4.21 Dexamethasone.

from 7 *d* to 9 *d* for Acuvue®, Night & Day™, and O2 Optix™, which is a 9- to 16-fold increase compared to the dexamethasone release duration by pure contact lens without Vitamin E loading (126).

The dexamethasone delivery by contact lens can be viewed as a one-dimensional transport by a flat thin film, and a mathematical model based on the drug diffusivity difference between Vitamin E and silicone hydrogel was also proposed to explain the dexamethasone release time increase by Vitamin E-loaded contact lens (126).

4.6.2.1 *Ceria Particles*

Ceria particles in contact lenses can eliminate reactive oxygen species and harmful radicals to treat and prevent eye diseases caused by the reactive oxygen species and harmful radicals (127). A method for manufacturing a contact lens containing ceria particles has been described. The method consists of (128):

1. Preparing the ceria particles,
2. Preparing poly-HEMA in a form of crosslinked hydrogel,
3. Mixing the ceria particles and the monomer mixture for poly-HEMA with each other to form a mixture,
4. Injecting the mixture in a mold having a contact lens shape,
5. Performing a photocuring polymerization of the mixture, wherein the preparation of the poly-HEMA includes: Mixing of HEMA, EGDMA and deionized water to form a mixed solution, adding a photoinitiator into the mixed solution, and applying ultraviolet rays to the mixed solution.

The preparation of the ceria particles includes (128):

Preparation 4–1: Dissolving 6-aminohexanoic acid in distilled water to form a first solution. Heating the first solution to 90–100°C. Dissolving hydrochloric acid in the first solution, adjusting pH of the first solution to 5 to 6. Dissolving cerium (III) nitrate hexahydrate in distilled water at room temperature to form a second solution. Mixing the heated first solution and the second solution to form a mixed solution, and stirring the mixed solution; then cooling the mixed solution to room temperature.

It was observed that the elimination rate of the hydrogen peroxide varied depending on the amount of the water-soluble ceria nanocomposite contained in the contact lens.

4.6.2.2 *Gold Nanoparticles*

It has been found that timolol loading by the conventional soaking method does not significantly alter the critical properties of a contact lens (129). However, there are challenges of low drug loading and high burst release.

The effect of gold nanoparticles on the loading and its release kinetics from the contact lens using the soaking method was investigated (129). In one approach, gold nanoparticles were loaded into the timolol soaking solution. In another approach, gold nanoparticles were incorporated into the contact lenses during fabrication. The contact lenses were soaked at two different concentrations of timolol (i.e., 2 $mg\,ml^{-1}$ and 4 $mg\,ml^{-1}$).

Swelling and optical transmittance were not significantly affected by the presence of gold nanoparticles in the contact lenses. A significant uptake/loading of timolol using the gold nanoparticles in both of the approaches was observed. The *in-vitro* flux data showed no significant improvement in the release rate profiles of timolol when using both approaches. However, the *in-vivo* study in the rabbit tear fluid showed a high timolol concentration with the gold nanoparticle-laden contact lens at all time points in comparison to the soaked contact lenses without gold nanoparticles.

The *in-vivo* pharmacodynamic study in rabbits showed a 2 $mmHg$ average fall in intraocular pressure (72 h) using the gold nanoparticle-laden contact lenses, while the soaked contact lenses without gold nanoparticles and eye drops solution (0.5% w/v) showed 2 $mmHg$. The drug distribution study in the ocular tissue showed a significant improvement in the drug deposition with the gold nanoparticle-laden contact lenses in the ciliary muscle and conjunctiva (129).

So, it could be successfully demonstrated that gold nanoparticles enhance the uptake of drug from the drug soaking solution to treat glaucoma without compromising the critical properties of the contact lens.

Furthermore, the limitation of the conventional soaking method of low drug loading and high burst release from the contact lenses could be overcome (129).

Drug-laden contact lenses that are prepared by traditional soaking technique show a poor drug uptake, high burst release, and altered critical lens properties (130). The effect of gold nanoparticles on ketotifen uptake from a drug-soaking solution and its release kinetics from the lens was investigated.

The Turkevich method was used to synthesize the gold-laden nanoparticles. This method involves the reduction of chloroauric acid (HAuCL4) with trisodium citrate dehydrate salt (131). First, 3.39 *mg* of chloroauric acid ($HAuCl_4$) was dissolved in 10 *ml* of purified water to obtain 1 *mM* chloroauric acid. Then, the solution of chloroauric acid was heated (100°C) using a hot plate, followed by the addition of 1 *ml* of trisodium citrate (1% w/v) under continuous stirring. Trisodium citrate is shown in Figure 4.22. The color of the solution mixture changed from pale yellow to ruby red, indicating the synthesis of the gold-laden nanoparticles (130).

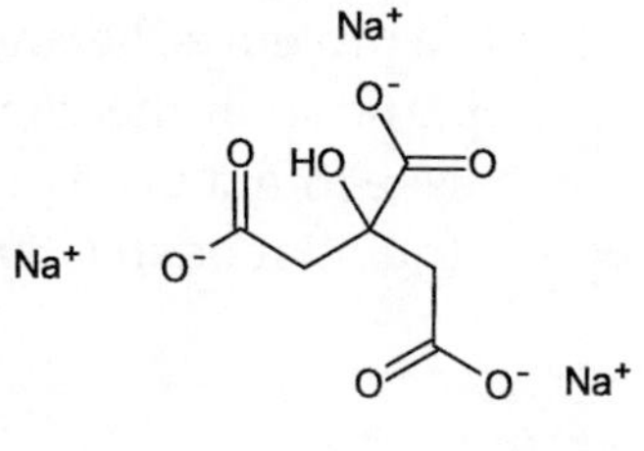

Figure 4.22 Trisodium citrate.

Blank silicone contact lenses were fabricated using a monomer mixture that is shown in Table 4.3. Poly(propylene) (PP) molds and an ultraviolet transilluminator were used to fabricate the contact lenses, with a diameter of 14.2 *mm* and a base curve of 6.5 *mm*. The excess monomer solution was added to the female mold and the

Table 4.3 monomer mixture for silicone contact lenses (130, 132).

Monomer	Amount/[% v/v]
Ethylene glycol dimethacrylate (EGDMA)	0.01
Dimethyl acrylamide (DMA)	30
N-Vinyl-2-pyrrolidone (NVP)	0.01
Siloxane	0.0025
Irgacure	0.02
2-Hydroxyethyl methacrylate (HEMA)	up to 100

male mold was placed over it, followed by curing at 360 *nm* for 20 *min*. The blank lenses were removed and stored in a desiccator at 45% humidity, until further treatment followed. To fabricate gold nanoparticle-laden contact lenses, 10 *mM* gold nanoparticles were added to the monomer mixture. The gold nanoparticles were spherical, with an average diameter of 17.2 *nm* and a zeta potential of $-21.2\,mV$.

Ketotifen was loaded into the blank contact lenses by soaking. Furthermore, ketotifen was loaded into blank contact lenses using drug-loaded gold nanoparticles soaking solution.

The swelling, oxygen permeability, and optical transmittance were improved when compared to lenses prepared by a traditional soaking method. The ability to sustain ketotifen release profile improved proportionally with an increase in the amount of gold nanoparticles in the lens. The protein adherence was reduced with the presence of gold nanoparticles in the contact lens. The gold nanoparticles-laden lenses were found to be safe in ocular irritation and histopathology reports (rabbit model) (130).

4.6.3 *Ketotifen Fumarate*

The successful *in-vivo* extended release of a small molecular weight therapeutic, ketotifen fumarate, from molecularly imprinted, therapeutic contact lenses could be demonstrated (133).

Ketotifen fumarate is the fumarate salt of ketotifen, a cycloheptathiophene derivative with anti-allergic activity. Ketotifen fumarate is shown in Figure 4.23.

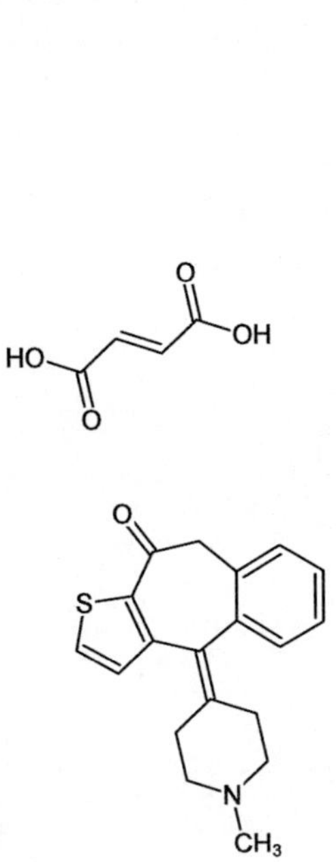

Figure 4.23 Ketotifen fumarate.

Here, a steady, effective concentration of drug is maintained in the tear film from a contact lens for an extended period of time for the entire duration of lens wear. Poly(HEMA-*co*-AA-*co*-AM-*co*-N-VP-co-PEG200DMA) soft contact lenses were prepared (100±5 μm thickness, diameter 11.8 mm, power zero), and a constant tear film concentration of 170±30 $\mu g\, ml^{-1}$ was measured for up to 26 h in a New Zealand white rabbit model.

The concentration of ketotifen fumarate in the tear fluid as a function of time for different lenses and eye drops is shown in Figure 4.24.

The results of the study showed a dramatic increase in ketotifen mean residence time and bioavailability compared to topical drop therapy and drug-soaked lenses. The mean residence time for imprinted lenses was 12.47±3.99 h, around 4- and 50-fold greater than non-imprinted lenses and 0.035% eye drops (Zaditor®), respectively. The results indicate that molecular imprinting provides an exciting rational engineering strategy for sustained release. It is clear that imprinted lenses are very promising combination devices and are much more effective and efficient delivery devices than eye drops (133).

In another study, the usefulness of silicone hydrogel contact lens-

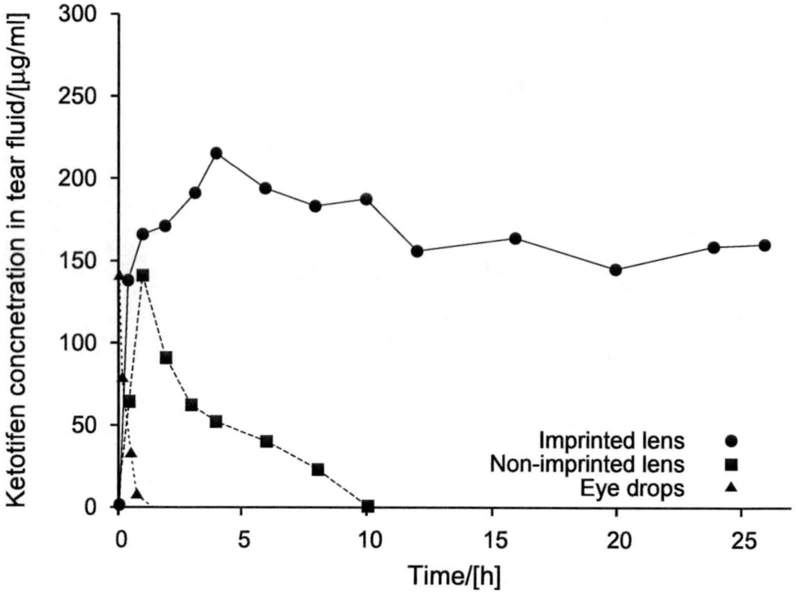

Figure 4.24 Ketotifen fumarate in the tear fluid as a function of time (133).

es loaded with ketotifen fumarate for ocular drug delivery was assessed (95).

First, silicone contact lenses were prepared by photopolymerization of a bitelechelic methacrylated poly(dimethyl siloxane)s macromonomer, TRIS, cf. Figure 4.27, and DMA using EGDMA as crosslinking agent and Darocur 1173 as an initiator. Then a surface plasma treatment was applied.

The formulations of the contact lenses are shown in Table 4.4.

The silicone hydrogel matrices of the contact lenses were characterized by equilibrium swelling ratio, tensile tests, ion permeability, and surface contact angle (95).

Finally, the contact lenses were loaded with ketotifen fumarate by presoaking in drug solution to evaluate drug loading capacity and *in-vitro* and *in-vivo* release behavior of the silicone contact lenses. The results showed that the equilibrium swelling ratio and the ion permeability increased, and the surface contact angle and tensile strength decreased with the increase of the DMA component in the silicone hydrogel. The drug loading and *in-vitro* releases were dependent on the hydrogel composition of hydrophilic/hydrophobic phase of the contact lenses. The cumulative release of ketotifen fu-

Table 4.4 Formulations of the contact lenses (95).

	Compound/[g]				
Sample	DMA	MA-PDMS-MA	TRIS	EGDMA	Hexanol
SCL 1	0.2472	0.3212	0.2498	0.0041	0.2046
SCL 2	0.2054	0.3212	0.2498	0.0039	0.1941
SCL 3	0.1408	0.3212	0.2498	0.0036	0.1780

DMA:	*N,N*-Dimethyl acrylamide
MA-PDMS-MA:	Bitelechelic methacrylated poly(dimethyl siloxane)
TRIS:	3-Methacryloxypropyltris(trimethylsiloxy)silane
EGDMA	Ethylene glycol dimethacrylate

marate from the silicone hydrogel contact lenses is shown in Figure 4.25.

In rabbit eyes, the presoaked contact lenses sustained ketotifen fumarate release for more than 24 h, which leads to a more stable drug concentration and a longer mean retention time in tear fluid than that of eye drops of 0.05% (95).

4.6.4 *Ciprofloxacin*

Model silicone hydrogel materials were created using a molecular imprinting strategy to deliver the antibiotic ciprofloxacin (84, 85).

Ciprofloxacin is an antibiotic used to treat a number of bacterial infections (134). It can be taken by mouth, as eye drops, as ear drops, or intravenously (135).

Ciprofloxacin or 1-cyclopropyl-6-fluoro-4-oxo-7-(1-piperazinyl)-1,4-dihydro-3-quinolinecarboxylic acid is shown in Figure 4.26.

As basic components, HEMA, EGDMA, AA, acetic acid, TRIS and ciprofloxacin-HCl were used. 3-Methacryloxypropyl-tris(trimethylsiloxy) silane is shown in Figure 4.27.

Model silicone hydrogel materials were created using a UV-induced polymerization process. Acetic acid and acrylic acid were used as functional monomers to interact with a ciprofloxacin template to efficiently create recognition cavities within the final polymerized material.

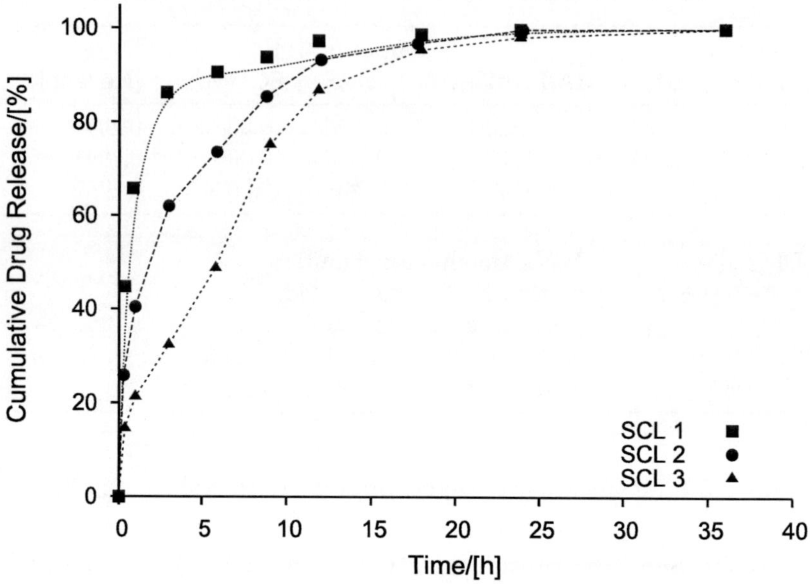

Figure 4.25 Cumulative release of ketotifen fumarate (95).

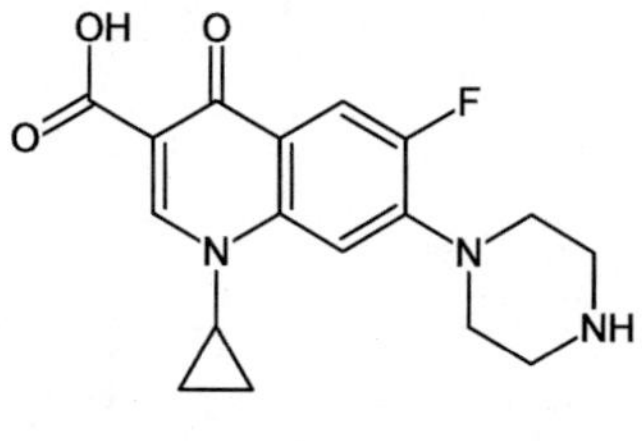

Figure 4.26 Ciprofloxacin.

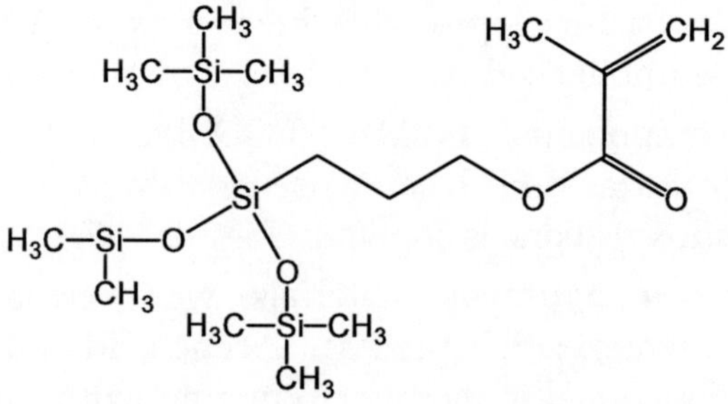

Figure 4.27 3-Methacryloxypropyltris(trimethylsiloxy) silane.

The synthesized materials were loaded with 9.06 *mM*, 0.10 *mM* and 0.025 *mM* solutions of ciprofloxacin, and the release of ciprofloxacin into an artificial tear solution was monitored over time.

The materials were shown to release for periods varying from 3 *d* to 14 *d*, depending on the loading solution, functional monomer concentration and the functional monomer:template ratio. Materials with a greater monomer:template ratio (8:1 and 16:1 imprinted) tended to release for longer periods of time. Materials with a lower monomer:template ratio (4:1 imprinted) tended to release comparatively greater amounts of ciprofloxacin into solution, but the release was somewhat shorter.

The total amount of drug released from the imprinted materials was sufficient to reach levels relevant to inhibit the growth of common ocular isolates of bacteria. This work is one of the first to demonstrate the feasibility of molecular imprinting in model silicone hydrogel-type material (84).

4.6.4.1 *Prototype Contact Lenses*

Prototype contact lenses were created by coating poly(lactic-*co*-glycolic acid) (PLGA) films containing test compounds with poly-*HEMA* by ultraviolet light polymerization. In detail, the preparation of the PLGA films can be done as follows (136):

Preparation 4–2: To create the drug-polymer film, PLGA was dissolved in 15 *ml* of ethyl acetate. Fluorescein was added to the solution and mixed to form a fine suspension inside the PLGA solution. Films were created with 118 *kDa* (high) and 18 *kDa* (low) molecular mass PLGA polymers and various ratios of PLGA to fluorescein. The suspension was poured into a fluoropolymer (Teflon) well. The ethyl acetate was removed by evaporation in a fume hood with laminar air flow overnight, then lyophilized for 48 *h*. Rings with a 14 *mm* outer diameter and a 5 *mm* central aperture were punched out of the fluorescein-PLGA film. Ciprofloxacin films were created by solvent casting, using PLGA 65:35 (118 *kDa* molecular mass) and a 1:1 ratio of medication to PLGA (20 *mg* ciprofloxacin and 20 *mg* PLGA).

Then, the drug-polymer film in poly-*HEMA* was coated by UV polymerization as follows (136):

Preparation 4–3: The monomer HEMA (11.6 *ml*) and the crosslinking agent EGDMA 44 μl were dissolved in 8.6 *ml* of deionized water. Then, 100

μl of 0.1 $g\,ml^{-1}$ photoinitiator (Irgacure 2959, Ciba) in dimethyl sulfoxide was added and the resulting solution was degassed under nitrogen for 40 *min*. Next, 160 μl of that solution was transferred into a 100 μm deep cylindrical rubber mold (16 *mm* diameter), covered with a glass slide, and placed in a nitrogen-filled plastic bag. The solution was then polymerized with a 305 *nm* UV lamp for 60 *min* to form the bottom poly-HEMA layer of the composite contact lens. The drug PLGA films were manually pressed onto the dried poly-HEMA gel. They were then placed together into a custom-made cylindrical rubber mold (450 μm deep by 16 *mm* in diameter), which was subsequently filled with the HEMA monomer photoinitiator solution and UV polymerized. The resultant contact lens prototype consisted of a thin drug PLGA film coated on all sides with poly-*HEMA* with a total thickness of 450 μm and a 16 *mm* outside diameter.

The films, containing encapsulated fluorescein or ciprofloxacin, were characterized by scanning electron microscopy.

Release studies were conducted in phosphate-buffered saline at 37°C with continuous shaking. The elution of ciprofloxacin from the contact lens was studied in an antimicrobial assay to verify antimicrobial effectiveness. After a brief and minimal initial burst, the prototype contact lenses demonstrated a controlled release of the molecules studied, with zero-order release kinetics under infinite sink conditions for over 4 weeks.

The rate of drug release was controlled by changing either the ratio of drug to PLGA or the molecular mass of the PLGA used. Both the PLGA and the poly-*HEMA* affected release kinetics. Ciprofloxacin released from the contact lenses inhibited ciprofloxacin-sensitive *Staphylococcus aureus* at all time points tested. So, a prototype contact lens for sustained drug release consisting of a thin drug-PLGA film coated with poly-*HEMA* could be used as a platform for ocular drug delivery with widespread therapeutic applications (136).

4.6.5 *Ofloxacin*

Ofloxacin is an antibiotic compound that is useful for the treatment of a number of bacterial infections (137). Ofloxacin was first patented in Japan (Daichi Laboratory) (138, 139). Ofloxacin (9-Fluoro-3-methyl-10-(4-methyl-1-piperazinyl)-7-oxo-2,3-dihydro-7H-[1,4]oxazino[2,3,4-ij]quinoline-6-carboxylic acid) is shown in Figure 4.28. It was shown in a previous study that two antibacterial ocular drugs, ofloxacin and neomycin, were only poorly loaded to poly-HEMA-based contact lenses (140). Neomycin is shown in Figure 4.28.

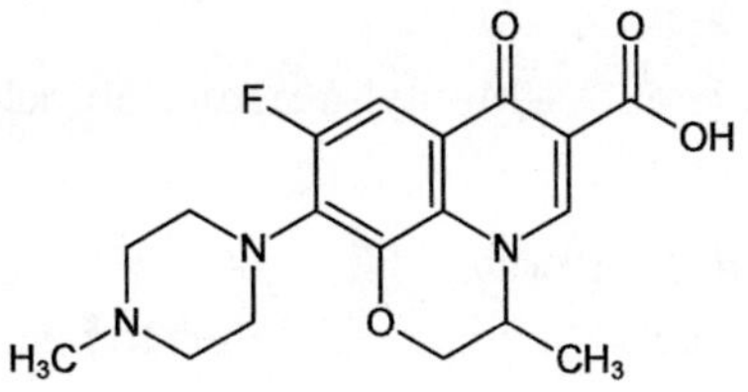

Ofloxacin

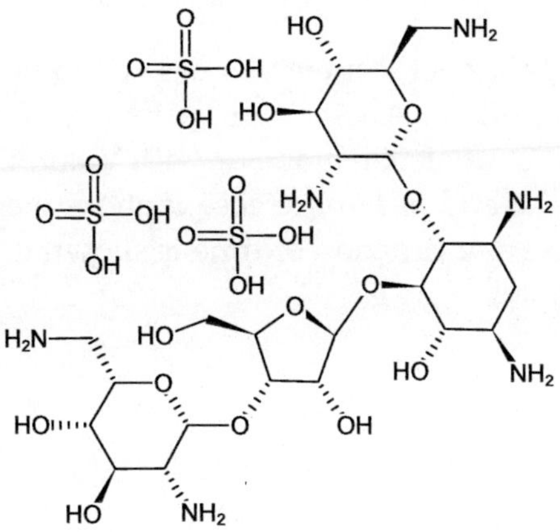

Neomycin

Figure 4.28 Antibacterial ocular drugs.

Then, it was investigated whether the alteration of the lens composition using several negatively charged comonomers can enhance loading of ocular drugs with a poor loadability of ofloxacin and neomycin. As comonomers, MA, AA, and 4-methyl-4-pentenoic acid were used for the synthesis of hydrogel-based contact lenses (140). 4-Methyl-4-pentenoic acid is shown in Figure 4.29.

Contact lenses containing these comonomers exhibited an increase in loading of ofloxacin and neomycin. In particular, compared with poly-HEMA contact lenses, contact lenses containing 2.5 mol% AA exhibited an enhanced loading of ofloxacin and neomycin,

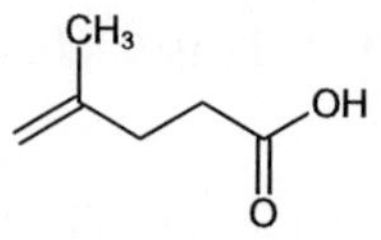

Figure 4.29 4-Methyl-4-pentenoic acid.

18 and 53 times, respectively. Charge interactions between the comonomers and the drug were considered to be the primary factors in the substantial increase of the drug loading (140).

The effectiveness of ofloxacin-loaded contact lenses as prolonged release devices for the treatment of bacterial keratitis was investigated (141).

Two silicone hydrogel contact lenses, Senofilcon A (Acuvue Oasys®) and Narafilcon A (Acuvue TruEye®) were modified by the incorporation of ofloxacin alone or with Vitamin E.

The drug uptake and *in-vitro* release kinetics were investigated. The *in-vitro* release as a function of time is shown in Figure 4.30.

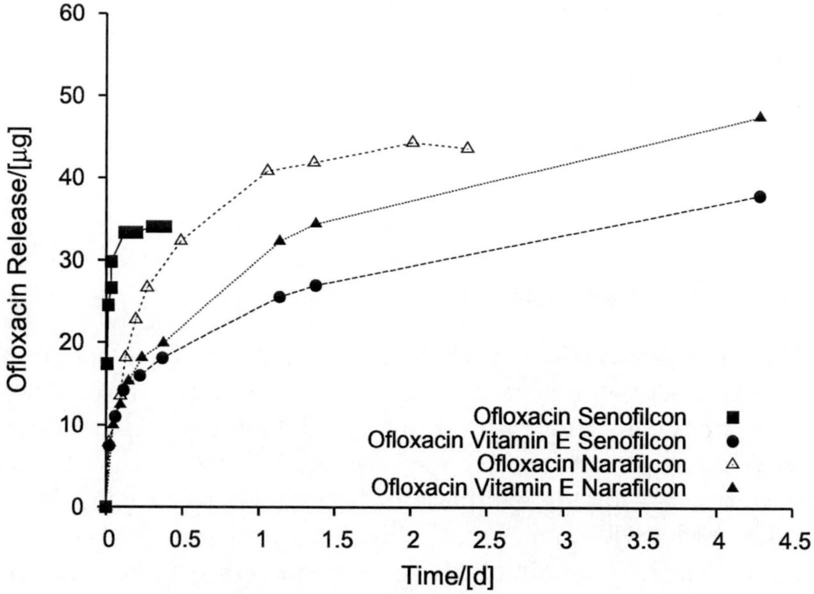

Figure 4.30 *In-vitro* release as a function of time (141).

The antibacterial efficacy was assessed against *Staphylococcus au-*

reus and *Pseudomonas aeruginosa* in an *ex-vivo* rabbit corneal model. The *in-vitro* studies showed a higher uptake ($p<0.05$) and a longer duration of release by Narafilcon A lenses compared to the Senofilcon A lenses. The addition of Vitamin E led to a significant increase in the duration of release ($p<0.05$) for both lenses (141).

The *ex-vivo* studies confirmed the effectiveness of the ofloxacin-loaded lenses in the reduction of bacterial load to clinically insignificant levels and ofloxacin-Vitamin E-loaded Narafilcon A lenses in the reduction of bacteria on the corneas to undetectable levels.

So, antibiotic-loaded lenses are effective in the treatment of ocular infections. Incorporation of Vitamin E will sustain this effect and eliminate the need for multiple instillations of eye drops (141).

4.6.6 *Polymyxin B and Vancomycin*

Drug-soft contact lens combination products were developed that are suitable for the controlled release of antimicrobial peptides on the ocular surface (101).

The incorporation of functional monomers and the application of molecular imprinting techniques were explored to endow HEMA hydrogels with the ability to load and to sustain the release of polymyxin B and vancomycin. Polymyxin B is shown in Figure 4.31. Vancomycin is shown in Figure 4.32.

Various ratios of HEMA and functional monomer crosslinking agents molar ratios were evaluated to prepare polymyxin B imprinted and non-imprinted hydrogels.

Acrylic acid functionalized and imprinted hydrogels loaded greater amounts of polymyxin B and led to more sustained release profiles, in comparison to non-functionalized and non-imprinted networks.

Polymyxin B-loaded hydrogels showed good biocompatibility in hen's egg chorioallantoic membrane tests. Functionalized hydrogels also loaded vancomycin and sustained its release, but the imprinting effect was only exhibited with polymyxin B, as demonstrated in rebinding tests.

Microbiological assays carried out with *Pseudomonas aeruginosa* allowed identification of the most suitable hydrogel composition for efficient bacteria eradication (101).

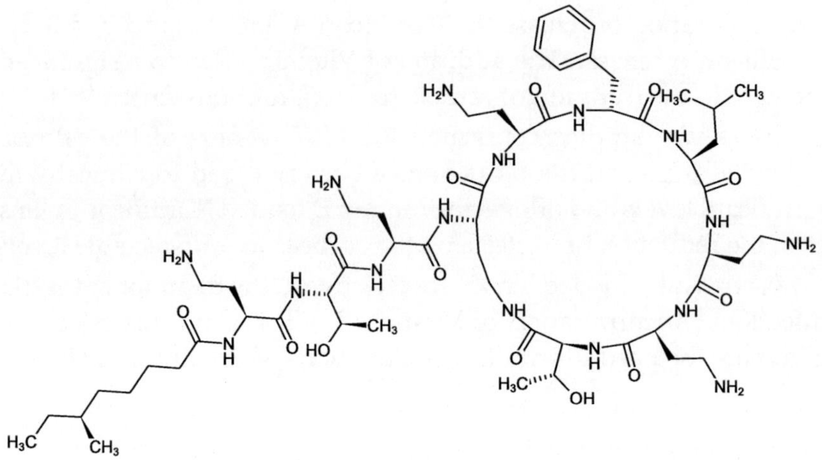

Figure 4.31 Polymyxin B.

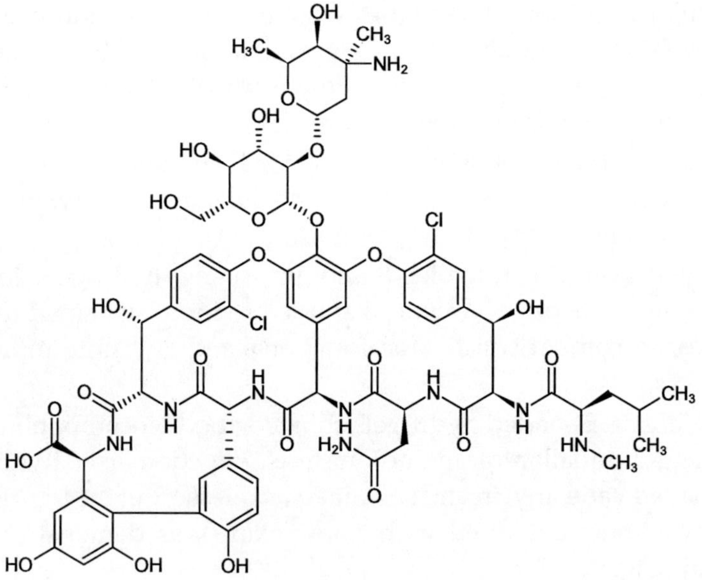

Figure 4.32 Vancomycin.

4.6.7 *Epinastine*

Epinastine is a second-generation antihistamine and mast cell stabilizer that is mainly used in eye drops to treat allergic conjunctivitis (142). Epinastine (9,13b-dihydro-1H-dibenzo[c,f]imidazo[1,5-a]azepin-3-amine) is shown in Figure 4.33.

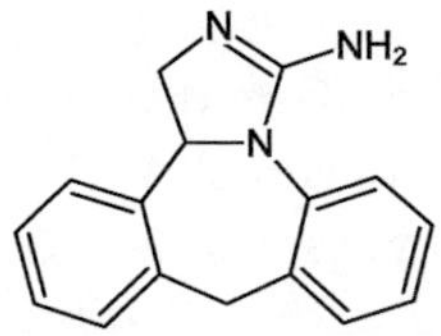

Figure 4.33 Epinastine.

Epinastine hydrochloride-releasing daily soft contact lenses for treatment of allergic conjunctivitis were developed (143).

Preformed soft contact lenses with or without ionic functional groups were soaked in a solution of epinastine hydrochloride in phosphate-buffered saline to prepare epinastine hydrochloride-releasing soft contact lenses.

Among these contact lenses with different ionicities, anionic lenses demonstrated the maximum, relatively linear epinastine hydrochloride release, *in-vitro*. The amount of epinastine hydrochloride release was directly proportional to the concentration of the epinastine hydrochloride solution used to prepare the contact lens.

The epinastine hydrochloride-releasing anionic soft contact lens also demonstrated a prolonged drug release and significantly greater efficacy compared with epinastine hydrochloride eye drops 12 *h* after treatment, *in-vivo* (143).

4.6.8 *Lactoferrin*

Lactoferrin is an iron-binding protein with an antioxidant activity. The amount of lactoferrin is significantly reduced in the lacrimal film of patients affected by keratoconus in comparison to healthy subjects. This is suspected to be the cause for tear iron increase and consequent iron deposition and oxygen free radical accumulation in the cornea (144). A study was conducted on whether lactoferrin-loaded contact lenses could exert an antioxidant activity on epithelial cells incubated in tears collected from patients affected by keratoconus.

Reflex tears were collected during the first 2 *min* of light or onion-induced lacrimation and stored at −20°C. After incubation in tears for 18 *h*, the mortality of epithelial cells was investigated by the trypan blue exclusion test. Epithelial cells incubated with reflex tears of keratoconus patients showed an increased mortality compared to epithelial cells maintained in control healthy tears. This difference in mortality was correlated with tear iron concentration.

The application of lactoferrin-loaded contact lenses counteracted keratoconus tear cytotoxicity, restoring viability obtained in the presence of control tears. Therapeutic contact lenses obtained by lactoferrin loading can reduce the oxidative stress induced by the tears of a patient and might represent an efficient device to arrest the progression of keratoconus (144).

4.6.9 *Bimatoprost*

Bimatoprost is widely used for the management of glaucoma. Bimatoprost is shown in Figure 4.34.

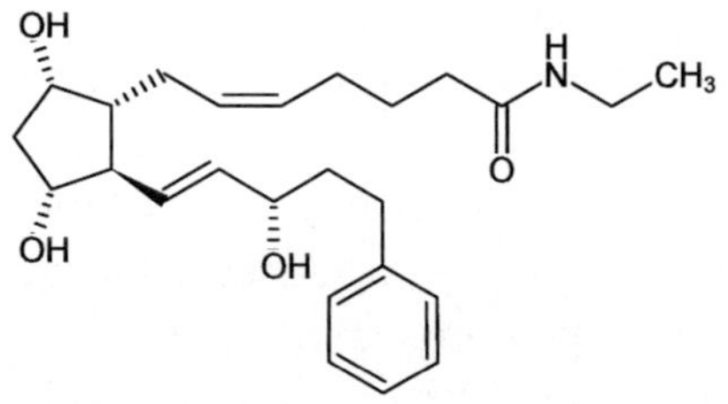

Figure 4.34 Bimatoprost.

Currently, bimatoprost is delivered via an eye drop solution, which is highly inefficient due to low bioavailability (100). To control the release of ocular drugs, contact lenses are used. However, the conventional soaking method showed a high burst release due to absence of any efficient controlling membrane.

A molecular imprinting technology was applied to improve the loading of bimatoprost from the soaking solution and to sustain the release of drug from the contact lens. The bimatoprost was loaded by conventional soaking method (BT-SM) and compared with the molecular imprinted contact lenses (BT-MP). The loading of bimatoprost by molecular imprinting technology affects the swelling of the contact lens. However, the batch BT-MP-10 did not show significant alterations.

The uptake study showed an improvement in the bimatoprost loading by the molecular imprinting technology in comparison to the conventional soaking technology. The *in-vitro* bimatoprost release data showed improvement in the bimatoprost release rate profiles with BT-MP contact lenses (up to 36–60 *h*) in comparison to BT-SM contact lenses (up to 24–36 *h*).

In-vivo rabbit tear fluid data with BT-MP batch showed an improvement in the bimatoprost retention time in comparison to BT-SM contact lens and eye drop solution (100).

The effect of a microemulsion on the bimatoprost uptake from the soaking solution and its effect on the drug release kinetics was investigated (99). The contact lenses were soaked in bimatoprost-microemulsion soaking solution and compared with the bimatoprost-soaking solution without microemulsion.

The uptake of bimatoprost-microemulsion in the contact lenses did not alter the swelling, transmittance and folding endurance properties. The two-fold increase in the uptake/loading of bimatoprost was noted from the bimatoprost-microemulsion soaking solution in comparison to bimatoprost soaking solution. The *in-vitro* flux data of microemulsion batches (up to 48–96 *h*) showed an improvement in the release rate profiles in comparison to soaking solution batches (up to 24–36 *h*). The *in-vivo* studies in the rabbit tear fluid showed low burst release and improvement in the bimatoprost retention time with microemulsion contact lens in comparison to the soaking solution contact lens and eye drop solution. The study demonstrates the potential of a microemulsion to improve the uptake of bimatoprost and sustain release kinetics without altering the critical lens properties of the contact lens (99).

4.6.10 Dipicolylamine

Corneal melting is an uncontrolled, excessive degradation of cellular and extracellular components of the cornea (145). This potential cause of corneal blindness is caused by excessive expression of zinc-dependent matrix metalloproteinases and as of now has no satisfying cure.

A therapeutic hydrogel was introduced that can be made into a contact lens to slow down the progression of corneal melting by deactivating matrix metalloproteinases. The hydrogel backbone contains a poly-HEMA, a main material for commercial contact lenses, and dipicolylamine, which has high affinity for and selectivity toward zinc ion. Dipicolylamine is shown in Figure 4.35.

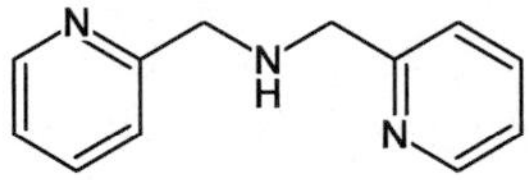

Figure 4.35 Dipicolylamine.

The dipicolylamine-conjugated poly- HEMA poly(dipicolylamine-HEMA) hydrogel selectively removes zinc ions from a physiological buffer and deactivates matrix metalloproteinase-1, matrix metalloproteinase-2, and matrix metalloproteinase-9 within 2 *h*.

The hydrogel also effectively prevents the degradation of porcine corneas by collagenase A, a zinc-dependent protease, whereas the cornea completely degrades within 15 *h* when incubated with poly-HEMA hydrogel.

The presence of this hydrogel does not affect the viability of keratocytes and corneal epithelial cells. Unlike the conventional matrix metalloproteinase inhibitors, the poly(dipicolylamine-HEMA) hydrogel minimizes the risk of serious nonspecific side effects and provides a method to slow down the progression of corneal melting and other related ocular diseases (145).

4.6.11 Gatifloxacin

The loading of gatifloxacin in contact lenses affects critical lens properties, such as optical and swelling properties, owing to drug precipitation in the contact lens matrix (146). Gatifloxacin is an antibiotic of the fluoroquinolone family (147). Gatifloxacin (1-cyclopropyl-6-fluoro-8-methoxy-7-(3-methyl-1-piperazinyl)-4-oxo-1,4-dihydro-3-quinolinecarboxylic acid) is shown in Figure 4.36.

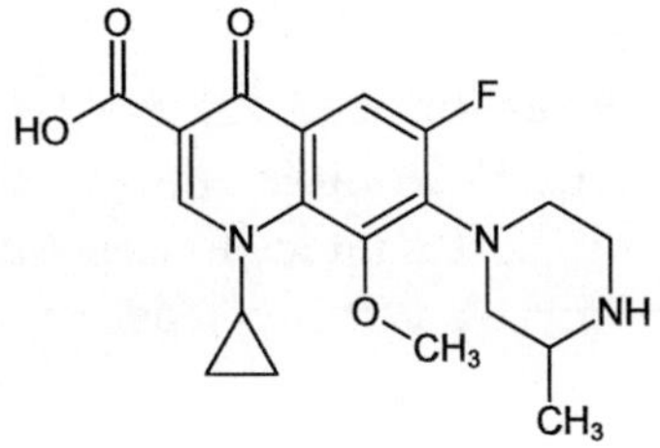

Figure 4.36 Gatifloxacin.

The presence of Pluronic® F-68 in the packaging solution creates *in situ* micelles in the contact lens to dissolve gatifloxacin precipitates and provide a sustained drug release (148).

The micelles can also improve the drug uptake from the drug-packaging solution to create an equilibrium of drug between the lens matrix and the packaging solution. Gatifloxacin-pluronic-loaded contact lenses were optimized to achieve the desired optical transmittance, swelling, and gatifloxacin loading capacity as well as sustained drug delivery (146).

The optimization of the gatifloxacin-pluronic-loaded contact lenses was carried out using a 32 factorial design by tailoring the concentration of Pluronic F-68 in the packaging solution and the amount of gatifloxacin in the monomer solution to achieve the desired lens properties.

The optimized batch with 0.3%w/v Pluronic F-68 in the packaging solution and 0.3%w/v gatifloxacin in the monomer solution showed an optical transmittance of 92.84%, a swelling of 92.36% and a gatifloxacin loading capacity of 92.56 μg. The *in-vitro* flux data of the optimized batch showed a sustained release up to 72 h, whereas soaked contact lenses and direct gatifloxacin-loaded contact lenses showed a sustained release of up to 48 h.

The *in-vivo* gatifloxacin release data for a rabbit tear fluid showed a sustained release with a high gatifloxacin level for the lens in comparison to the soaked contact lenses and the eye drop solution (146).

4.6.12 *Hydroxypropyl Methylcellulose*

Symptoms of contact lenses-induced dry eye (CLIDE) can be treated through the application of macromolecular rewetting agents via eye drops (91). Therapeutic soft contact lenses can be formulated to alleviate CLIDE symptoms by slowly releasing a comfort agent from the lens.

An extended wear silicone hydrogel contact lens has been developed with extended, controllable release of 120 *kDa* HPMC using a molecular imprinting strategy.

A commercial silicone hydrogel lens was tailored to release approximately 1000 μg of HPMC over a period of up to 60 d in a constant manner at a rate of 16 $\mu g\, d^{-1}$ under physiological flow rates, releasing over the entire range of continuous wear. The release rates could be significantly varied by the imprinting effect and functional monomer to template ratio (M/T) with M/T values 0, 0.2, 2.8, and 3.4 corresponding to HPMC release durations of 10, 13, 23, and 53 days, respectively. The lenses had a high optical quality and adequate mechanical properties for their usage as contact lenses (91).

Thus, silicone hydrogel lenses have a potential for imprinting procedures to release macromolecules for the duration of wear, which may lead to decreased CLIDE symptoms and more comfortable contact lenses (91).

4.6.13 *Dorzolamide*

Dorzolamide is a carbonic anhydrase inhibitor. It lowers the intraocular pressure by reducing aqueous humor formation. It is formulated as a 2% eye drop for use in the management of glaucoma and ocular hypertension (149). Dorzolamide is shown in Figure 4.37.

A series of imprinted and non-imprinted hydrogels were prepared using HEMA as a backbone monomer, *EGDMA* as crosslinking monomer, MA as a functional monomer and dorzolamide as the template molecule (88).

Different concentrations of MA (0, 100, 200, 400 *mM*) were used for the preparation of the non-imprinted hydrogels. Two

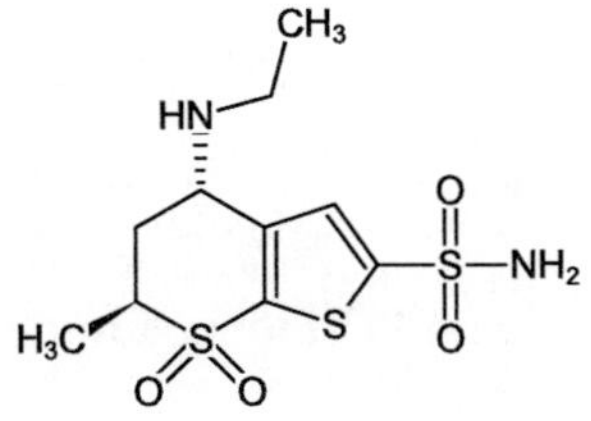

Figure 4.37 Dorzolamide.

dorzolamide:MA molar ratios of 1:8 and 1:4 and 400 *mM M.A* were also applied in the imprinting process.

The hydrogels with a thickness of 0.4 *mm* were synthesized by a thermal polymerization at 50°C in 24 *h* in a PP mold. The mold was made from two PP plates. Then, the swelling and binding properties of hydrogels were evaluated in water. The monomer-template interactions provide specific binding sites in imprinted cavities for the dorzolamide template molecule.

Their loading and releasing properties were also studied in 0.9% NaCl and in an artificial lachrymal fluid. The results showed that using MA as comonomer and applying the molecular imprinting technique increased loading capacity of the hydrogels. The optimized imprinted hydrogel (MIP1:4), prepared with 400 *mM* MA and dorzolamide:MA molar ratio of 1:4, had the highest affinity for dorzolamide and the greatest ability to control the release process in aqueous media.

These data indicated that the use of suitable comonomer and applying a molecular imprinting technique had important influence on loading and releasing properties of hydrogels (88).

4.6.14 *Ethoxzolamide*

Ethoxzolamide is a sulfonamide that inhibits the carbonic anhydrase activity in proximal renal tubules to decrease reabsorption of water, sodium, potassium, and bicarbonate (150). Ethoxzolamide (6-ethoxy-1,3-benzothiazole-2-sulfonamide) is shown in Figure 4.38.

The reduction in carbonic anhydrase also reduces the intraocular pressure in the eye by decreasing aqueous humor (150).

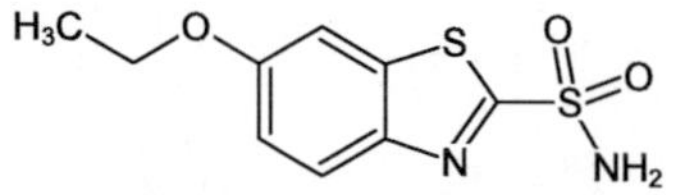

Figure 4.38 Ethoxzolamide.

It was found that partitioning of drugs into networks synthesized from multiple functional monomers was 8 times greater than networks synthesized from single monomers (83).

One-dimensional permeation studies showed that the gel with maximum incorporated chemical functionality had the lowest diffusion coefficient, which was one to two orders of magnitude lower than all other gels studied. All imprinted networks showed significantly lower diffusion coefficients than non-imprinted networks, in spite of comparable mesh sizes and equilibrium polymer volume fractions in the swollen state (83).

Hydrogels with high affinity for carbonic anhydrase inhibitor drugs have been designed that try to mimic the active site of the physiological metallo-enzyme receptor (89).

Using HEMA as the backbone component, zinc methacrylate, 1-vinylimidazole or 4-vinylimidazole, and *N*-hydroxyethyl acrylamide, cf. Figure 4.39, were combined in different ratios to reproduce in the hydrogels the cone-shaped cavity of the carbonic anhydrase, which contains a Zn^{2+} ion coordinated to three histidine residues. *L*-Histidine is shown in Figure 4.39. 4-Vinylimidazole resembles the histidine functionality better than 1-vinylimidazole, and, consequently, pHEMA-ZnMA2 hydrogels bearing 4-vinylimidazole moieties were those with the greatest ability to host acetazolamide or ethoxzolamide (2 to 3 times greater network/water partition coefficient) and to sustain the release of these antiglaucoma drugs (50% lower release rate estimated by fitting to the square root kinetics) (89).

The use of acetazolamide as template during polymerization did not enhance the affinity of the network for the drugs. In addition to the remarkable improvement in the performance as controlled release systems, the biomimetic hydrogels were highly cytocompatible and possessed adequate oxygen permeability to be used as medicated soft contact lenses or inserts (89).

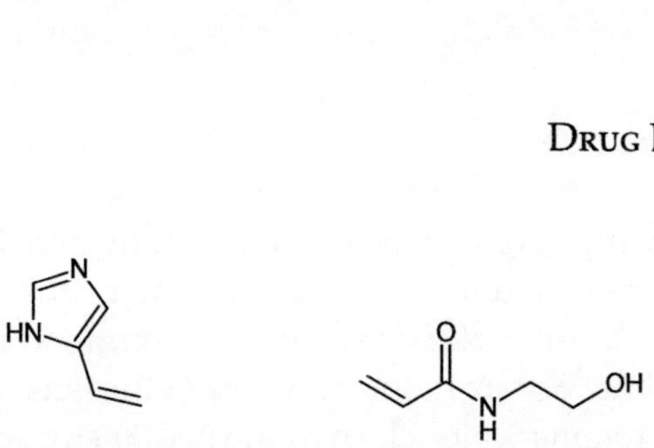

4-Vinylimidazole *N*-Hydroxyethyl acrylamide

Figure 4.39 Monomers for hydrogels.

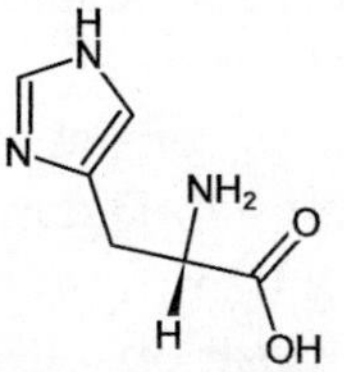

Figure 4.40 *L*-Histidine.

4.6.15 *Hyaluronic Acid*

Hyaluronic acid (HA) has been used as a topically delivered artificial tear solution for over 20 years (151), and it has a proven track record for the treatment of ocular discomfort and dry eye syndrome (152–154). HA is shown in Figure 4.41.

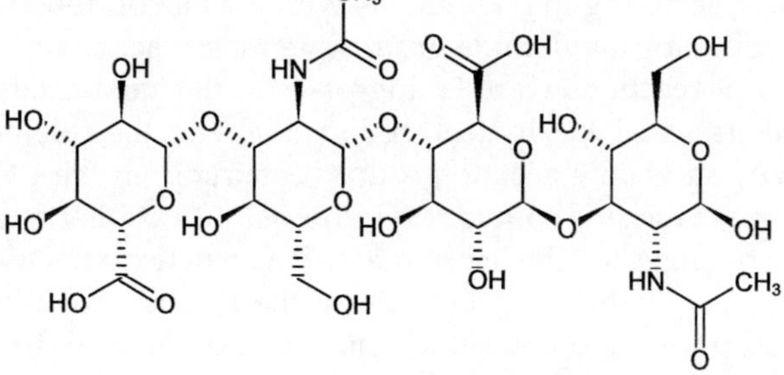

Figure 4.41 Hyaluronic acid.

The viscoelasticity of HA enhances the tear stability, and it slows tear removal by decreasing the flow rate. HA is also mucoadhesive and interacts with ocular mucins when delivered to the surface of the eye. When a contact lens is present in the eye, HA may cover the lens as an *artificial mucin* and counteract the tear film destabilization that occurs in the presence of the lens. Because HA is hygroscopic, it retains water close to the ocular surface and reduces the dehydration.

Biomimetic soft contact lenses were produced using functional monomers and a commercial lens formulation known as nelfilcon A (155). Nelfilcon A contact lenses are daily disposable lenses, although such lenses have been tested with wear over multiple days (156).

Nelfilcon A hydrogel lenses consist of biocompatible poly(vinyl alcohol) (PVA) macromers crosslinked into a network structure (90). PVA contains hydroxyl (–OH) groups attached to a repeating polymeric backbone in the 1,3 position. It is synthesized by the acid hydrolysis of poly(vinyl acetate). The 1,3-hydroxyl groups are positioned to undergo a cyclic acetal formation upon the reaction with aldehydes. This is a highly useful mechanism for the attachment of moieties necessary for the hydrogel formation. The synthesis was described as follows (90):

Preparation 4–4: First, a diacetal with acrylate functionality, *N*-acryloylaminoacetaldehyde dimethylacetal, was synthesized by reacting aminoacetaldehyde with acryloyl chloride in a low-temperature alkaline aqueous solution. After neutralization and extraction, the crude product was purified through molecular distillation. In the second step, PVA was transacetylized with *N*-acryloylaminoacetaldehyde dimethylacetal, cf. Figure 4.42, resulting in PVA chains with a well-controlled number of pendant crosslinking acrylamide groups per macromer chain.

A number of reactions were taking place at this acid catalyzed stage: The crosslinkers acetal was hydrolyzed to aldehyde, the aldehyde reacted with the PVA, and some acetate groups remaining on the PVA from its synthesis were converted to hydroxyl groups. Atmospheric oxygen was used as the stabilizer for the acrylamide. The reaction was quenched by neutralizing with alkali. The polymer was then purified by ultrafiltration to the desired purity and concentration. As photoinitator, Irgacure 2959 was then added to the purified polymer.

To prepare a prepolymer mixture, 5 *g* of the nelfilcon A formulation, containing the modified PVA macromer, was mixed with 32.5 *mg* of HA sodium salt in a 15 *ml* centrifuge tube (the ratio of 6.5 *mg* HA per *g* nelfilcon A was the same for all gels studied). The functional monomers acrylamide, *N*-vinyl pyrrolidone and 2-(diethylamino)ethyl methacrylate were added to prepare the imprinted hydrogels. The mixture was repeatedly stirred, centrifuged (30 *min* to 1 *h* at a time, a minimum of four times), and rested overnight to dissolve the HA in the prepolymer until homogeneous. The mixture was finally centrifuged for 5 *min* to 10 *min* to remove air bubbles.

Some compounds that are used in Preparation 4–4 are shown in Figure 4.42. Irgacure 2959 is also known as 2-hydroxy-1-[4-(2-hydroxyethoxy)phenyl]-2-methyl-1-propanone.

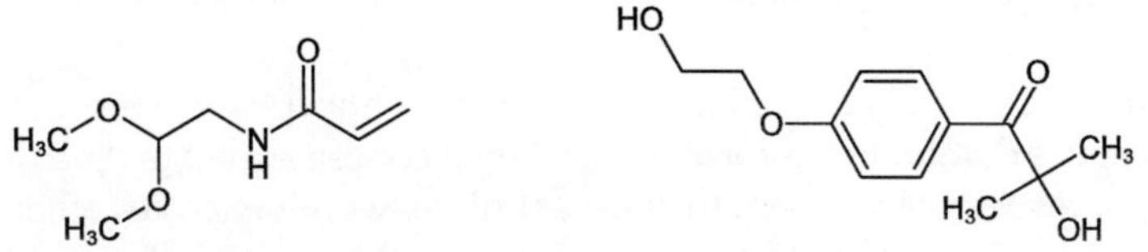

N-Acryloylaminoacetaldehyde dimethylacetal

Irgacure 2959

Figure 4.42 Compounds used in Preparation 4–4.

The cumulative release of HA from non-imprinted Nelfilcon A hydrogel is shown in Figure 4.43.

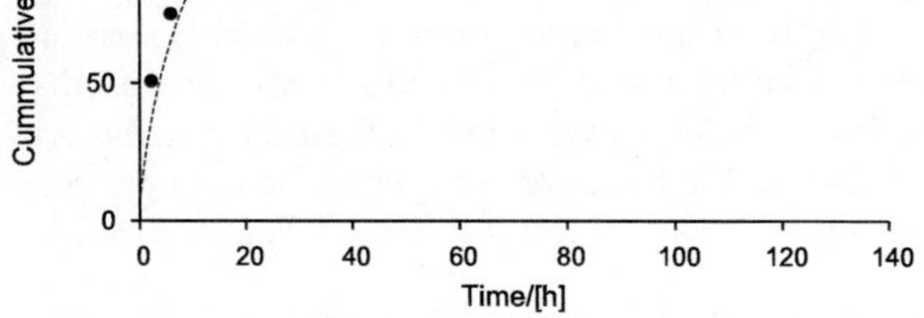

Figure 4.43 Cumulative release of hyaluronic acid (90).

The release profile demonstrates a Fickian kinetics over 5 *d*, with three distinct release rates (90).

The initial rate lasts about 6 *h* to 10 *h* with a release rate of around 12 $\mu g h^{-1}$. The intermediate region from 6 to 30 *h* shows a nearly linear release profile, delivering around 4 $\mu g\,h^{-1}$. After about 2 *d*, the release rate significantly tapers off until it is negligible (90).

A ring-implanted PVA contact lens was fabricated and evaluated as a therapeutic contact lens with respect to the potential of sustained release of HA (157). HA was loaded on chitosan nanoparticles and then the HA-loaded nanoparticles were dispersed in a ring-shaped PVA hydrogel which is implanted in the final PVA contact lens.

HA-loaded nanoparticles were formed by an ionotropic gelation technique (158) as follows:

Preparation 4–5: Hyaluronic acid and tripolyphosphate were dissolved in ultrapure distilled water to achieve a final concentration of 0.625 and 0.5 $mg\,ml^{-1}$, respectively. Then, the two solutions were mixed together in the mass ratio of 7.5:1. The chitosan solution with 0.625 $mg\,ml^{-1}$ concentration was prepared by dissolving a certain amount of the polymer in a 2% w/v acid acetic solvent (at a pH of 4 and 5), then it was slowly mixed with HA-tripolyphosphate solutions in a mass ratio of 1:1. After constant stirring for 15 *min* at room temperature, the nanoparticles were isolated by centrifugation (15 000 *g*, 20 *min*). The weight ratio of the loaded HA to nanoparticle was 0.21. The nanoparticles were collected and kept at 4°C for further experiments and analysis.

The nanoparticles-loaded ring implant was fabricated by dispersing a certain amount of nanoparticles in the PVA solution.

Preparation 4–6: Here, a 8% PVA solution was prepared by dissolving a given amount of the polymer in distilled water at 90°C for 3 *h*. Next, 1.4 *mg* of nanoparticles containing 0.3 *mg* HA were dispersed into the solution by mild stirring, and the solution was cast into a designed ring-shaped mold and exposed to three freeze-thaw cycles: 8 *h* freeing at −20°C and 4 *h* thawing at 20°C. The ring-shaped Teflon mold with 6 *mm* inner diameter and 8 *mm* outer diameter and 50 μm width was prepared by the CNC method based on a design presented in a study by Maulvi and others (159). After finishing the freeze-thaw cycles, the nanoparticle-embedded hydrogel ring implant was carefully removed from the mold.

The fabrication and the preparation of the ring-implanted contact lenses and and the hydrogel-based ring implant are illustrated in Figure 4.44.

The results of the study showed that HA was successfully loaded on nanoparticles (520 ± 18 *nm*) with a loading efficacy of 87% and a loading capacity of 50%. The contact lens hydrogel has a

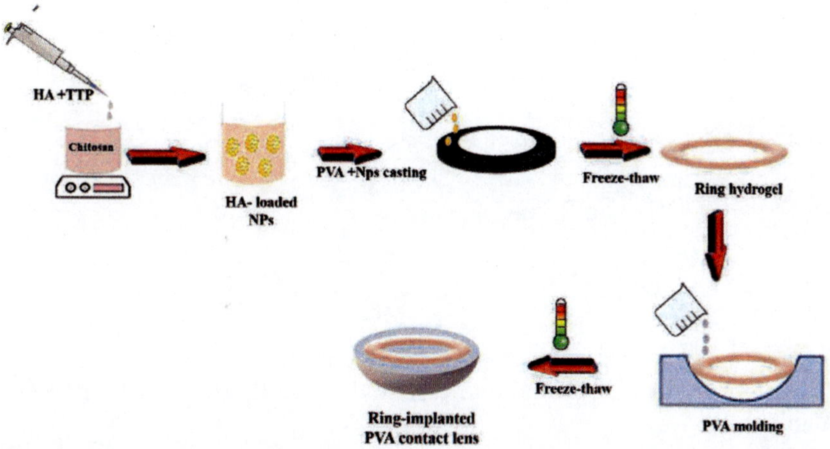

Figure 4.44 Preparation of the ring-implanted contact lenses, reprinted from *Macromolecular Bioscience* (157).

275% swelling ratio, no degradation during 14 *d*, 97% light transmittance, and desirable rheological stability under physiological shear force. The release data showed a sustained release for HA from the ring-implanted contact lens up to 14 *d*. The cellular study revealed no corneal epithelial cell cytotoxicity and cell attachment on the contact lens. So, the study demonstrated the successful application of the ring-implanted contact lens to sustain the delivery of HA for treating dry eye syndrome (157).

4.6.16 *Lifitegrast*

Lifitegrast is an FDA-approved drug that inhibits T-cell mediated inflammation associated with dry eye syndrome (160). This compound is shown in Figure 4.45.

Lifitegrast is a potent inhibitor of the interaction between LFA-1 on T-cells and ICAM-1 on endothelial cells at the ocular surface. It is effective in treating dry eye syndrome, but 5% (81.2 *mM*) lifitegrast has low drug utilization and elicits off-target effects.

Contact lenses have been developed to release therapeutically relevant doses of lifitegrast to every tear film for up to 10 *h*. Here, lifitegrast is coupled to the polymer of the soft hydrogel lens via a photolabile crosslinking agent. Exposures of the lens to wavelengths of 400–430 *nm* of indoor daylight excite the caged molecules

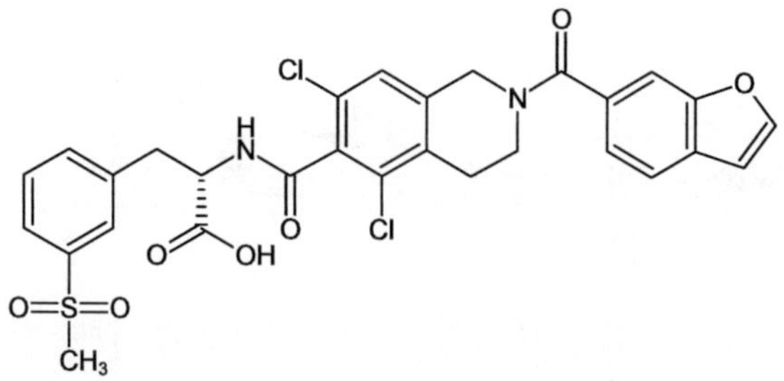

Figure 4.45 Lifitegrast (*N*-[[2-(6-Benzofuranylcarbonyl)-5,7-dichloro-1,2,3,4-tetrahydro-6-isoquinolinyl]carbonyl]-3-(methylsulfonyl)-*L*-phenylalanine).

and trigger a bond-cleavage reaction that releases authentic lifitegrast passively to the tear film. The photoproduct of the reaction remains chemically linked to the polymer of the single-use lens. The studies show that passive exposures of the lens to indoor light would generate an average of 990 *nM* lifitegrast to every tear film in a zero-order reaction for up to 10 *h*.

The amount of released lifitegrast from the lens increases during exposure to outdoor sunlight. Over a 10 *h* exposure to indoor light, a single lens would release 0.44% of the lifitegrast present in two drops of commercial 5% lifitegrast. Compared to tear-drop approaches, such engineered lenses would sustain the passive delivery of therapeutically relevant doses of lifitegrast over a longer period, and exhibit improved drug utilization at a lower cost. This technology can be easily integrated into daily-use contact lenses in order to prevent inflammation at the ocular surface, dry eye and contact lens-mediated discomfort (160).

4.6.17 Diclofenac Sodium

Molecularly imprinted, therapeutic contact lenses capable of controlled release of non-steroidal anti-inflammatory diclofenac sodium were synthesized, exploiting ionic non-covalent interactions (161). Diclofenac sodium (sodium 2-[(2,6-dichlorophenyl)amino]phenylacetate) is shown in Figure 4.46.

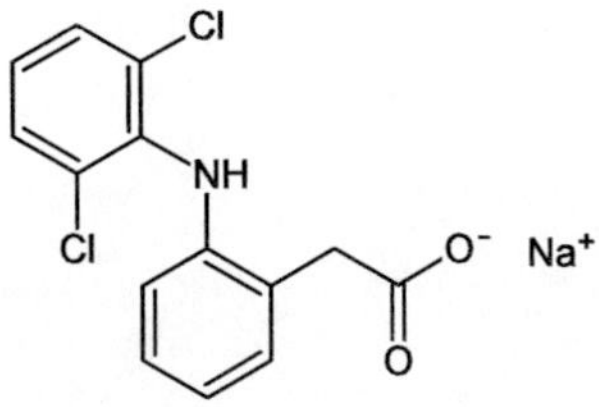

Figure 4.46 Diclofenac sodium.

Poly(HEMA-*co*-DEAEM-*co*-PEG200DMA) soft contact lenses were prepared with 105±0.2 *mm* thickness, a diameter of 15.0±0.2 *mm*, and base curve of 8.6±0.2 *mm* with different monomer to template ratios. Dynamic release studies were conducted in artificial lacrimal solution using two different *in-vitro* methods.

Under infinite sink conditions, imprinted contact lenses demonstrated concentration-dependent release kinetics. Under physiological flow rates, by increasing the monomer to template (M/T) ratio from 1 to 10.5, the release rate decreased from 11.72 $\mu g\, h^{-1}$ to 6.75 $\mu g\, h^{-1}$ (161) during the first 48 *h*. The release rate was more constant, moving toward zero-order release. To use these lenses as daily disposable lenses, the first 24 *h* of release was studied and found to be linear with a rate of 17.27, 11.99, and 8.74 $\mu g\, h^{-1}$ for M/T ratios of 1, 3.5, and 10.5, respectively.

The release of diclofenac sodium as a function of the monomer to template (M/T) ratio is shown in Figure 4.47.

Furthermore, the lenses prepared with a M/T ratio of 10.5 released diclofenac at a rate close to the maximum dose delivered by commercial eye drops, making them ideal for use as daily disposable lenses, and potentially leading to better patient benefit with substantially increased efficacy (161).

The *in-vitro* release of diclofenac sodium from contact lenses based on poly-HEMA hydrogels containing an embedded microemulsion to extend release duration was evaluated (162).

The oil-in-water microemulsion systems are prepared with two non-ionic surfactants, Brij 97 or Tween 80, together with a long-alkyl chain cationic surfactant, cetalkonium chloride. Cetalkonium chloride is shown in Figure 4.48. Without cetalkonium chloride, Brij 97

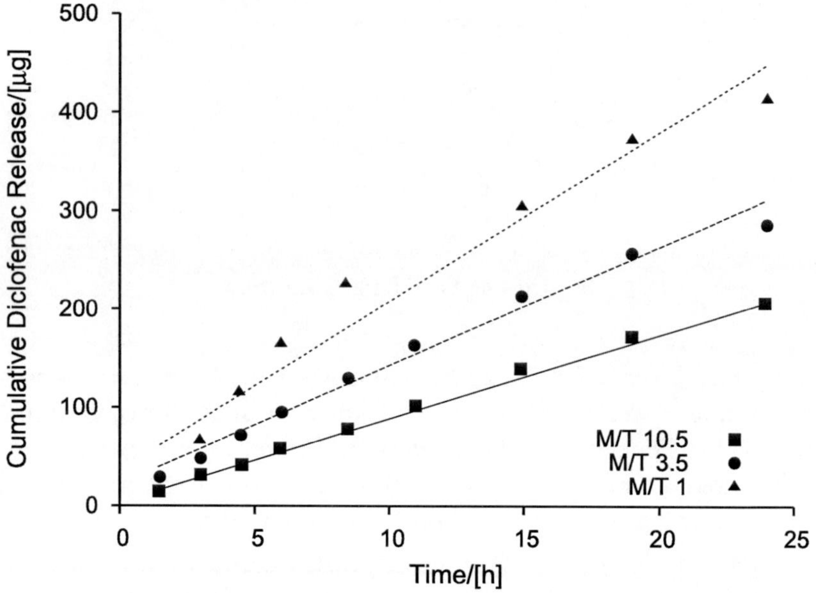

Figure 4.47 Release of diclofenac sodium vs. (M/T) ratio (161).

or Tween 80-based microemulsions showed average droplet sizes of 12 *nm* and 18 *nm*, respectively. The addition of cetalkonium chloride decreased the average droplet sizes to 2 *nm* to 5 *nm* for both non-ionic surfactants (162).

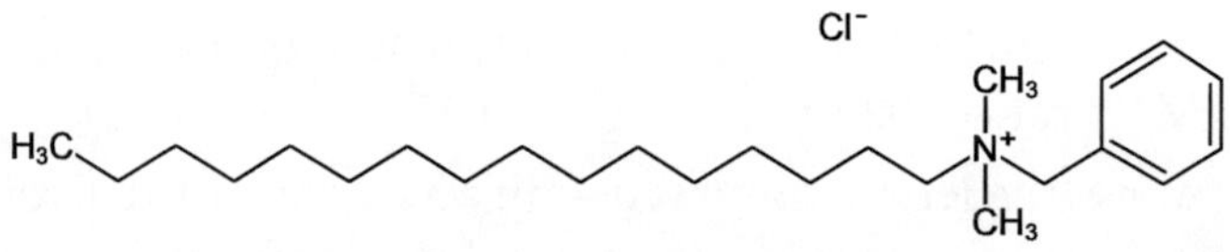

Figure 4.48 Cetalkonium chloride.

Such a significant reduction in the average droplet size corresponds to an increase in the diclofenac sodium release duration, as revealed by the *in-vitro* experiments. The optical transparency and water content of Brij 97-based contact lenses with cationic microemulsions were excellent. However, the optical transparency of the corresponding Tween 80-based contact lenses was unsatisfactory.

These results indicate that cationic microemulsion-laden contact lenses can benefit from combinatory effects of microemulsions and cationic surfactant at low cetalkonium chloride weight percentage.

4.6.18 *Moxifloxacin*

Moxifloxacin is an antibiotic drug that is used to treat a number of bacterial infections. Moxifloxacin is shown in Figure 4.49.

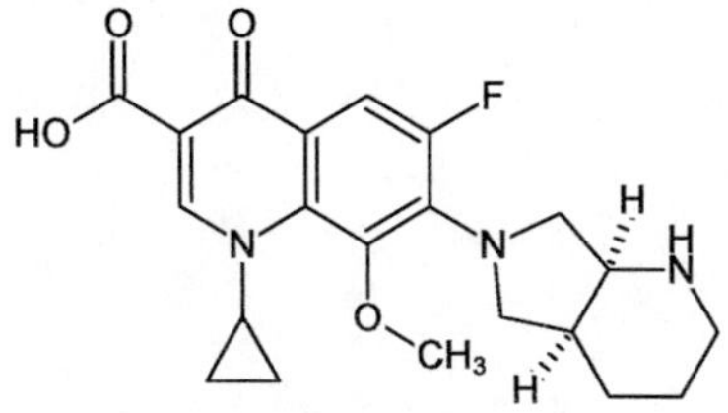

Figure 4.49 Moxifloxacin.

A silicon-based (TRIS) hydrogel was prepared as reported (163). A composition containing TRIS (*N*-[Tris(trimethylsiloxy) silylpropyl]acrylamide), acrylic acid, and a functional monomer that may establish potential interactions with moxifloxacin hydrochloride was also prepared (164). *N*-[Tris(trimethylsiloxy)silylpropyl]acrylamide is shown in Figure 4.50.

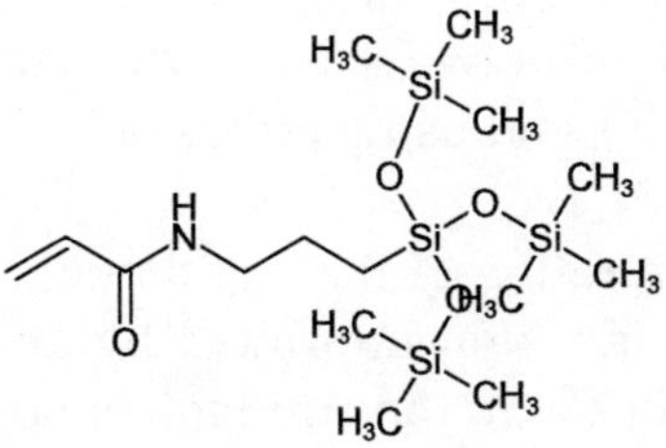

Figure 4.50 *N*-[Tris(trimethylsiloxy)silylpropyl]acrylamide.

The other employed co-monomers that were used are NVP, HEMA and AA, and moxifloxacin was used as the antibiotic drug.

After extensive washing, all hydrogels were loaded with the drug by soaking in moxifloxacin hydrochloride solution (2.5 $mg\,ml^{-1}$) at room temperature for 72 h. Release kinetics was investigated under sink conditions in NaCl solution. Transmittance, swelling and oxygen permeability were recorded.

Imprinted silicone hydrogels bearing acrylic acid were demonstrated to be able to host a large amount of moxifloxacin hydrochloride and provide a controlled release (164).

4.6.19 *Norfloxacin*

Poly(2-hydroxyethyl methacrylate) lenses with the ability to load norfloxacin and to control its release have been fabricated (98). Norfloxacin is shown in Figure 4.51.

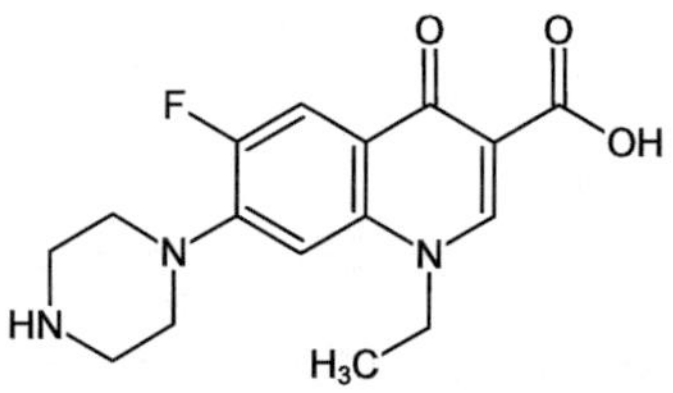

Figure 4.51 Norfloxacin.

Isothermal titration calorimetry studies revealed that a maximum binding interaction between norfloxacin and acrylic acid occurs at a 1:1 molar ratio, and that the process saturates at 1:4 molar ratio. Hydrogels were synthesized using different norfloxacin:acrylic acid molar ratios (1:2 to 1:16) at two fixed acrylic acid total concentrations (100 *mM* and 200 *mM*), and using molds of different thicknesses (0.4 *mm* and 0.9 *mm*).

The molar concentration of the crosslinking agent was 1.6 times of that of acrylic acid. Non-imprinted hydrogels as control were prepared similarly but with the omission of norfloxacin. All hydrogels showed a similar degree of swelling (55%) and, once hydrated, presented adequate optical and viscoelastic properties. After immersion in 0.025 *mM*, 0.050 *mM* and 0.10 *mM* drug solutions, imprinted hydrogels loaded greater amounts of norfloxacin than the non-imprinted ones.

Imprinted hydrogels synthesized using molar ratios of norfloxacin to acrylic acid of 1:3 and 1:4 have the greatest ability to control the release process, sustaining it for more than 24 *h*.

These results also prove that isothermal titration calorimetry is a useful tool for the optimization of the structure of the imprinted cavities in order to obtain efficient therapeutic soft contact lenses (98).

4.6.20 *Sparfloxacin*

Sparfloxacin is a fluoroquinolone antibiotic that is used in the treatment of bacterial infections. Sparfloxacin (5-Amino-1-cyclopropyl-7-(3,5-dimethyl-1-piperazinyl)-6,8-difluoro-4-oxo-1,4-dihydro-3-quinolinecarboxylic acid) is shown in Figure 4.52.

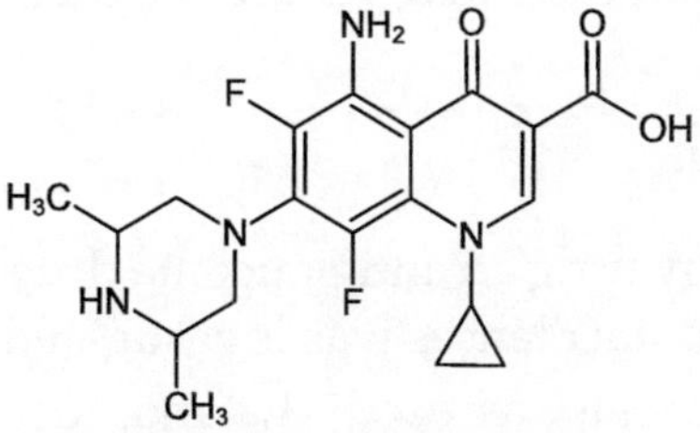

Figure 4.52 Sparfloxacin.

Currently, conjunctivitis is treated by frequent high-dose administration of a sparfloxacin eye drop solution (165).

However, such eye drops are inconvenient because of low bioavailability, short ocular drug residence time, and the need for frequent instillation, which lead to patient noncompliance affecting the routine lifestyle of patients.

Silicone contact lenses can be used to sustain the release of sparfloxacin (165). However, the presence of sparfloxacin alters the optical and physical properties of the contact lens.

To overcome these problems, a poly(*N*-vinyl-2-pyrrolidone) (PVP)-coated sparfloxacin-laden ring contact lens was designed to provide sustained ocular drug delivery without altering the optical and swelling properties of the contact lens. The ring was implanted within the periphery of the lens. Sparfloxacin was loaded by soaking, direct loading, and a ring casting method.

The PVP was coated on the surface of the contact lens by a novel short surface curing technique. The *in-vitro* sparfloxacin release data of soaking (up to 12-36 *h*) and loading batches directly (up to 12-24 *h*) showed high burst release, whereas a ring casting batch showed sustained release up to 36-48 *h* without significant ($p > 0.05$) alteration of the optical and swelling properties. All the batches showed sustained release of PVP up to 48 *h*. The *in-vivo* release studies in the rabbit tear fluid showed improvement in the sparfloxacin [>MIC for *Staphylococcus aureus*] and PVP retention time in comparison to an eye drop solution. The *in-vivo* efficacy study in the *S. aureus*-induced conjunctivitis showed improved healing effect with the single PVP-coated ring contact lens in comparison to the frequent high-dose sparfloxacin eye drop therapy. The study demonstrated the successful application to co-deliver sparfloxacin and PVP from the contact lens for an extended period to treat conjunctivitis (165).

4.6.21 Latanoprost

The potential of delivering an antiglaucoma drug using commercial silicone hydrogel contact lenses was investigated (166).

As drug, latanoprost was used. Latanoprost is sold under the brand name Xalatan, among others (167). It is used to treat increased pressure inside the eye. This includes ocular hypertension and open angle glaucoma. It is also applied as eye drops to the eyes. The onset of effects is usually within 4 *h*, and they last for up to 1 *d* (168). Common side effects include blurry vision, redness of the eye, itchiness, and darkening of the iris. Latanoprost is in the prostaglandin analogue family of medication. It works by increasing the outflow of aqueous fluid from the eyes through the uveoscleral tract (169). Latanoprost (isopropyl (5Z)-7-(1R,2R,3R,5S)-3,5-dihydroxy-2-[(3R)-3-hydroxy-5-phenylpentyl]cyclopentyl-5-heptenoate) is shown in Figure 4.53.

The moderately hydrophobic drug latanoprost was rapidly loaded in 4 *min* by swelling contact lenses in a solution of the drug in *n*-propanol.

A fraction of the drug was radiolabeled, thus allowing measurement of the uptake and subsequent release of drug into artificial tear fluid. The following issues were addressed (166):

1. How much drug can be loaded into each type of lens,
2. How fast is drug release, and

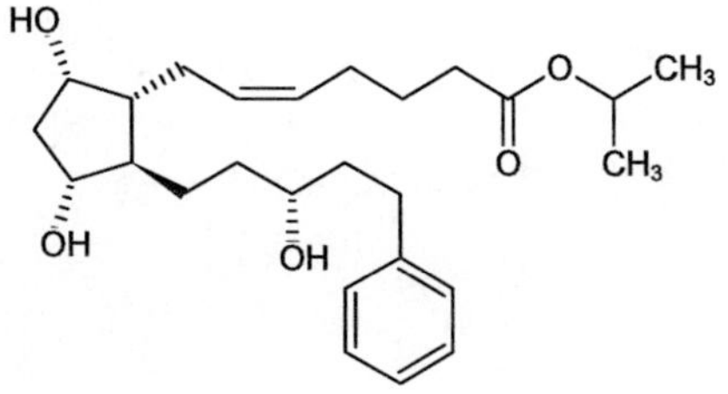

Figure 4.53 Latanoprost.

3. How are these values related to the contact lens chemistry.

The results showed that much more latanoprost could be loaded into silicone hydrogel lenses than a conventional contact lens of poly-HEMA. The drug uptake correlated with the amount of swelling in *n*-propanol, with Galyfilcon lenses having the greatest swelling and highest drug uptake (166).

The drug release from the silicone hydrogel lenses occurred over days, whereas the conventional lens released nearly all the drug in a burst over a few hours. To assess the correlations between lens chemistry, drug chemistry and uptake, and solvent chemistry, the Hansen solubility parameters were calculated using estimates of contact lens chemistry. The results showed that the drug uptake in silicone hydrogel lenses correlated with favorable solubility parameter interactions between the *n*-propanol and the lens material, but did not correlate with interactions between the drug and the lens materials (166).

4.6.22 *Loteprednol*

Loteprednol etabonate is a corticosteroid used to treat inflammations of the eye. Loteprednol etabonate is shown in Figure 4.54.

Topical corticosteroids are effective in reducing postoperative pain and inflammation following ocular surgery and have become a standard of care (170). However, ophthalmic use of these drugs can be associated with adverse effects, including elevation of intraocular pressure, cataract formation with prolonged use, infections, and delayed wound healing (171–174).

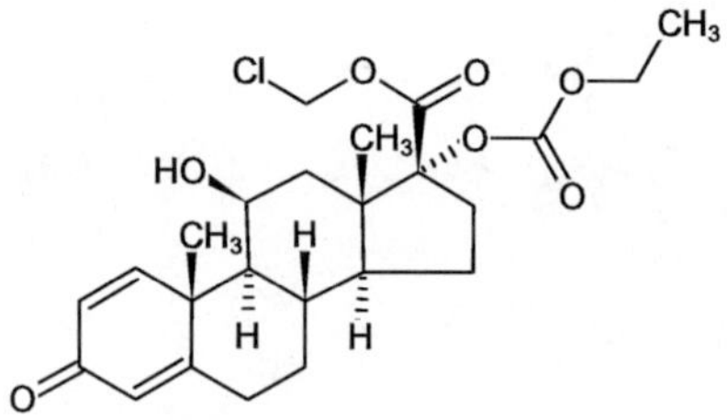

Figure 4.54 Loteprednol etabonate.

Loteprednol etabonate is a C_{20} ester-based topical ophthalmic corticosteroid that was retrometabolically designed to undergo a rapid hydrolysis into inactive metabolites after binding to the glucocorticoid receptor and exerting its anti-inflammatory effects (175, 176). This results in a corticosteroid with potent anti-inflammatory activity with a reduced risk of undesirable effects (170).

4.6.23 *Release of Multiple Therapeutics*

4.6.23.1 *Trehalose, Ibuprofen, Prednisolone, Hydroxypropyl methylcellulose*

The simultaneous release of four molecules from a new contact lens to ensure high level of lens wear comfort were assessed (92).

Silicone hydrogel contact lenses were engineered via molecular imprinting strategies to simultaneously release up to four template molecules including hydroxypropyl methylcellulose, trehalose, ibuprofen, and prednisolone. These compounds are shown in Figure 4.55.

Trehalose is an ingredient, along with HA, in an artificial tears product used to treat dry eye (177, 178). Prednisolone can be used for the treatment of severe acute and chronic allergic and inflammatory processes involving the eye (179).

By adjusting the ratio of functional monomer to the comfort molecule, a high level of control was demonstrated concerning the release rate. Hydroxypropyl methylcellulose, trehalose, ibuprofen, and prednisolone could be released in therapeutically relevant concentrations with varying rates from a single lens.

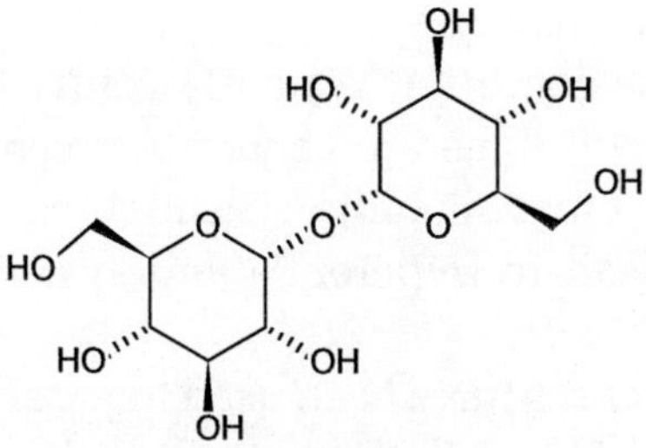

Trehalose

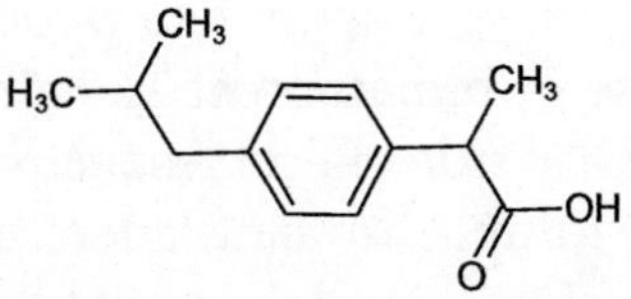

Ibuprofen

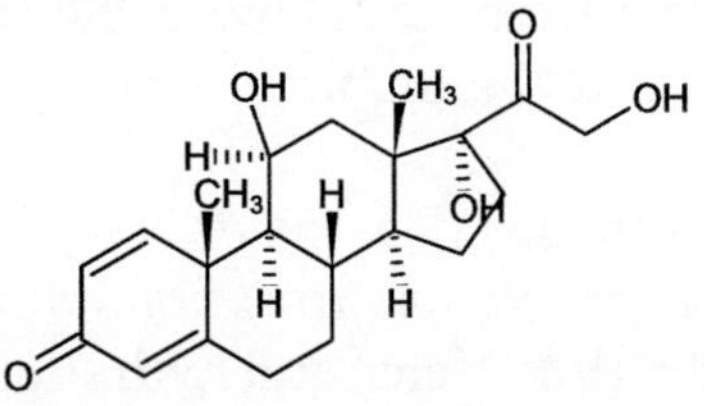

Prednisolone

Figure 4.55 Template molecules.

The results of the study indicate the use of the materials as daily disposable lenses for single day release or extended wear lenses with multiple day release. Imprinted lenses are expected to lead to a higher efficacy for patients compared to topical eye drops by improving compliance and mitigating concentration peaks and valleys associated with multiple drops (92).

4.6.23.2 *Timolol, Bimatoprost, Hyaluronic Acid*

A fixed combination of bimatoprost/timolol eye drop solution is used to manage the elevated intraocular pressure in glaucoma patients, including individuals whose condition is poorly controlled by monotherapy (132). Eye drop solutions are generally given in high dose, due to their poor ocular bioavailability. The high ocular dose of bimatoprost and timolol lead to hyperemia and systemic cardiac side effects respectively.

Multiple implant-laden contact lenses have been used to passively deliver timolol, bimatoprost and HA at therapeutically relevant doses without a high burst release. The drug-loaded implants were individually implanted in the outer periphery of the silicone contact lenses. Atomic force microscopy showed the smooth surface of the implant contact lens, as the implants were inside the contact lens matrix.

The implant lens showed a major loss of drugs during the monomer extraction and wet sterilization, while the option of dry radiation sterilization (IM-R lens) and hydration for 24 *h* prior to use showed a relatively lower loss of drugs. The loss of drugs is shown in Table 4.5.

Table 4.5 Loss of drugs (132).

Implant lens		Dry radiation sterilization lens	
Compound	Amount/[%]	Compound	Amount/[%]
Timolol	60.60	Timolol	16.87
Bimatoprost	61.75	Bimatoprost	47.95
Hyaluronic acid	46.03	Hyaluronic acid	24.41

The *in-vitro* drug release data of IM-R lens showed a sustained release for 72 *h*, with low burst release in comparison to the soaked and direct drug-laden contact lenses. The *in-vivo* drug release data in the rabbit tear fluid showed sustained release using IM-R lens in comparison to the soaked lens and eye drop therapy. The burst release with the IM-R lens was many folds reduced, which could bypass the side effects associated with multiple eye drop therapy.

The *in-vivo* pharmacodynamic study in the rabbit model showed peak and valley profile with multiple eye drop therapy, while IM-R lens showed prolonged reduction in intraocular pressure for 120 *h*. So, the application of implantation technology to deliver multiple drugs through contact lenses to treat glaucoma could be demonstrated (132).

References

1. J.B. Ciolino, C.H. Dohlman, and D.S. Kohane, Contact lenses for drug delivery, *Seminars in Ophthalmology*, Vol. 24, p. 156, 2009.
2. K. Singh, A.B. Nair, A. Kumar, and R. Kumria, Novel approaches in formulation and drug delivery using contact lenses, *Journal of Basic and Clinical Pharmacy*, Vol. 2, p. 87, March 2011.
3. C.J. White, A. Tieppo, and M.E. Byrne, Controlled drug release from contact lenses: A comprehensive review from 1965-present, *Journal of Drug Delivery Science and Technology*, Vol. 21, p. 369, 2011.
4. K.-H. Hsu, S. Gause, and A. Chauhan, Review of ophthalmic drug delivery by contact lenses, *Journal of Drug Delivery Science and Technology*, Vol. 24, p. 123, 2014.
5. H. Gupta and M. Aqil, Contact lenses in ocular therapeutics, *Drug Discovery Today*, Vol. 17, p. 522, 2012.
6. J. Xu, Y. Xue, G. Hu, T. Lin, J. Gou, T. Yin, H. He, Y. Zhang, and X. Tang, A comprehensive review on contact lens for ophthalmic drug delivery, *Journal of Controlled Release*, Vol. 281, p. 97, 2018.
7. F.A. Maulvi, T.G. Soni, and D.O. Shah, A review on therapeutic contact lenses for ocular drug delivery, *Drug Delivery*, Vol. 23, p. 3017, 2016.
8. F. Sartini, M. Menchini, C. Posarelli, G. Casini, and M. Figus, In vivo efficacy of contact lens drug-delivery systems in glaucoma management. A systematic review, *Applied Sciences*, Vol. 11, 2021.
9. X. Zhang, X. Cao, and P. Qi, Therapeutic contact lenses for ophthalmic drug delivery: Major challenges, *Journal of Biomaterials Science, Polymer Edition*, Vol. 31, p. 549, 2020.
10. Z. Mutlu, S. Shams Es-Haghi, and M. Cakmak, Recent trends in advanced contact lenses, *Advanced Healthcare Materials*, Vol. 8, p. 1801390, 2019.

11. S.B. Vedaga, S.B. Gondkar, and R.B. Saudagar, Contact lenses: A promising drug delivery system, *Journal of Drug Delivery and Therapeutics*, Vol. 9, p. 1105, June 2019.
12. G. Kim and H. Noh, Water soluble drug releasing soft contact lens in response to pH of tears, *Journal of Pharmaceutical Sciences and Research*, Vol. 36, p. 012057, 2016.
13. A. Hendi, M.U. Hassan, M. Elsherif, B. Alqattan, S. Park, A.K. Yetisen, and H. Butt, Healthcare applications of pH-sensitive hydrogel-based devices: A review, *International Journal of Nanomedicine*, Vol. 15, p. 3887, 2020.
14. G. Kim, H.J. Kim, and H. Noh, pH sensitive soft contact lens for selective drug-delivery, *Macromolecular Research*, Vol. 26, p. 278, 2018.
15. C. Wang and J. Park, Magnetic micropump embedded in contact lens for on-demand drug delivery, *Micro and Nano Systems Letters*, Vol. 8, p. 1, 2020.
16. J. Mun, J. won Mok, S. Jeong, S. Cho, C.-K. Joo, and S.K. Hahn, Drug-eluting contact lens containing cyclosporine-loaded cholesterol-hyaluronate micelles for dry eye syndrome, *RSC Advances*, Vol. 9, p. 16578, 2019.
17. C. Torres-Luna, N. Hu, X. Fan, R. Domszy, J. Yang, R.M. Briber, and A. Yang, Extended delivery of cationic drugs from contact lenses loaded with unsaturated fatty acids, *European Journal of Pharmaceutics and Biopharmaceutics*, Vol. 155, p. 1 , 2020.
18. I.S. Kurniawansyah, S.R. Mita, and K. Ravi, Drug delivery system by hydrogel soft contact lens materials: A review, *Journal of Pharmaceutical Sciences and Research*, Vol. 10, p. 254, 2018.
19. L. Yao and X. Niu, Polyolefin contact lens molds and uses thereof, US Patent 8 003 024, assigned to CooperVision International Holding Co. LP, August 23, 2011.
20. G. Jha and A. Kumar, Drug delivery through soft contact lenses: An introduction, *Chronicles of Young Scientists*, Vol. 2, p. 3, 2011.
21. X. Hu, L. Hao, H. Wang, X. Yang, G. Zhang, G. Wang, and X. Zhang, Hydrogel contact lens for extended delivery of ophthalmic drugs, *International Journal of Polymer Science*, Vol. 2011, p. 814163, 2011.
22. C. Alvarez-Lorenzo, H. Hiratani, and A. Concheiro, Contact lenses for drug delivery, *American Journal of Drug Delivery*, Vol. 4, p. 131, 2006.
23. R.C. Cooper and H. Yang, Hydrogel-based ocular drug delivery systems: Emerging fabrication strategies, applications, and bench-to-bedside manufacturing considerations, *Journal of Controlled Release*, Vol. 306, p. 29, 2019.
24. Q. Zhu and S. Mao, Enhanced drug loading efficiency of contact lenses via salt-induced modulation, *Asian Journal of Pharmaceutical Sciences*, Vol. 14, p. 204, 2019.

25. C.-C. Lin and A.T. Metters, Hydrogels in controlled release formulations: Network design and mathematical modeling, *Advanced Drug Delivery Reviews*, Vol. 58, p. 1379, 2006. Computational Drug Delivery.
26. A. Chauhan and C.-C. Li, Modeling ophthalmic drug delivery by soaked contact lenses, *Industrial & Engineering Chemistry Research*, Vol. 45, p. 3718, 2006.
27. R. Peterson, J. Wolffsohn, J. Nick, L. Winterton, and J. Lally, Clinical performance of daily disposable soft contact lenses using sustained release technology, *Contact Lens and Anterior Eye*, Vol. 29, p. 127, 08 2006.
28. L. Xinming, C. Yingde, A.W. Lloyd, S.V. Mikhalovsky, S.R. Sandeman, C.A. Howel, and L. Liewen, Polymeric hydrogels for novel contact lens-based ophthalmic drug delivery systems: A review, *Contact Lens and Anterior Eye*, Vol. 31, p. 57, 2008.
29. P. Andrade-Vivero, E. Fernandez-Gabriel, C. Alvarez-Lorenzo, and A. Concheiro, Improving the loading and release of NSAIDs from pHEMA hydrogels by copolymerization with functional monomers, *Journal of Pharmaceutical Sciences*, Vol. 96, p. 802, April 2007.
30. S.L. Willis, J.L. Court, R.P. Redman, J.-H. Wang, S.W. Leppard, V.J. O'Byrne, S.A. Small, A.L. Lewis, S.A. Jones, and P.W. Stratford, A novel phosphorylcholine-coated contact lens for extended wear use, *Biomaterials*, Vol. 22, p. 3261, 2001.
31. C.C.S. Karlgard, N.S. Wong, L.W. Jones, and C. Moresoli, In vitro uptake and release studies of ocular pharmaceutical agents by silicon-containing and p-HEMA hydrogel contact lens materials, *International Journal of Pharmaceutics*, Vol. 257, p. 141, 2003.
32. J. Kim, A. Conway, and A. Chauhan, Extended delivery of ophthalmic drugs by silicone hydrogel contact lenses, *Biomaterials*, Vol. 29, p. 2259, 2008.
33. R. Gaudana, J. Jwala, S.H.S. Boddu, and A.K. Mitra, Recent perspectives in ocular drug delivery, *Pharmaceutical Research*, Vol. 26, p. 1197, 2008.
34. S.K. Sahoo, F. Dilnawaz, and S. Krishnakumar, Nanotechnology in ocular drug delivery, *Drug Discovery Today*, Vol. 13, p. 144, 2008.
35. O. Kayser, A. Lemke, and N. Hernandez-Trejo, The impact of nanobiotechnology on the development of new drug delivery systems, *Current Pharmaceutical Biotechnology*, Vol. 6, p. 3, 2005.
36. J. Vandervoort and A. Ludwig, Ocular drug delivery: Nanomedicine applications, *Nanomedicine*, Vol. 2, p. 11, 2007.
37. D. Gulsen and A. Chauhan, Ophthalmic Drug Delivery through Contact Lenses, *Investigative Ophthalmology & Visual Science*, Vol. 45, p. 2342, 07 2004.

38. D. Gulsen and A. Chauhan, Dispersion of microemulsion drops in HEMA hydrogel: A potential ophthalmic drug delivery vehicle, *International Journal of Pharmaceutics*, Vol. 292, p. 95, 2005.
39. Y. Kapoor and A. Chauhan, Drug and surfactant transport in Cyclosporine A and Brij 98 laden p-HEMA hydrogels, *Journal of Colloid and Interface Science*, Vol. 322, p. 624, 2008.
40. Y. Kapoor, J.C. Thomas, G. Tan, V.T. John, and A. Chauhan, Surfactant-laden soft contact lenses for extended delivery of ophthalmic drugs, *Biomaterials*, Vol. 30, p. 867, 2009.
41. R. Uchida, T. Sato, H. Tanigawa, and K. Uno, Azulene incorporation and release by hydrogel containing methacrylamide propyltrimenthylammonium chloride, and its application to soft contact lens, *Journal of Controlled Release*, Vol. 92, p. 259, 2003.
42. T. Sato, R. Uchida, H. Tanigawa, K. Uno, and A. Murakami, Application of polymer gels containing side-chain phosphate groups to drug-delivery contact lenses, *Journal of Applied Polymer Science*, Vol. 98, p. 731, 2005.
43. V. Dulong, D. Le Cerf, L. Picton, and G. Muller, Carboxymethylpullulan hydrogels with a ionic and/or amphiphilic behavior: Swelling properties and entrapment of cationic and/or hydrophobic molecules, *Colloids and Surfaces A: Physicochemical and Engineering Aspects*, Vol. 274, p. 163 , 2006.
44. J.-F. Rosa dos Santos, C. Alvarez-Lorenzo, M. Silva, L. Balsa, J. Couceiro, J.-J. Torres-Labandeira, and A. Concheiro, Soft contact lenses functionalized with pendant cyclodextrins for controlled drug delivery, *Biomaterials*, Vol. 30, p. 1348, 2009.
45. J. Xu, X. Li, and F. Sun, Cyclodextrin-containing hydrogels for contact lenses as a platform for drug incorporation and release, *Acta Biomaterialia*, Vol. 6, p. 486, 2010.
46. T.R. Thatiparti, A.J. Shoffstall, and H.A. von Recum, Cyclodextrin-based device coatings for affinity-based release of antibiotics, *Biomaterials*, Vol. 31, p. 2335, 2010.
47. T.R. Thatiparti and H.A. von Recum, Cyclodextrin complexation for affinity-based antibiotic delivery, *Macromolecular Bioscience*, Vol. 10, p. 82, 2010.
48. Y.-R. Hsieh, D.-M. Liu, and Y.-C. Jian, Amphiphilic polymer and manufacturing method thereof, use of amphiphilic polymer as contact lens material, contact lens material including amphiphilic polymer, US Patent 10 961 325, assigned to National Chiao Tung University NCTU, March 30, 2021.
49. Y.-R. Hsieh, D.-M. Liu, and Y.-C. Chien, Amphiphilic macromolecules, contact lens thereof and preparing methods thereof, US Patent 10 851 209, assigned to National Chiao Tung University, December 01, 2020.

50. C.-C. Peng and A. Chauhan, Extended cyclosporine delivery by silicone-hydrogel contact lenses, *Journal of Controlled Release*, Vol. 154, p. 267, 2011.
51. N.-P.-D. Tran and M.-C. Yang, Synthesis and characterization of silicone contact lenses based on TRIS-DMA-NVP-HEMA hydrogels, *Polymers*, Vol. 11, p. 944, May 2019.
52. T. Matsunaga, T. Tashiro, T. Sato, T. Funaki, and A. Murakami, Development of soft contact lens for drug delivery using zwitter ionic hydrogel, *Investigative Ophthalmology & Visual Science*, Vol. 55, p. 6050, 2014.
53. Wikipedia contributors, Cromoglicic acid — Wikipedia, the free encyclopedia, https://en.wikipedia.org/w/index.php?title=Cromoglicic_acid&oldid=980212768, 2020. [Online; accessed 16-December-2020].
54. A. Danion, H. Brochu, Y. Martin, and P. Vermette, Fabrication and characterization of contact lenses bearing surface-immobilized layers of intact liposomes, *Journal of Biomedical Materials Research Part A*, Vol. 82A, p. 41, 2007.
55. Wikipedia contributors, Avidin — Wikipedia, the free encyclopedia, https://en.wikipedia.org/w/index.php?title=Avidin&oldid=950251449, 2020. [Online; accessed 19-September-2020].
56. R.C. Smith, M. Riollano, A. Leung, and P.T. Hammond, Layer-by-layer platform technology for small-molecule delivery, *Angewandte Chemie International Edition*, Vol. 48, p. 8974, 2009.
57. X. Su, B.-S. Kim, S.R. Kim, P.T. Hammond, and D.J. Irvine, Layer-by-layer-assembled multilayer films for transcutaneous drug and vaccine delivery, *ACS Nano*, Vol. 3, p. 3719, 2009.
58. C.J. Ochs, G.K. Such, Y. Yan, M.P. van Koeverden, and F. Caruso, Biodegradable click capsules with engineered drug-loaded multilayers, *ACS Nano*, Vol. 4, p. 1653, 2010.
59. R. Li, X. Guan, X. Lin, P. Guan, X. Zhang, Z. Rao, L. Du, J. Zhao, J. Rong, and J. Zhao, Poly(2-hydroxyethyl methacrylate)/β-cyclodextrin-hyaluronan contact lens with tear protein adsorption resistance and sustained drug delivery for ophthalmic diseases, *Acta Biomaterialia*, Vol. 110, p. 105 , 2020.
60. C. Alvarez-Lorenzo, S. Anguiano-Igea, A. Varela-García, M. Vivero-Lopez, and A. Concheiro, Bioinspired hydrogels for drug-eluting contact lenses, *Acta Biomaterialia*, Vol. 84, p. 49, 2019.
61. Wikipedia contributors, Tobramycin — Wikipedia, the free encyclopedia, https://en.wikipedia.org/w/index.php?title=Tobramycin&oldid=953605587, 2020. [Online; accessed 3-June-2020].
62. J. Fischer and C. Ganellin, (Eds.), *Analogue-based Drug Discovery*, Wiley, 2006.

63. I. Postic and H. Sheardown, Altering the release of tobramycin by incorporating poly(ethylene glycol) into model silicone hydrogel contact lens materials, *Journal of Biomaterials Science, Polymer Edition*, Vol. 30, p. 1115, 2019.
64. A. Chan, D. Myung, D.J. Waters, C.W. Frank, and C.N. Ta, Drug release of Vancomycin and Tobramycin from a soft contact lens based system, *Investigative Ophthalmology & Visual Science*, Vol. 49, p. 3189, 2008.
65. J. Aveyard, R.C. Deller, R. Lace, R.L. Williams, S.B. Kaye, K.N. Kolegraff, J.M. Curran, and R.A. D'Sa, Antimicrobial nitric oxide releasing contact lens gels for the treatment of microbial keratitis, *ACS Applied Materials & Interfaces*, Vol. 11, p. 37491, 2019.
66. R. Arshady and K. Mosbach, Synthesis of substrate-selective polymers by host-guest polymerization, *Die Makromolekulare Chemie*, Vol. 182, p. 687, 1981.
67. C.-M. Phan, H. Walther, H. Gao, J. Rossy, L.N. Subbaraman, and L.W. Jones, Insights to using contact lenses for drug delivery, *UWSpace*, 2013.
68. F. Tashakori-Sabzevar and S.A. Mohajeri, Development of ocular drug delivery systems using molecularly imprinted soft contact lenses, *Drug Development and Industrial Pharmacy*, Vol. 41, p. 703, 2015.
69. S.A. Zaidi, Molecular imprinted polymers as drug delivery vehicles, *Drug Delivery*, Vol. 23, p. 2262, 2016.
70. Wikipedia contributors, Molecular imprinting — Wikipedia, the free encyclopedia, https://en.wikipedia.org/w/index.php?title=Molecular_imprinting&oldid=958779375, 2020. [Online; accessed 3-June-2020].
71. S.A. Zaidi, Molecular imprinting: A useful approach for drug delivery, *Materials Science for Energy Technologies*, Vol. 3, p. 72, 2020.
72. S.A. Zaidi and W.J. Cheong, Robust open tubular layer of S-ketoprofen imprinted polymer for chiral LC separation, *Journal of Separation Science*, Vol. 31, p. 2962, 2008.
73. S.A. Zaidi, K.M. Han, D.G. Hwang, and W.J. Cheong, Preparation of open tubular molecule imprinted polymer capillary columns with various templates by a generalized procedure and their chiral and non-chiral separation performance in CEC, *Electrophoresis*, Vol. 31, p. 1019, 2010.
74. S.A. Zaidi, S.M. Lee, and W.J. Cheong, Open tubular capillary columns with basic templates made by the generalized preparation protocol in capillary electrochromatography chiral separation and template structural effects on chiral separation capability, *Journal of Chromatography A*, Vol. 1218, p. 1291, 2011.

75. S.A. Zaidi and J.H. Shin, Molecularly imprinted polymer electrochemical sensors based on synergistic effect of composites synthesized from graphene and other nanosystems, *Int. J. Electrochem. Sci.*, Vol. 9, p. 4598, 2014.
76. S.A. Zaidi, Recent developments in molecularly imprinted polymer nanofibers and their applications, *Analytical Methods*, Vol. 7, p. 7406, 2015.
77. R. Gui, H. Jin, H. Guo, and Z. Wang, Recent advances and future prospects in molecularly imprinted polymers-based electrochemical biosensors, *Biosensors and Bioelectronics*, Vol. 100, p. 56, 2018.
78. C.J. White and M.E. Byrne, Molecularly imprinted therapeutic contact lenses, *Expert Opinion on Drug Delivery*, Vol. 7, p. 765, 2010.
79. A. Chauhan, Ocular drug delivery role of contact lenses, *The Official Scientific Journal of Delhi Ophthalmological Society*, Vol. 26, p. 131, 2015.
80. C. Alvarez-Lorenzo, F. Yañez, and A. Concheiro, Ocular drug delivery from molecularly-imprinted contact lenses, *Journal of Drug Delivery Science and Technology*, Vol. 20, p. 237, 2010.
81. P. Dixon, C. Shafor, S. Gause, K.-H. Hsu, K.C. Powell, and A. Chauhan, Therapeutic contact lenses: A patent review, *Expert Opinion on Therapeutic Patents*, Vol. 25, p. 1117, 2015.
82. A. Chauhan and Y. Kapoor, Contact lens based bioactive agent delivery system, US Patent 8 075 909, assigned to University of Florida Research Foundation, Incorporated (Gainesville, FL), December 13, 2011.
83. S. Venkatesh, J. Saha, S. Pass, and M.E. Byrne, Transport and structural analysis of molecular imprinted hydrogels for controlled drug delivery, *European Journal of Pharmaceutics and Biopharmaceutics*, Vol. 69, p. 852, 2008.
84. A. Hui, H. Sheardown, and L. Jones, Acetic and acrylic acid molecular imprinted model silicone hydrogel materials for ciprofloxacin-HCl delivery, *Materials*, Vol. 5, p. 85, January 2012.
85. A. Hui, M. Willcox, and L. Jones, In vitro and in vivo evaluation of novel ciprofloxacin-releasing silicone hydrogel contact lenses, *Investigative Ophthalmology & Visual Science*, Vol. 55, p. 4896, August 2014.
86. F. Yañez, L. Martikainen, M.E.M. Braga, C. Alvarez-Lorenzo, A. Concheiro, C.M.M. Duarte, M.H. Gil, and H.C. de Sousa, Supercritical fluid-assisted preparation of imprinted contact lenses for drug delivery, *Acta Biomaterialia*, Vol. 7, p. 1019, 2011.
87. H. Hiratani, Y. Mizutani, and C. Alvarez-Lorenzo, Controlling drug release from imprinted hydrogels by modifying the characteristics of the imprinted cavities, *Macromolecular Bioscience*, Vol. 5, p. 728, 2005.

88. B.M. Nikouei, S.A. Vahabzadeh, and S.A. Mohajeri, Preparation of a molecularly imprinted soft contact lens as a new ocular drug delivery system for dorzolamide, *Current Drug Delivery*, Vol. 10, p. 279, 2013.
89. A. Ribeiro, F. Veiga, D. Santos, J.J. Torres-Labandeira, A. Concheiro, and C. Alvarez-Lorenzo, Bioinspired imprinted PHEMA-hydrogels for ocular delivery of carbonic anhydrase inhibitor drugs, *Biomacromolecules*, Vol. 12, p. 701, 2011.
90. M. Ali and M.E. Byrne, Controlled release of high molecular weight hyaluronic acid from molecularly imprinted hydrogel contact lenses, *Pharmaceutical Research*, Vol. 26, p. 714, 2009.
91. C.J. White, M.K. McBride, K.M. Pate, A. Tieppo, and M.E. Byrne, Extended release of high molecular weight hydroxypropyl methylcellulose from molecularly imprinted, extended wear silicone hydrogel contact lenses, *Biomaterials*, Vol. 32, p. 5698, 2011.
92. C.J. White, S.A. DiPasquale, and M.E. Byrne, Controlled release of multiple therapeutics from silicone hydrogel contact lenses, *Optometry and Vision Science: Official Publication of the American Academy of Optometry*, Vol. 93, p. 377, April 2016.
93. M. Ali, S. Horikawa, S. Venkatesh, J. Saha, J.W. Hong, and M.E. Byrne, Zero-order therapeutic release from imprinted hydrogel contact lenses within in vitro physiological ocular tear flow, *Journal of Controlled Release*, Vol. 124, p. 154, 2007.
94. G. Vasapollo, R.D. Sole, L. Mergola, M.R. Lazzoi, A. Scardino, S. Scorrano, and G. Mele, Molecularly imprinted polymers: Present and future prospective, *International Journal of Molecular Sciences*, Vol. 12, p. 5908, September 2011.
95. J. Xu, X. Li, and F. Sun, In vitro and in vivo evaluation of ketotifen fumarate-loaded silicone hydrogel contact lenses for ocular drug delivery, *Drug Delivery*, Vol. 18, p. 150, 2011.
96. F. Hadizadeh, A. Zakerian, and S.A. Mohajeri, Non-covalently lactose imprinted polymers and recognition of saccharides in aqueous solutions, *Journal of the Iranian Chemical Society*, Vol. 10, p. 207, 2013.
97. F. Hadizadeh, M. Hassanpour Moghadam, and S.A. Mohajeri, Application of molecularly imprinted hydrogel for the preparation of lactose-free milk, *Journal of the Science of Food and Agriculture*, Vol. 93, p. 304, 2013.
98. C. Alvarez-Lorenzo, F. Yañez, R. Barreiro-Iglesias, and A. Concheiro, Imprinted soft contact lenses as norfloxacin delivery systems, *Journal of Controlled Release*, Vol. 113, p. 236, 2006.
99. W. Xu, W. Jiao, S. Li, X. Tao, and G. Mu, Bimatoprost loaded microemulsion laden contact lens to treat glaucoma, *Journal of Drug Delivery Science and Technology*, Vol. 54, p. 101330, 2019.

100. F. Yan, Y. Liu, S. Han, Q. Zhao, and N. Liu, Bimatoprost imprinted silicone contact lens to treat glaucoma, *AAPS PharmSciTech*, Vol. 21, p. 63, 2020.
101. N. Malakooti, C. Alexander, and C. Alvarez-Lorenzo, Imprinted contact lenses for sustained release of polymyxin B and related antimicrobial peptides, *Journal of Pharmaceutical Sciences*, Vol. 104, p. 3386, 2015.
102. B. Malaekeh-Nikouei, F.A. Ghaeni, V.S. Motamedshariaty, and S.A. Mohajeri, Controlled release of prednisolone acetate from molecularly imprinted hydrogel contact lenses, *Journal of Applied Polymer Science*, Vol. 126, p. 387, 2012.
103. H. Hiratani and C. Alvarez-Lorenzo, Timolol uptake and release by imprinted soft contact lenses made of *N,N*-diethylacrylamide and methacrylic acid, *Journal of Controlled Release*, Vol. 83, p. 223, 2002.
104. H. Hiratani, A. Fujiwara, Y. Tamiya, Y. Mizutani, and C. Alvarez-Lorenzo, Ocular release of timolol from molecularly imprinted soft contact lenses, *Biomaterials*, Vol. 26, p. 1293, 2005.
105. C.-C. Li and A. Chauhan, Ocular transport model for ophthalmic delivery of timolol through p-HEMA contact lenses, *Journal of Drug Delivery Science and Technology*, Vol. 17, p. 69 , 2007.
106. S.A. Mohajeri, G. Karimi, and M.R. Khansari, Clozapine imprinted polymers: Synthesis, characterization and application for drug assay in human serum, *Analytica Chimica Acta*, Vol. 683, p. 143, 2010.
107. C.-C. Peng, M.T. Burke, B.E. Carbia, C. Plummer, and A. Chauhan, Extended drug delivery by contact lenses for glaucoma therapy, *Journal of Controlled Release*, Vol. 162, p. 152, 2012.
108. S.A. Mohajeri, S.A. Sajadi Tabassi, M. Hassanpour Moghadam, and S.A. Mohajeri, Preparation of a pH-sensitive pantoprazole-imprinted polymer and evaluation of its drug-binding and -releasing properties, *Science China Chemistry*, Vol. 57, p. 857, 2014.
109. A. Sahebnasagh, G. Karimi, and S.A. Mohajeri, Preparation and evaluation of histamine imprinted polymer as a selective sorbent in molecularly imprinted solid-phase extraction coupled with high performance liquid chromatography analysis in canned fish, *Food Analytical Methods*, Vol. 7, p. 1, 2014.
110. M.E. Byrne, K. Park, and N.A. Peppas, Molecular imprinting within hydrogels, *Advanced Drug Delivery Reviews*, Vol. 54, p. 149, 2002.
111. D. Cunliffe, A. Kirby, and C. Alexander, Molecularly imprinted drug delivery systems, *Advanced Drug Delivery Reviews*, Vol. 57, p. 1836, 2005.
112. M.E. Byrne and V. Salian, Molecular imprinting within hydrogels II: Progress and analysis of the field, *International Journal of Pharmaceutics*, Vol. 364, p. 188, 2008. Future Perspectives in Pharmaceutics Contributions from Younger Scientists.

113. N.M. Bergmann and N.A. Peppas, Molecularly imprinted polymers with specific recognition for macromolecules and proteins, *Progress in Polymer Science*, Vol. 33, p. 271, 2008.
114. E.M. Alapi and J. Fischer, Table of selected analogue classes in J. Fischer and C.R. Ganellin, (Eds.), *Analogue-based Drug Discovery*, chapter Part III, pp. 443–552. Wiley, 2006.
115. C. Alvarez-Lorenzo, H. Hiratani, J.L. Gómez-Amoza, R. Martínez-Pacheco, C. Souto, and A. Concheiro, Soft contact lenses capable of sustained delivery of timolol, *Journal of Pharmaceutical Sciences*, Vol. 91, p. 2182, 2002.
116. AHFS DI Essentials, Timolol (EENT), Technical report, American Society of Health-System Pharmacists, 4500 East-West Highway, Suite 900, Bethesda, Maryland 20814, 2019. electronic: https://www.drugs.com/monograph/timolol-eent.html.
117. H. Hiratani and C. Alvarez-Lorenzo, The nature of backbone monomers determines the performance of imprinted soft contact lenses as timolol drug delivery systems, *Biomaterials*, Vol. 25, p. 1105, 2004.
118. J. Deng, S. Chen, J. Chen, H. Ding, D. Deng, and Z. Xie, Self-reporting colorimetric analysis of drug release by molecular imprinted structural color contact lens, *ACS Applied Materials & Interfaces*, Vol. 10, p. 34611, 2018.
119. F. Yañez, A. Chauhan, A. Concheiro, and C. Alvarez-Lorenzo, Timolol-imprinted soft contact lenses: Influence of the template: Functional monomer ratio and the hydrogel thickness, *Journal of Applied Polymer Science*, Vol. 122, p. 1333, 2011.
120. S.R. Flaxman, R.R.A. Bourne, S. Resnikoff, P. Ackland, T. Braithwaite, M.V. Cicinelli, A. Das, J.B. Jonas, J. Keeffe, J.H. Kempen, et al., Global causes of blindness and distance vision impairment 1990–2020: A systematic review and meta-analysis, *The Lancet Global Health*, Vol. 5, p. e1221, 2017.
121. R.N. Weinreb and P.T. Khaw, Primary open-angle glaucoma, *The Lancet*, Vol. 363, p. 1711, 2004.
122. D.M. Eddy, L.E. Sanders, and J.F. Eddy, The value of screening for glaucoma with tonometry, *Survey of Ophthalmology*, Vol. 28, p. 194, 1983.
123. A. Sommer, J.M. Tielsch, J. Katz, H.A. Quigley, J.D. Gottsch, J. Javitt, and K. Singh, Relationship between intraocular pressure and primary open angle glaucoma among white and black Americans: The Baltimore eye survey, *Archives of Ophthalmology*, Vol. 109, p. 1090, 1991.
124. N. Wei, H. Dang, C. Huang, and Y. Sheng, Timolol loaded microemulsion laden silicone contact lens to manage glaucoma: In vitro and in

vivo studies, *Journal of Dispersion Science and Technology*, Vol. 0, p. 1, 2020.

125. X. Ding, G. Ben-Shlomo, and L. Que, Soft contact lens with embedded microtubes for sustained and self-adaptive drug delivery for glaucoma treatment, *ACS Applied Materials & Interfaces*, Vol. 12, p. 45789, 2020.

126. J. Kim, C.-C. Peng, and A. Chauhan, Extended release of dexamethasone from silicone-hydrogel contact lenses containing vitamin E, *Journal of Controlled Release*, Vol. 148, p. 110, 2010. 11th European Sumposium on Controlled Drug Delivery.

127. S.W. Choi, B.G. Cha, and J. Kim, Therapeutic contact lens for scavenging excessive reactive oxygen species on the ocular surface, *ACS Nano*, Vol. 14, p. 2483, 2020.

128. J.Y. Kim, B.G. Cha, and S.W. Choi, Contact lens comprising ceria particles and method of fabricating the same, US Patent Application 20 190 129 069, assigned to Research & Business Foundation Sungkyunkwan University, Suwon-si (KR), May 2, 2019.

129. F.A. Maulvi, R.J. Patil, A.R. Desai, M.R. Shukla, R.J. Vaidya, K.M. Ranch, B.A. Vyas, S.A. Shah, and D.O. Shah, Effect of gold nanoparticles on timolol uptake and its release kinetics from contact lenses: In vitro and in vivo evaluation, *Acta Biomaterialia*, Vol. 86, p. 350 , 2019.

130. Q. Guo, L. Jia, Qinggeletu, R. Zhang, and X. Yang, In vitro and in vivo evaluation of ketotifen-gold nanoparticles laden contact lens for controlled drug delivery to manage conjunctivitis, *Journal of Drug Delivery Science and Technology*, p. 102538, 2021.

131. R. Herizchi, E. Abbasi, M. Milani, and A. Akbarzadeh, Current methods for synthesis of gold nanoparticles, *Artificial Cells, Nanomedicine, and Biotechnology*, Vol. 44, p. 596, 2016.

132. A.R. Desai, F.A. Maulvi, D.M. Desai, M.R. Shukla, K.M. Ranch, B.A. Vyas, S.A. Shah, S. Sandeman, and D.O. Shah, Multiple drug delivery from the drug-implants-laden silicone contact lens: Addressing the issue of burst drug release, *Materials Science and Engineering: C*, Vol. 112, p. 110885, 2020.

133. A. Tieppo, C.J. White, A.C. Paine, M.L. Voyles, M.K. McBride, and M.E. Byrne, Sustained in vivo release from imprinted therapeutic contact lenses, *Journal of Controlled Release*, Vol. 157, p. 391, 2012.

134. Wikipedia contributors, Ciprofloxacin — Wikipedia, the free encyclopedia, https://en.wikipedia.org/w/index.php?title=Ciprofloxacin&oldid=956429084, 2020. [Online; accessed 28-May-2020].

135. AHFS DI Essentials, Ciprofloxacin hydrochloride, Technical report, American Society of Health-System Pharmacists, 4500 East-West

Highway, Suite 900, Bethesda, Maryland 20814, 2015. electronic: http://www.drugs.com/monograph/ciprofloxacin-hydrochloride.html.

136. J.B. Ciolino, T.R. Hoare, N.G. Iwata, I. Behlau, C.H. Dohlman, R. Langer, and D.S. Kohane, A Drug-Eluting Contact Lens, *Investigative Ophthalmology & Visual Science*, Vol. 50, p. 3346, 07 2009.
137. Wikipedia contributors, Ofloxacin — Wikipedia, the free encyclopedia, https://en.wikipedia.org/w/index.php?title=Ofloxacin&oldid=960082828, 2020. [Online; accessed 6-June-2020].
138. I. Hayakawa, T. Hiramitsu, and Y. Tanaka, Benzoxazine derivatives, US Patent 4 382 892, assigned to Daiichi Seiyaku Co. Ltd. (Tokyo, JP), May 10, 1983.
139. Y. Mouton and O. Leroy, Ofloxacin, *International Journal of Antimicrobial Agents*, Vol. 1, p. 57, 1991.
140. D. Lee, N. Lee, and I. Kwon, Efficient loading of ophthalmic drugs with poor loadability into contact lenses using functional comonomers, *Biomaterials Science*, Vol. 6, p. 2639, 2018.
141. U. Ubani-Ukoma, D. Gibson, G. Schultz, B.O. Silva, and A. Chauhan, Evaluating the potential of drug eluting contact lenses for treatment of bacterial keratitis using an ex vivo corneal model, *International Journal of Pharmaceutics*, Vol. 565, p. 499, 2019.
142. Wikipedia contributors, Epinastine — Wikipedia, the free encyclopedia, https://en.wikipedia.org/w/index.php?title=Epinastine&oldid=939201807, 2020. [Online; accessed 6-June-2020].
143. T. Minami, W. Ishida, T. Kishimoto, I. Nakajima, S. Hino, R. Arai, T. Matsunaga, A. Fukushima, and S. Yamagami, In vitro and in vivo performance of epinastine hydrochloride-releasing contact lenses, *PONE*, Vol. 14, p. e0210362, 2019.
144. V. Pastori, S. Tavazzi, and M. Lecchi, Lactoferrin-loaded contact lenses counteract cytotoxicity caused in vitro by keratoconic tears, *Contact Lens and Anterior Eye*, Vol. 42, p. 253 , 2019.
145. C. Lopez, S. Park, S. Edwards, S. Vong, S. Hou, M. Lee, H. Sauerland, J.-J. Lee, and K.J. Jeong, Matrix metalloproteinase-deactivating contact lens for corneal melting, *ACS Biomaterials Science & Engineering*, Vol. 5, p. 1195, 2019.
146. F.A. Maulvi, R.J. Parmar, A.R. Desai, D.M. Desai, M.R. Shukla, K.M. Ranch, S.A. Shah, and D.O. Shah, Tailored gatifloxacin Pluronic® F-68-loaded contact lens: Addressing the issue of transmittance and swelling, *International Journal of Pharmaceutics*, Vol. 581, p. 119279, 2020.
147. Wikipedia contributors, Gatifloxacin — Wikipedia, the free encyclopedia, https://en.wikipedia.org/w/index.php?title=Gatifloxacin&oldid=950862698, 2020. [Online; accessed 4-June-2020].

148. F.A. Maulvi, R.J. Parmar, M.R. Shukla, A.R. Desai, D.T. Desai, K.M. Ranch, S.A. Shah, S. Sandeman, and D.O. Shah, Plackett-Burman design for screening of critical variables and their effects on the optical transparency and swelling of gatifloxacin-pluronic-loaded contact lens, *International Journal of Pharmaceutics*, Vol. 566, p. 513, 2019.
149. J.A. Balfour and M.I. Wilde, Dorzolamide, *Drugs & Aging*, Vol. 10, p. 384, 1997.
150. Wikipedia contributors, Ethoxzolamide — Wikipedia, the free encyclopedia, https://en.wikipedia.org/w/index.php?title=Ethoxzolamide&oldid=737428255, 2016. [Online; accessed 1-June-2020].
151. J.C. Stuart and J.G. Linn, Dilute sodium hyaluronate (Healon) in the treatment of ocular surface disorders, *Annals of Ophthalmology*, Vol. 17, p. 190, 1985.
152. P. Aragona, V. Papa, A. Micali, M. Santocono, and G. Milazzo, Long term treatment with sodium hyaluronate-containing artificial tears reduces ocular surface damage in patients with dry eye, *British Journal of Ophthalmology*, Vol. 86, p. 181, 2002.
153. P. Aragona, G. Di Stefano, F. Ferreri, R. Spinella, and A. Stilo, Sodium hyaluronate eye drops of different osmolarity for the treatment of dry eye in Sjögren's syndrome patients, *British Journal of Ophthalmology*, Vol. 86, p. 879, 2002.
154. F. Brignole, P.-J. Pisella, B. Dupas, V. Baeyens, and C. Baudouin, Efficacy and safety of 0.18% sodium hyaluronate in patients with moderate dry eye syndrome and superficial keratitis, *Graefe's Archive for Clinical and Experimental Ophthalmology*, Vol. 243, p. 531, 2005.
155. N. Bühler, H.-P. Haerri, M. Hofmann, C. Irrgang, A. Mühlebach, B. Müller, and F. Stockinger, Nelfilcon A, a new material for contact lenses, *Chimia International Journal for Chemistry*, Vol. 53, p. 269, 1999.
156. L. Michaud and C.J. Giasson, Overwear of contact lenses: Increased severity of clinical signs as a function of protein adsorption, *Optometry and Vision Science*, Vol. 79, p. 184, 2002.
157. E. Akbari, R. Imani, P. Shokrollahi, and S. Heidari keshel, Preparation of nanoparticle-containing ring-implanted poly(vinyl alcohol) contact lens for sustained release of hyaluronic acid, *Macromolecular Bioscience*, Vol. n/a, p. 2100043, 2021.
158. X. Deng, M. Cao, J. Zhang, K. Hu, Z. Yin, Z. Zhou, X. Xiao, Y. Yang, W. Sheng, Y. Wu, et al., Hyaluronic acid-chitosan nanoparticles for co-delivery of MiR-34a and doxorubicin in therapy against triple negative breast cancer, *Biomaterials*, Vol. 35, p. 4333, 2014.
159. F.A. Maulvi, D.H. Lakdawala, A.A. Shaikh, A.R. Desai, H.H. Choksi, R.J. Vaidya, K.M. Ranch, A.R. Koli, B.A. Vyas, and D.O. Shah, In vitro

and in vivo evaluation of novel implantation technology in hydrogel contact lenses for controlled drug delivery, *Journal of Controlled Release*, Vol. 226, p. 47, 2016.
160. C. Mu, V. Lee, Y. Liu, Y. Han, and G. Marriott, An engineered contact lens for passive and sustained release of lifitegrast, an anti-dry eye syndrome drug, *bioRxiv*, 2021.
161. A. Tieppo, K.M. Pate, and M.E. Byrne, In vitro controlled release of an anti-inflammatory from daily disposable therapeutic contact lenses under physiological ocular tear flow, *European Journal of Pharmaceutics and Biopharmaceutics*, Vol. 81, p. 170, 2012.
162. C. Torres-Luna, N. Hu, A. Koolivand, X. Fan, Y. Zhu, R. Domszy, J. Yang, A. Yang, and N.S. Wang, Effect of a cationic surfactant on microemulsion globules and drug release from hydrogel contact lenses, *Pharmaceutics*, Vol. 11, p. 262, June 2019.
163. D. Silva, L.F.V. Pinto, D. Bozukova, L.F. Santos, A.P. Serro, and B. Saramago, Chitosan/alginate based multilayers to control drug release from ophthalmic lens, *Colloids and Surfaces B: Biointerfaces*, Vol. 147, p. 81, 2016.
164. D. Silva, H.C. de Sousa, M.H. Gil, C. Alvarez-Lorenzo, A. Concheiro, B. Saramago, and A.P. Serro, Moxifloxacin imprinted silicon based hydrogels for sustained ocular release, *Annals of Medicine*, Vol. 51, p. 103, 2019.
165. W. Ran, H. Ma, and M. Li, In-vitro and in-vivo studies of polyvinyl pyrrolidone-coated sparfloxacin-loaded ring contact lens to treat conjunctivitis, *Journal of Pharmaceutical Sciences*, Vol. 109, p. 1951, 2020.
166. R.R. Horne, J.T. Rich, M.W. Bradley, and W.G. Pitt, Latanoprost uptake and release from commercial contact lenses, *Journal of Biomaterials Science, Polymer Edition*, Vol. 31, p. 1, 2020.
167. Wikipedia contributors, Latanoprost — Wikipedia, the free encyclopedia, https://en.wikipedia.org/w/index.php?title=Latanoprost&oldid=960703420, 2020. [Online; accessed 5-June-2020].
168. Drugs.com, Latanoprost, Technical report, American Society of Health-System Pharmacists, 4500 East-West Highway, Suite 900, Bethesda, Maryland 20814, 2019. electronic: https://www.drugs.com/monograph/latanoprost.html.
169. S.S. Patel and C.M. Spencer, Latanoprost, *Drugs & Aging*, Vol. 9, p. 363, 1996.
170. M.E. Cavet, S. Glogowski, E.R. Lowe, and E. Phillips, Rheological properties, dissolution kinetics, and ocular pharmacokinetics of loteprednol etabonate (submicron) ophthalmic gel 0.38%, *Journal of Ocular Pharmacology and Therapeutics*, Vol. 35, p. 291, 2019.
171. C.N.J. McGhee, S. Dean, and H. Danesh-Meyer, Locally administered ocular corticosteroids, *Drug Safety*, Vol. 25, p. 33, 2002.

172. E.R. James, The etiology of steroid cataract, *Journal of Ocular Pharmacology and Therapeutics*, Vol. 23, p. 403, 2007.
173. C.E. Pavesio and H.H. DeCory, Treatment of ocular inflammatory conditions with loteprednol etabonate, *British Journal of Ophthalmology*, Vol. 92, p. 455, 2008.
174. U. Pleyer, P.G. Ursell, and P. Rama, Intraocular pressure effects of common topical steroids for post-cataract inflammation: Are they all the same?, *Ophthalmology and Therapy*, Vol. 2, p. 55, 2013.
175. N. Bodor, N. Bodor, and W.-M. Wu, A comparison of intraocular pressure elevating activity of loteprednol etabonate and dexamethasone in rabbits, *Current Eye Research*, Vol. 11, p. 525, 1992.
176. N. Bodor, Recent advances in retrometabolic design approaches, *Journal of Controlled Release*, Vol. 62, p. 209, 1999.
177. J.C. Pinto-Bonilla, A. Del Olmo-Jimeno, F. Llovet-Osuna, and E. Hernández-Galilea, A randomized crossover study comparing trehalose/hyaluronate eyedrops and standard treatment: Patient satisfaction in the treatment of dry eye syndrome, *Therapeutics and Clinical Risk Management*, Vol. 11, p. 595, April 2015.
178. A.D. Pucker, S.M. Ng, and J.J. Nichols, Over the counter (OTC) artificial tear drops for dry eye syndrome, *The Cochrane Database of Systematic Reviews*, Vol. 2, p. CD009729, February 2016.
179. Drugs.com, Prednisolone, Technical report, American Society of Health-System Pharmacists, 4500 East-West Highway, Suite 900, Bethesda, Maryland 20814, 2019. electronic: https://www.drugs.com/monograph/prednisolone.html.

5

Medical Problems

An easy to use reference in an A-Z format on the instrumentation, fitting, complications, and therapeutics of contact lenses has been published (1).

The *Clinical Manual of Contact Lenses*, can help both students and practitioners to fit, evaluate, and troubleshoot contact lens issues in everyday practice (2). Here, chapters are available concerning scleral lens fitting, clinical management of keratoconus, postsurgical fitting, myopia control, orthokeratology, presbyopia, extended wear, and correction of astigmatism.

Also, a comprehensive guide to the field of contact lenses for optometrists and ophthalmic assistants has been presented (3). Complications associated with wearing contact lenses and also the fitting of lenses after refractive surgery have been discussed.

5.1 Eye Diseases

A lot of eye diseases have been classified (4). Some of these diseases that can be treated with modified contact lenses, or are caused by contact lenses, are listed in Table 5.1.

5.2 Corneal Edema

Corneal edema is a swelling behavior of the cornea. The issues of corneal edema have been described in some monographs (5, 6).

Table 5.1 Eye diseases.

Desease	References
Scleritis	(4)
Keratitis	(4)
Corneal ulcer	(4)
Snow blindness	(4)
Corneal neovascularization	(4)
Fuchs' dystrophy	(4)
Keratoconjunctivitis sicca	(4)
Iritis	(4)
Uveitis	(4)
Dacryoadenitis	(4)
Epiphora	(4)
Dysthyroid exophthalmos	(4)
Dry eye disease	(7–9)
Stevens-Johnson syndrome	(8)
Sjögren's syndrome	(8)
Keratomileusis	(8)
Acanthamoeba keratitis	(10)
Microbial keratitis	(11)
Ocular medicamentosa	(12)
Conjunctivochalasis	(12)
Pinguecula	(12)
Hyperkeratinization	(12)
Salzmann's nodular degeneration	(12)
Presbyopia	(13)
Papillary conjunctivitis	(14)

5.2.1 *PMMA Lenses*

An evaluation was made of the incidence of corneal edema with poly(methyl methacrylate) (PMMA) contact lenses and Polycon (Silafocon A) lenses of identical design. Edema occurred significantly more frequently with PMMA than with Polycon lenses (15).

In another study (16), a short-term study of the physiologic response of the cornea to PMMA contact lenses and hard, gas-permeable contact lenses of different materials such as Polycon and Menicon O_2, thicknesses, and fittings, was carried out on nine unadapted subjects using one eye as the experimental eye and the other as the control eye with no lens.

Changes in corneal thickness were monitored at seven locations across the cornea using an electronic micropachymeter. It was found that gas-permeable lenses produced less corneal swelling than the PMMA lenses (16).

However, lens thickness and the fit of the lens were still important control variables with these gas-permeable lenses. The thin gas-permeable lens produced less swelling than thicker lenses, and the flatter-fitting gas-permeable lenses produced less swelling than the steeper-fitting lenses. The swelling with all the hard lenses studied was confined primarily to the central 6 *mm* of the cornea (16).

5.2.2 *Thickness Changes*

Isolated rabbit corneas bathed in Krebs-Ringer bicarbonate solution (17) were observed for thickness changes after a 90 *min* equilibration period (18). Control corneas swelled an average of 0.5 $\mu m\, hr^{-1}$ and placement of a PMMA contact lens on the epithelial surface caused the corneas to swell 24.5, $\mu m\, hr^{-1}$, an effect similar to 0.5 *mM* epithelial cyanide exposure. The pronounced swelling induced by PMMA lens placement was much less, however, in the epithelial presence of 3.2 *mM* sodium oxalate (3.22 $\mu m\, hr^{-1}$) or 3.2 *mM* sodium oxamate (5.38 $\mu m\, hr^{-1}$). An equiosmotic excess of 4.8 *mM* NaCl was least active (15.89 $\mu m\, hr^{-1}$). Oxamic acid is also known as oxalic acid monoamide, cf. Figure 5.1. On normal isolated corneas (without contact lenses), the Ringer containing an excess of 4.8 *mM* NaCl significantly deswelled the corneas (-13.44 $\mu m\, hr^{-1}$), which contrasted with oxalate and oxamate containing Ringer solutions.

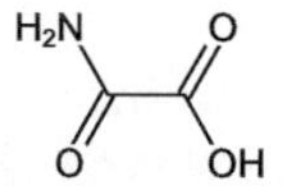

Figure 5.1 Oxamic acid.

So, the study supports the notion that contact lens-induced edema results from stromal lactate accumulation, and suggests a potential alternative to osmotic therapy for its amelioration. These lactate dehydrogenase inhibitors, in the concentrations used, have no acute osmotic or toxic effect on normal corneas *in vitro* (18).

5.2.3 *Corneal Swelling*

The corneal swelling response to Polycon and Menicon O_2, lenses was monitored over 6 *h* of eye closure. The properties of these lenses are listed in Table 5.2.

Table 5.2 Properties of the lenses (19).

Property	Lens material	
	Menicon O_2	Polycon
Oxygen permeability /[$cm \times ml\, O_2 s^{-1} ml^{-1} mmHg^{-1}$]	9.0×10^{-11}	5.8×10^{-11}
Wetting Angle/[°]	16	25
Water content/[%]	16	25
Refractive index	1.481	1.490
Lens thickness/[*mm*]	0.155	0.146

For five subjects (4 females and 1 male aged 18–21 *y*), the average corneal swelling with the Polycon and Menicon O_2 lenses was 15.9±4.8% and 15.2±4.3% respectively.

The average corneal swelling with respect to time is shown in Figure 5.2.

Two of the subjects experienced more than 19% edema with both lenses.

In view of the high levels of edema, neither lens is considered capable of supporting extended wear and patients should be advised accordingly. Patients should also be cautioned regarding napping

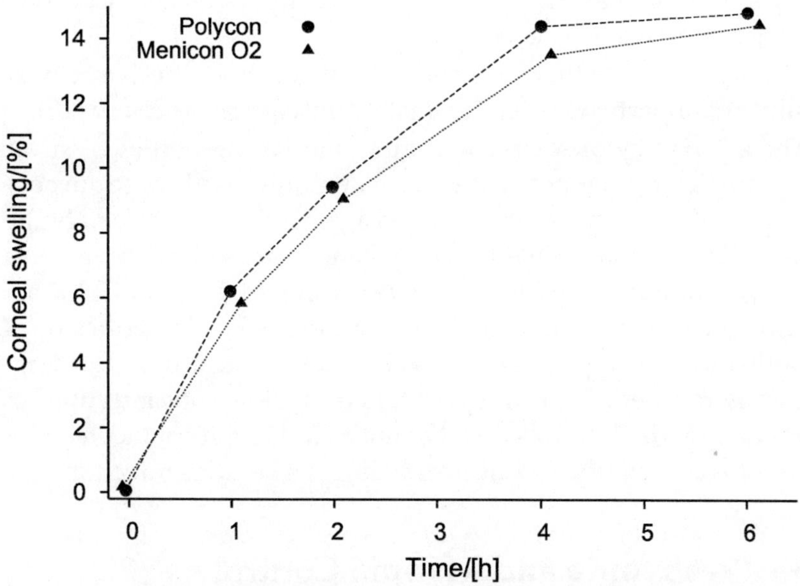

Figure 5.2 Average corneal swelling vs. time (19).

with these lenses in, as they can induce approximately 6% edema in 1 *h* and 9% edema in 2 *h*.

So, it has been suggested that in order for a gas-permeable lens to be considered for extended wear it should have an oxygen transmissibility of at least 25×10^{-9} $cm \times ml\ O_2 s^{-1} ml^{-1} mmHg^{-1}$ (19).

5.2.4 *Acanthamoeba Keratitis*

Acanthamoeba keratitis is a severe sight-threatening corneal infection that has become a significant medical problem, especially among contact lens wearers. The disease manifests as eye pain, congestion, blurred vision, lachrymation, and ring-shaped infiltrates of the cornea, and can lead to permanent blindness (20).

Inappropriate habits of contact lens users may result in an increased risk of Acanthamoeba keratitis infection. The anti-amoebic efficiency of popular multipurpose contact lens solutions is insufficient to reduce this risk. The prevention of Acanthamoeba keratitis is crucial to reduce the number of Acanthamoeba keratitis infections.

Nanoparticles are known to be active agents against bacteria, viruses, and fungi and have also been recently tested against protozoa, including *Acanthamoeba* spp.

It could be shown that an anti-amoebic and anti-adhesive activity of silver nanoparticles exists against *Acanthamoeba castellanii* (20).

The activity, cytotoxicity, and anti-adhesive properties of silver nanoparticles conjugated with five commonly used multipurpose contact lens solutions were evaluated against the *A. castellanii* NEFF strain. The results showed a significant increase in anti-amoebic activity, without increasing the overall cytotoxicity, of SoloCare Aqua and Opti-Free conjugated with nanoparticles. The adhesion of Acanthamoeba trophozoites to the contact lens surface was also significantly reduced. So, it was concluded that low concentrations of silver nanoparticles can be used as an ingredient in contact lens solutions to decrease the risk of Acanthamoeba keratitis infection (20).

5.3 Presbyopia and Myopia Control

Presbyopia is a condition associated with the aging of the eye that results in progressively worsening ability to focus clearly on close objects. The symptoms include difficulty of reading small print, having to hold reading material farther away, headaches, and eyestrain (21).

To assess the fit success of three Alcon multifocal contact lens materials with the same optical design (Lotrafilcon B, Nelfilcon A, Delefilcon A) in presbyopic patients a common fitting guide was used (22). Fitting guides have been detailed (23). A modified fitting guide required fewer lenses to fit each eye at the screening visit than the previous fitting guide.

Myopia is an eye disorder, where light focuses in front of the retina, instead of on the retina. This causes distant objects to be blurry while close objects appear normal (24).

Myopia can be easily corrected with optical and surgical interventions, however, pathological myopia is known to increase the risk of eye diseases such as cataracts, glaucoma and macular degeneration (25, 26).

The genesis of myopia remains uncertain, but is generally considered to have a multifactorial origin composed of optical, genetic and environmental factors (26).

One popular theory regarding myopia progression is the accommodative lag theory. During near work people may under-accommodate due to poor accommodative response, and therefore introduce hyperopic defocus in the fovea, stimulating eye growth. This theory was supported by studies in which children with higher myopia are associated with more near work activities, such as reading (27, 28).

Furthermore, myopic eyes were found to have a greater amount of accommodative lag. Peripheral hyperopia might be a precursor for myopia progression (26)

The use of multifocal and bifocal contact lenses for presbyopia and myopia control has been reviewed (29).

Bifocal and multifocal optical devices are intended to get images into focus from objects placed at different distances from the observer. Glasses, contact lenses, and intraocular lenses can meet these requirements to provide such a solution. In addition, contact lenses provide unique characteristics as a platform for implementing bifocality and multifocality. Compared to glasses, they are closer to the eye, providing a wider field of view, less distortion, and their use is more consistent as they are not so easily removed throughout the day. In addition, contact lenses are also minimally invasive, can be easily exchangeable, and, therefore, suitable for conditions in which surgical procedures are not indicated. Contact lenses can remain centered with the eye despite eye movements, providing the possibility for simultaneous imaging from different object distances.

The recent developments in material platforms, optical designs, simulated visual performance, and the clinical performance assessment of bifocal and multifocal contact lenses for presbyopia correction and/or myopia progression control have been detailed (29).

5.4 Toxic Soft Lenses

Complications associated with the use of contact lenses have been described in a chapter of a monograph (30). The basic reasons for complications are:

1. Inadequate lens-to-cornea fitting,
2. Insufficient oxygen transmissibility of the contact lens,
3. A preexisting ocular pathology,

4. Interference with environmental factors,
5. Poorly maintained contact lenses,
6. Contaminated contact lenses, and
7. Use of incorrect contact lenses.

More recently, a review appeared concerning the existing literature describing complications with contemporary contact lenses and their management (31).

5.4.1 *Allergic and Toxic Reactions*

5.4.1.1 *Thimerosal*

The allergic and toxic effects of preservatives found in soft contact lens solutions have been reviewed (32). Thimerosal, a preservative commonly found in soft contact lens solutions, may cause ocular delayed hypersensitivity. Thimerosal is shown in Figure 5.3.

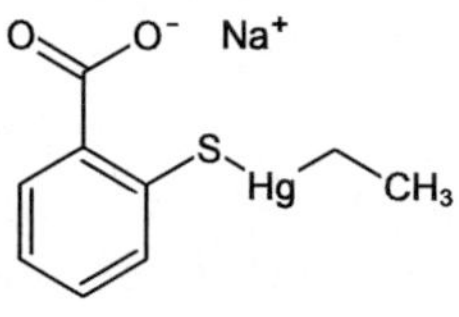

Figure 5.3 Thimerosal.

Patients with delayed hypersensitivity to thimerosal may develop conjunctival hyperemia, corneal infiltrates and intolerance to lens wear with the use of soft contact lens solutions containing thimerosal. Delayed hypersensitivity to thimerosal can be demonstrated by an occlusive patch test or intradermal injection. Discontinuation of chemical disinfection with substitution of thermal disinfection using unit-dose, non-preserved saline causes resolution of signs and symptoms. Another cause of lens wear intolerance is contact lens associated giant papillary conjunctivitis.

Protein deposits on the lens may act as antigens and initiate an allergic condition which disappears when the lens is discontinued. Alternatively, the giant papillae may be the result of mechanical irritation induced by the contact lenses. The chemical preservatives that are found in soft contact lens solutions cause epithelial toxicity when applied to isolated rabbit corneas. However, corneal toxicity in a clinical setting has not been demonstrated (32).

5.4.1.2 *Benzalkonium Chlorides*

Benzalkonium chlorides are generally known to be bactericidal and are not toxic to the eye at levels below about 0.01 % (33). Therefore, a benzalkonium chloride compound is a commonly used preservative in ophthalmic preparations and hard contact lens care products. However, the same levels of benzalkonium chlorides are toxic to the eye when used with soft contact lenses because of the tendency of the benzalkonium chloride and other quaternary amines to concentrate in the soft lens.

It has been found that soft contact lenses may be effectively sterilized and used without damage to the lenses or injury to the eyes of the user by contacting the soft lens with a sterile, aqueous, substantially isotonic solution containing an active ingredient (33). A preferred compound is alkyl (tallow) triethanol ammonium chloride.

5.4.1.3 *Acanthamoeba Infections*

Acanthamoeba castellanii has been recognized as an opportunistic human pathogen capable of causing severe lesions during eye infections, which are mainly associated with contact lens users (34).

Free-living amebae belonging to the genus Acanthamoeba are the causative agents of granulomatous amebic encephalitis, a chronic progressive disease of the central nervous system, and of amebic keratitis, a chronic eye infection. Granulomatous amebic encephalitis occurs more frequently in immunocompromised patients while keratitis occurs in healthy individuals.

The recent increased incidence in Acanthamoeba infections is due in part to infection in patients with acquired immune deficiency syndrome, while that for keratitis is due to the increased use of contact lenses (35).

During periods of stress, trophozoites of Acanthamoeba undergo a cellular differentiation process (termed encystment) resulting in the formation of double-walled cysts with their associated increased *in-vitro* resistance to antimicrobial agents used both in therapy and in contact lens disinfection systems (36).

In order to describe the early morphological events observed during the invasion of two pathogenic strains of Acanthamoeba (genotype T4), *A. castellanii* and *A. culbertsoni*, at the olfactory meatus and cerebral, pulmonary, renal, hepatic and splenic tissue levels, an *in-vivo* invasion study was done (37).

A. castellanii showed a higher invasion rate than *A. culbertsoni*, which was only able to reach lung and brain tissue in the *in-vivo* model. This study supports the previous evidence of lack of inflammatory response during the early stages of infection. Acanthamoeba invasion of the central nervous system (CNS) and other organs is a slow and contact-dependent process. The early morphological events during the invasion of amoebae include the penetration of trophozoites into different epithelia: olfactory, respiratory, alveolar space, and renal tubule, which resemble the process of amoebae invasion described in corneal tissue. The data suggest that after reaching the nasal epithelium, trophozoites continued invading, separating and lifting the most superficial cells, then migrate and penetrate between the cell junctions without causing a cytolytic effect on adjacent cells. These results reaffirm the idea that contact-dependent mechanisms are relevant for amoebae of the genus Acanthamoebagenus regardless of the invasion site (37).

Acanthamoeba keratitis is a rare, vision-threatening condition, which has increased in recent years due to the wearing of soft contact lenses (38). Acanthamoeba is a protozoa found in soil, fresh and sea water, and in contact lens cleaning solutions (39).

Riboflavin and UVA therapy can be used as an adjuvant treatment for medically refractive Acanthamoeba keratitis (40). Two treatment sessions involving the topical application of a 0.1% B2 solution to the ocular surface combined with 30 *min* of UVA irradiation focused on the corneal ulcer.

All the treated patients showed a rapid reduction in their symptoms and a decreased ulcer size after the first treatment session. The progress of the clinical improvement began to slow after 1 to 3 weeks of the first application and was then renewed after the second application (40).

Acanthamoeba keratitis with total necrosis and dislodgment of cornea, iris, and crystalline lens with exposure of vitreous hyaloids face was investigated (41).

In the case of a patient, a slit-lamp examination revealed ring infiltration and stromal edema with haziness. The patient was prescribed anti-acanthamoeba treatment.

At the last examination, the left eye was pthysic due to a ciliary shut down and visual acuity remained light perception.

So, early awareness of Acanthamoeba keratitis, especially in contact lens wearers, and applying diagnostic modalities, like confocal microscopy and early appropriate management with cysticide agents, such as poly(hexamethylene) biguanide, may prevent such untoward complications (41).

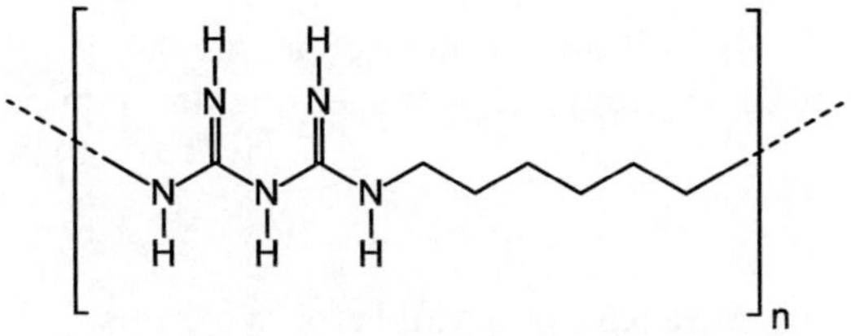

Figure 5.4 Poly(hexamethylene) biguanide.

5.4.1.4 *Acanthamoeba Infections*

Free-living amoeba of the *Acanthamoeba* spp. genus is the causal agent of Acanthamoeba keratitis, an ocular infection that poses a risk to corneal integrity. The number of reported cases worldwide is increasing yearly, especially among contact lens users, and the rate of successful treatment is low, despite advances in antimicrobial chemotherapy and supportive care (38).

The ophthalmic toxicity profile of chlorhexidine and propamidine isethionate eye drops was assessed by an *in-vitro* evaluation method (42). Chlorhexidine (1,1′-hexamethylenebis[5-(4-chlorophenyl)biguanide]) and propamidine isethionate (a mixture of 2-Hydroxyethanesulfonic acid and 4,4′-[1,3-Propanediyl bis(oxy)] dibenzenecarboximidamide in a ratio of 1:2) are shown in Figure 5.5.

Both eye drop formulations showed a time-dependent and concentration-dependent toxicity profile, in which long periods of time

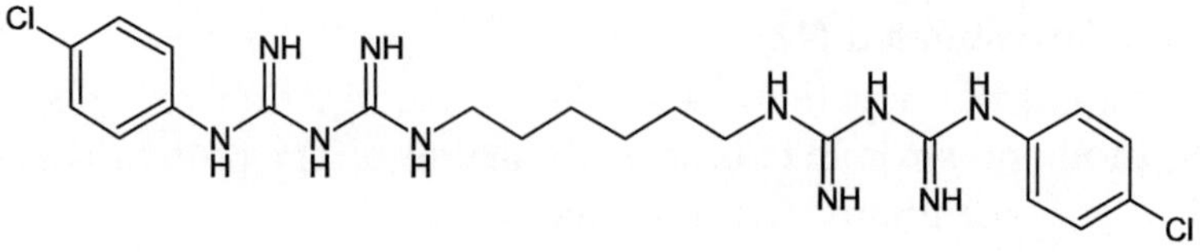

Chlorhexidine
1,1′-Hexamethylenebis[5-(4-chlorophenyl)biguanide]

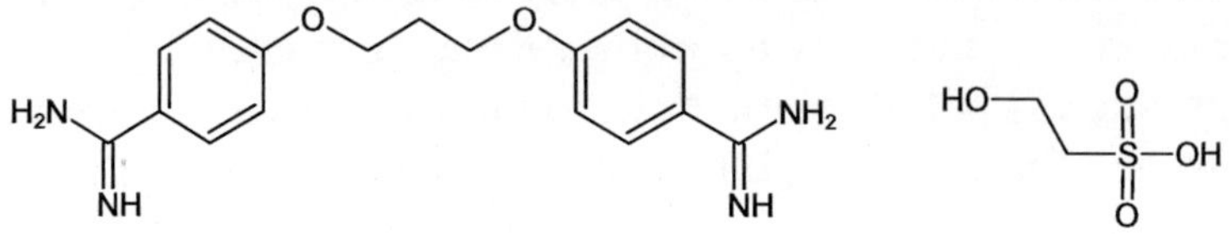

Propamidine isethionate
4,4′-[1,3-Propanediyl bis(oxy)] dibenzenecarboximidamide
2-Hydroxyethanesulfonic acid

Figure 5.5 Compounds for eye drops.

and high concentrations were more detrimental to cells. In prolonged times of exposure, propamidine is more harmful to cells than chlorhexidine. In contrast, no irritation has been detected in using the hen's egg chorioallantoic membrane test and no alterations in the corneal transparency nor permeability was produced by the treatment with both eye drops (42).

5.5 Disinfection Agents

There are many known compounds that can act as a disinfecting agent. For example, solutions of 70-85% (volume/volume) ethanol are commonly used as disinfectants (43). There are two forms of ethanol generally available: Denatured ethanol and potable alcohol. Both denatured and potable ethanol compounds are used in the preparation of such solutions.

Denatured ethanol contains additives for the purpose of preventing or reducing abuse or consumption of the alcohol. Such additives may include aviation fuel, emetics, various organic solvents and mercury salts.

Bitrex® (denatonium benzoate, cf. Figure 5.6) is an example of an additive that is commonly present in ethanol in varying amounts. For instance, Bitrex is present in specially denatured alcohol grade-3 (SDAG-3) at 700 *mg* per 100 *l*, and is present in specially denatured alcohol grade-6 (SDAG-6) at 1,000 *mg* per 100 *l*. Solutions of 70-85% ethanol are effective in inactivating most vegetative bacteria-, fungi-, and lipid-containing viruses. However, ethanol is not effective against bacterial spores (43).

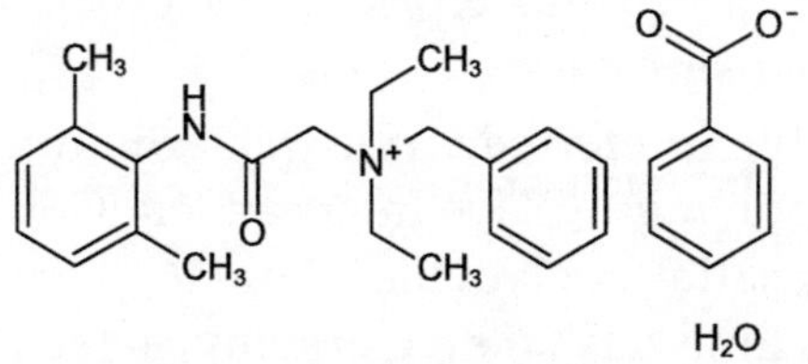

Figure 5.6 Denatonium benzoate.

Combinations of disinfecting agents can compound the risks associated with the use of any of those agents individually. Due to interactions between disinfecting agents, the combination may introduce new hazards in use, such as reduced efficacy of the disinfecting agents, irritation to the user, environmental risks such as flammability, and reduced residual effects of the disinfecting agents.

5.5.1 *Polymeric Biguanide and Vinylimidazole*

A disinfecting solution for contact lenses consists of the combination of a polymeric biguanide and a quaternized vinylimidazole polymer (44). Unlike hard contact lenses, soft-type contact lenses have a tendency to bind and concentrate fluids, environmental pollutants, water impurities, as well as antimicrobial agents and other active ingredients commonly found in lens care solutions. In most instances, the low levels of the ingredients in these do not lead to eye tissue irritation when used properly.

Nevertheless, especially due to the inherent binding action of protein deposits to soft lens materials, some disinfecting agents and preservatives tend to build up on lens surfaces and may become concentrated to potentially hazardous levels. Thus, when released they could cause corneal inflammation and other eye tissue irritation.

Poly(hexamethylene biguanide) (PHMB) and related polymers have been shown to be effective biocidal agents. PHMB, however, is less effective against fungi than bacteria. In contrast, quaternized polymers are effective against fungi and less effective against bacteria.

The combination of a biguanide polymer and a copolymer from *N*-vinyl-2-pyrrolidone and quaternized vinylimidazole has been found to result in a strong antimicrobial activity across the entire range of microorganisms typically associated with ophthalmic preservation and disinfection.

A particularly preferred polyquaternium copolymer is Luviquat® 370 polymer (CTFA International Cosmetic Ingredient Dictionary designation polyquaternium-16, commercially available from BASF, Ludwigshafen, Germany) which is the polymerization product of a mixture of comonomers of which 70% is *N*-vinyl-2-pyrrolidone and 30% is vinylimidazolium methochloride, commercially available as a composition with a solids content of about 40% by weight in water. These compounds are shown in Figure 5.7.

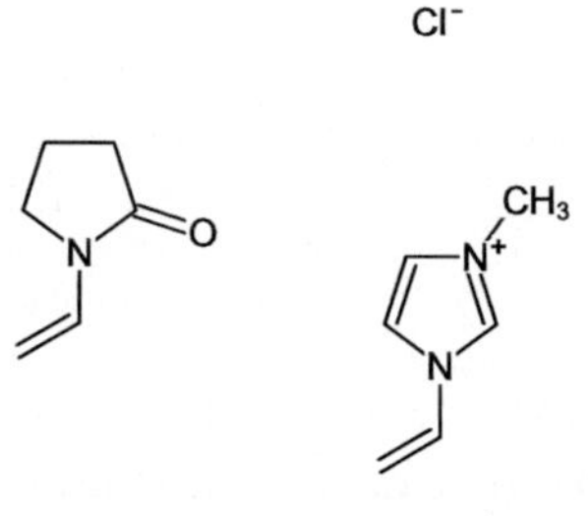

Figure 5.7 *N*-Vinyl-2-pyrrolidone and Vinylimidazolium methochloride.

5.5.2 *Saccharides*

Ophthalmic solutions have been described that have a preservative efficacy and comfort after prolonged use (45). These ophthalmic solutions have been used for some period of time and are available as over-the-counter products.

There is a need to ensure that solutions that are used in direct contact with corneal tissue, such as the delivery of active pharmaceutical agent to the eye, or indirectly, such as the cleaning, conditioning or storage of devices that will come in contact with corneal tissue, such as contact lenses, do not introduce sources of bacterial or other microbial infection.

Thus, preservatives are included to reduce the viability of microbes in the solution and to lessen the chance of contamination of the solution by the user since many of the solutions are bought, opened, used, sealed and then reused.

These ophthalmic solutions employ inositol, i.e., cyclohexanhexol, and other simple saccharides in order to more effectively preserve solutions and reduce the degree to which cationic preservatives will deposit on contact lenses. Some simple saccharides are detailed in Table 5.3. Also, some compounds are shown in Figure 5.8.

Table 5.3 Saccharides (45).

Compound	Compound	Compound	Compound
Inositol	Mannitol	Sorbitol	Sucrose
Dextrose	Glycerin	Propylene Glycol	Ribose
Triose	Tetrose	Erythrose	Threose
Pentose	Arabinose	Ribulose	Xylose
Xylulose	Lyxose	Hexose	Allose
Altrose	Fructose	Galactose	Glucose
Gulose	Idose	Mannose	Sorbose
Talose	Tagatose	Adlose	Ketose
Heptose	Sedoheptulose	Xylitol	Polyol

Preservatives that are specifically useful include PHMB, Polyquad™, chlorhexidine, and benzalkonium chloride, as well as other cationic preservatives that may prove useful in the present invention as well. The cationic preservatives are used at effective amounts as preservatives, and in the instance of PHMB from 0.0001% to higher levels of about 0.01%.

Ophthalmologically acceptable chelating agents that are useful are listed in Table 5.4 and some compounds are shown in Figure 5.9.

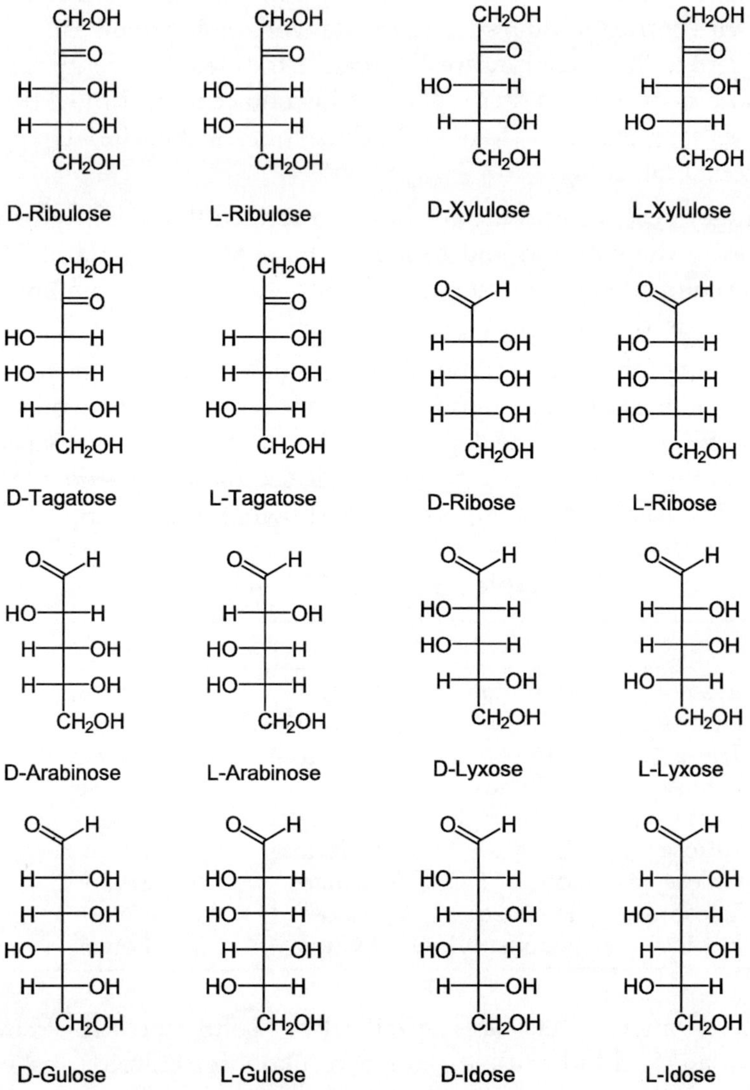

Figure 5.8 Saccharides (46).

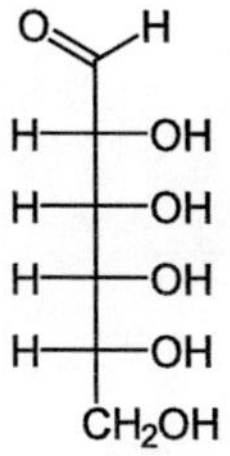

D-Allose

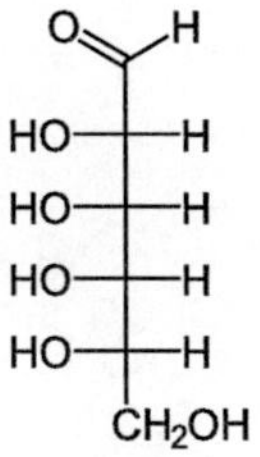

L-Allose

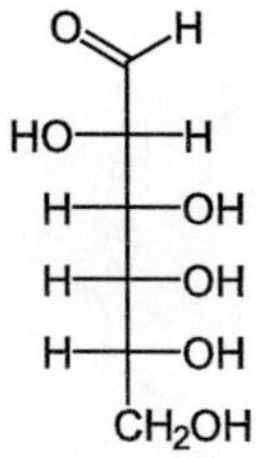

D-Altrose

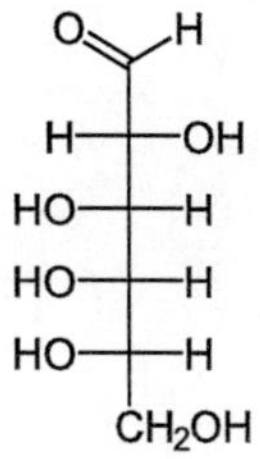

L-Altrose

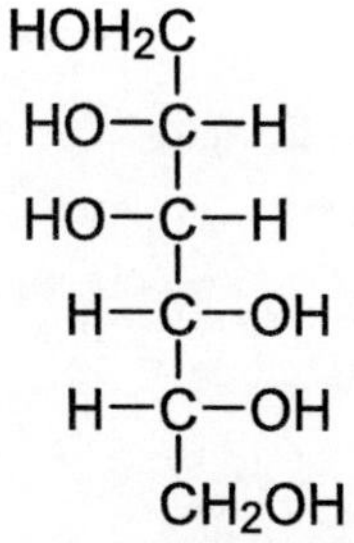

D-Mannit(ol)

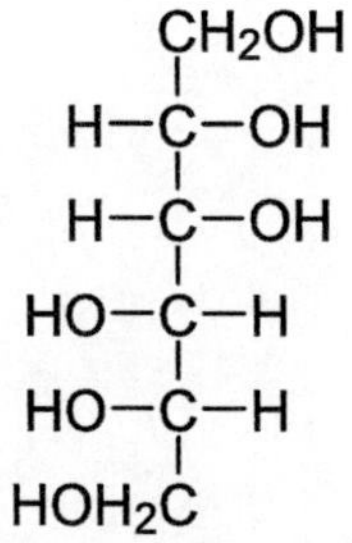

L-Mannit(ol)

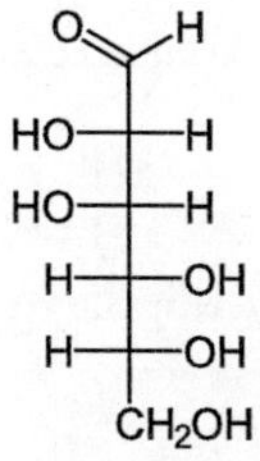

D-Mannose

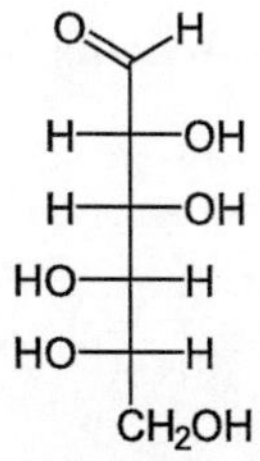

L-Mannose

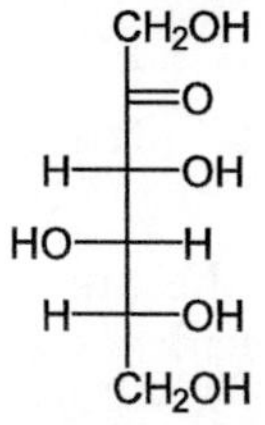

D-Sorbose

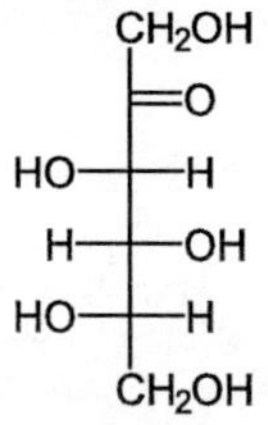

L-Sorbose

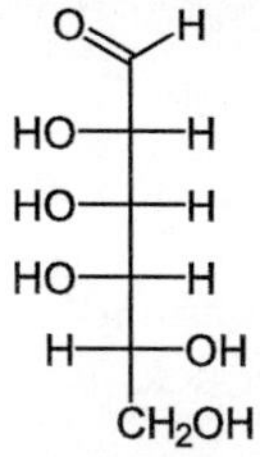

D-Talose

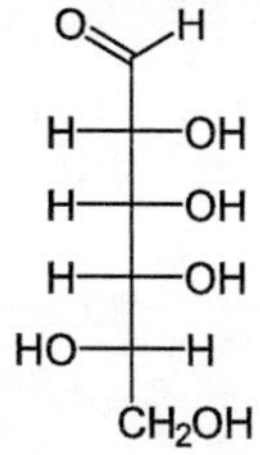

L-Talose

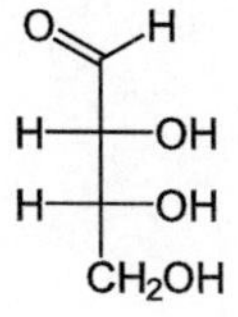

D-Erythrose

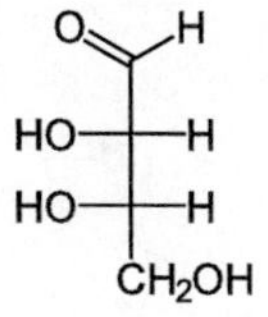

L-Erythrose

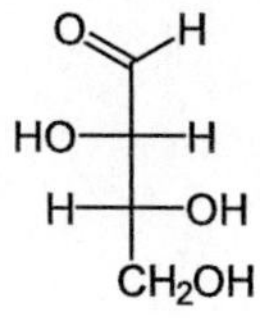

D-Threose

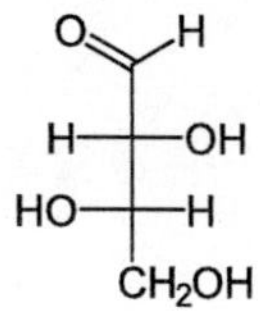

L-Threose

Figure 5.8 (cont) Saccharides (46).

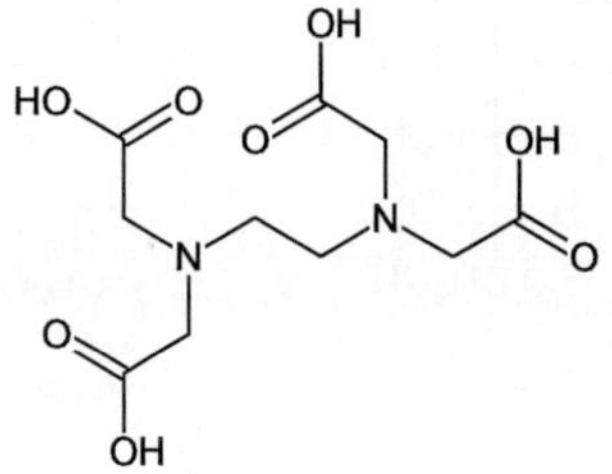

Ethylenediaminetetraacetic acid

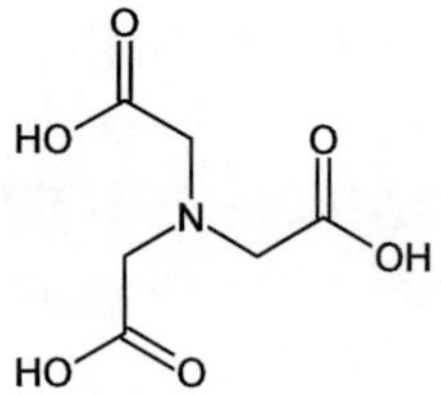

Nitrilotriacetic acid

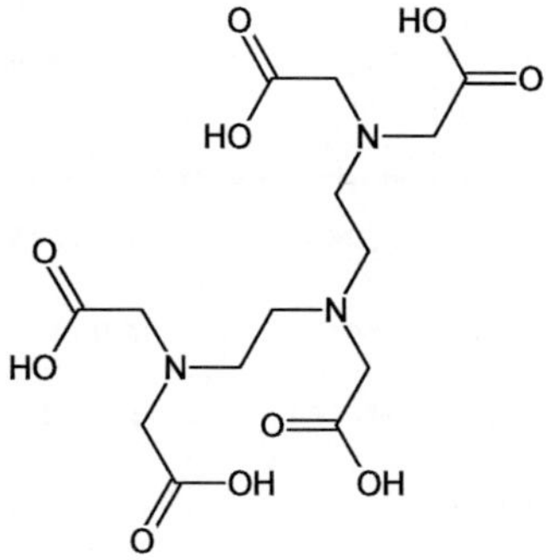

Diethylenetriamine pentaacetic acid

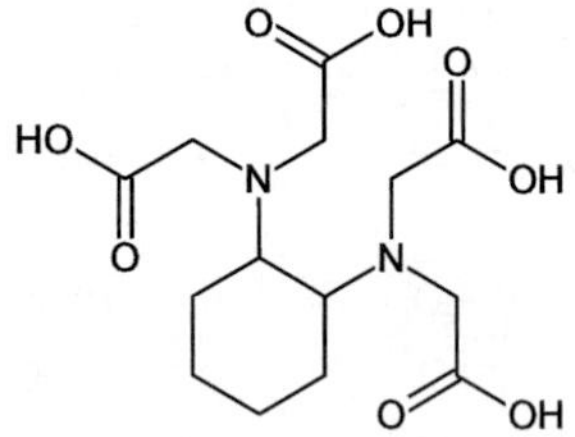

1,2-Diaminocyclohexane tetraacetic acid

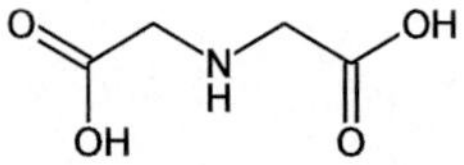

Amino diacetic acid

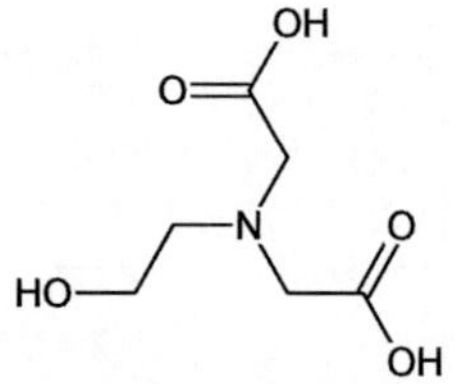

Hydroxyethylamino diacetic acid

Figure 5.9 Chelating agents.

Table 5.4 Chelating agents (45).

Compound
Ethylenediaminetetraacetic acid
Nitrilotriacetic acid
Diethylenetriamine pentaacetic acid
Hydroxyethylethylenediamine triacetic acid
1,2-Diaminocyclohexane tetraacetic acid
Aminodiacetic acid
Hydroxyethylamino diacetic acid

These acids can be used in the form of their water-soluble salts, particularly their alkali metal salts.

The pH of the solutions should be adjusted to be compatible with the eye and the contact lens, preferably between 7.0 to 7.6. Significant deviations from neutral (pH 7.3) will cause changes in the physical parameters (i.e., diameter) in some contact lenses. A low pH of less than 5.5 can cause burning and stinging of the eyes. A very low or very high pH of less than 3.0 or greater than 10 can cause ocular damage.

Additional preservatives that can be employed are Poly(hexamethylene) biguanide, *N*-alkyl-2-pyrrolidone, chlorhexidine, alexidine, polyquaternium-1, hexetidine, bronopol and a very low concentration of hydrogen peroxide of 30–200 *ppm* (45). Some of these compounds are shown in Figure 5.10

5.5.3 *Amphipathic Peptides*

The term *amphipathic* in application to peptides refers to peptides which contain hydrophilic and hydrophobic amino acid moieties as side chains, which are oriented in relation to one another so that the peptides have discrete hydrophilic and hydrophobic faces or regions defined by a multiplicity of the respective hydrophilic and hydrophobic side chains (47).

For example, when the peptide is in an amphipathic α-helix conformation, the hydrophobic amino acid side chains are oriented on one face of the α-helix while the hydrophilic amino acid side chains are oriented on the other face of the α-helix. When the peptide is amphipathic and exists in solution in a β-pleated sheet confor-

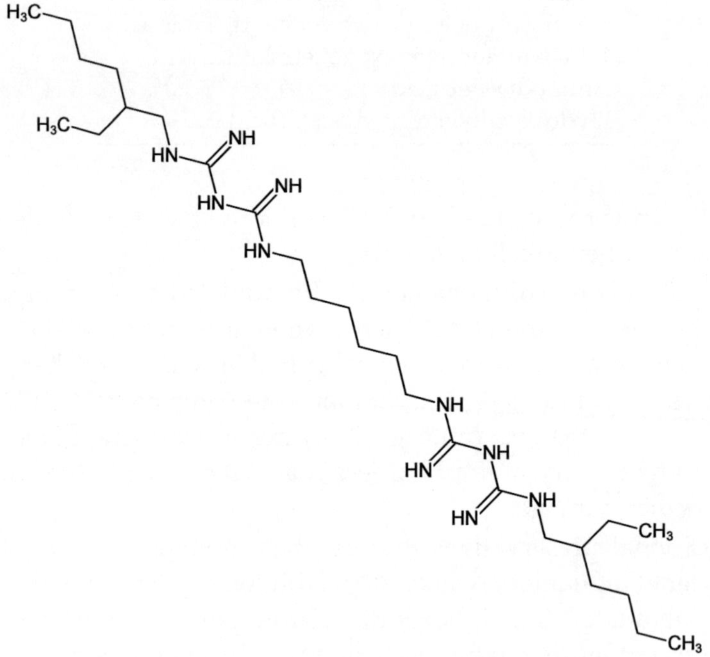

Alexidine

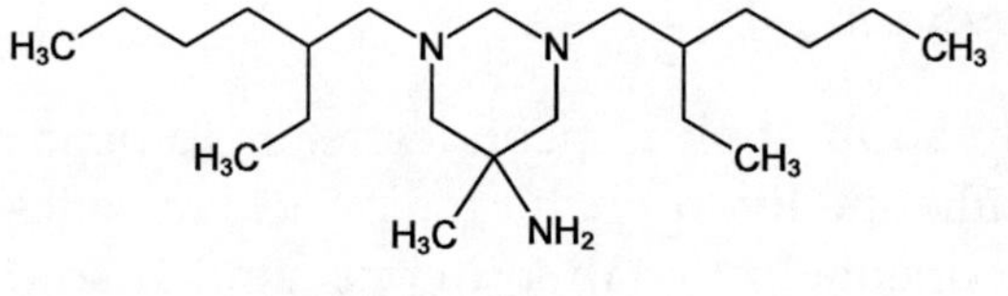

Hexetidine

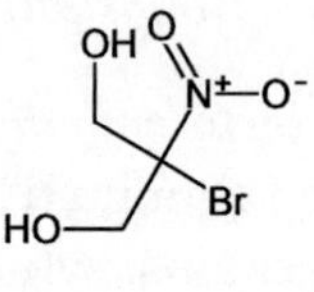

Bronopol

Figure 5.10 Preservatives.

mation, the peptide likewise exhibits hydrophobic and hydrophilic faces derived from the alignment of the oriented amino acid side chains of the molecule.

A wide variety of amphipathic peptides may be effectively utilized, including the natural and synthetic melittin-class, the cecropin-class, the magainin-class, and defensin-class peptides.

The β-pleated sheet conformation of peptides potentially usefully employed may be readily determined by the circular dichroism technique (48). The preparation of polymeric biguanides from a diamine and salts thereof and a diamine salt of dicyanimide has been detailed (49–51). The preparation runs as:

Preparation 5–1: First, 29.2 parts of hexamethylenediamine are dissolved in 200 parts of water and 49.4 parts of zinc dicyanimide are added to the solution. The mixture is heated to 60°C, the pH of the mixture at this stage being about 11. Carbon dioxide gas is passed through the mixture until the pH is 8–7. The mixture is cooled, filtered and the insoluble residue washed with water to extract the optimum amount of the hexamethylenediamine salt of dicyanimide, which is obtained in substantially quantitative yield from the zinc dicyanimide used. Then, 29.0 parts of hexamethylenediamine are added to the mixture of filtrates and washes and about 50.7 parts of 36% aqueous hydrochloric acid are added until the solution is at pH 8-7. The solution is then distilled at atmospheric pressure to remove water until the temperature of the mixture is 150–155°C. It is then stirred at 150–155°C for 4 *h*.

The product is obtained as an aqueous solution containing 107 parts of poly(hexamethylene biguanide hydrochloride) by adding water to the reaction mixture and cooling.

The monomer, hexamethylene biguanide, is shown in Figure 5.11.

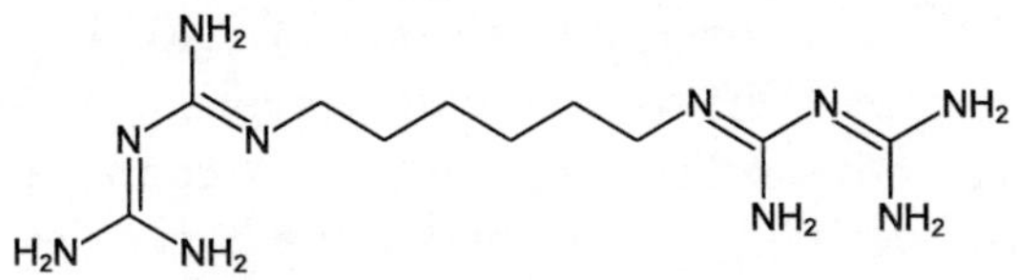

Figure 5.11 Hexamethylene biguanide.

5.5.4 *Antibacterial Properties*

Compared with traditional glasses, the comfortable and convenient contact lens has seen an upsurge among the public (52). However, due to the lack of antibacterial properties of ordinary contact lenses, the risk of eye infection is greatly increased accordingly. On the other hand, ordinary contact lenses also cannot effectively reduce the short-wavelength blue light emitted from electronic products, such as mobile phones and computers. Aiming at the above two problems, zinc oxide (ZnO)/cyclized poly(acrylonitrile) (CPAn) composites were developed for the modification of contact lenses. After loading with this composition, the contact lens showed a broad spectrum of antibacterial properties.

Staphylococcus aureus and *Escherichia coli* were selected as the representatives of Gram-positive bacteria and Gram-negative bacteria to conduct antibacterial experiments. In the CPAn group, the bacterial survival rate of *S. aureus* was around 88% via the plate count method, which indicated that CPAn had no significant antibacterial effect. However, the ZnO group exhibited an excellent antibacterial activity with only about 8% of the bacteria surviving.

Further experiments also showed that this composition can block UVB, UVA, as well as blue light selectively, under the premise of ensuring hydrophilicity and certain transparency (52).

CPAn has a strong absorption effect in the visible range, while ZnO almost none. Therefore, the absorption capacity of ZnO/CPAn to visible light was greatly increased due to the introduction of CPAn. The energy band gaps of ZnO (3.16 *eV*), CPAn (2.20 *eV*), and ZnO/CPAn (2.40 *eV*) were calculated according to the UV-vis absorption curves (52).

For ZnO/CPAn, the energy band gap of 2.40 *eV* meant that it could be excited by light sources with wavelengths less than 516 *nm* to produce active substances with antibacterial ability, which had been partly verified by the Rhodamine B dye degradation experiment. Moreover, the contact angle of ZnO/CPAn was less than 90°, which was considered hydrophilic, revealing that it could be added to many commercially available contact lenses composed of a hydrophilic material (52).

5.6 Silicone Hydrogels

Many authors defend the high permeability of silicone hydrogels due to the great advantage of these lenses compared to conventional hydrogels since, by allowing greater passage of oxygen to the cornea, they reduce hypoxia, corneal edema, and limbal and conjunctival redness, making these types of lenses especially suitable for prolonged use (53–55).

However, in a study, the worst results with respect to non-wearers were found in those who wore silicone hydrogel contact lenses and were exposed to the computer for more than 6 $h\,d^{-1}$ (56).

Due to their high elastic modulus, highly hydrophobic surfaces, and the tendency to accumulate lipid deposits, silicone hydrogel lenses in some cases may not completely satisfy criteria of biocompatibility with the ocular surface, leading to various kinds of complications and reduced comfort (57–60).

Moreover, the risk of infection increases if these lenses (most for biweekly or monthly use) are not adequately cleaned or disinfected (61–64).

5.7 Limbal Stem Cell Deficiency

The corneal epithelium is constantly renewed throughout life (65). Corneal epithelial stem cells reside at the limbus, a distinct anatomical structure at the corneo-conjunctival junction (66–70). In cases of mild corneal surface damage, the limbal stem cells are activated, proliferate, and migrate to the central cornea, assisting tissue regeneration and homeostasis (65).

Extensive damage to the limbal region of the cornea leads to a severe form of corneal blindness termed limbal stem cell deficiency (LSCD) (65). Whereas most cases of corneal opacity can be treated with full thickness corneal transplants, LSCD requires a stem cell transplantation for successful ocular surface reconstruction.

Current treatments for LSCD using limbal stem cell transplantation involve the use of murine NIH 3T3 cells and human amniotic membranes as culture substrates, which pose the threat of transmission of animal-derived pathogens and donor tissue-derived cryptic infections. In this study, the aim was to produce surface-modified therapeutic contact lenses for the culture and delivery of corneal epithelial cells for the treatment of LSCD. This approach avoids the possibility of suture-related complications and is completely synthetic.

Plasma polymerization was used to deposit acid functional groups onto the lenses at various concentrations. Before plasma polymerization, acrylic acid (AA) and 1,7-octadiene monomers were processed with three freeze-thaw cycles to remove any dissolved gas. Silicone hydrogel contact lenses (Efrofilcon A and Contamac) were placed concave side facing upward within the chamber on a culture plate as a support base. A cleaned glass coverslip was also inserted for X-ray photoelectron spectroscopy analysis of the deposited plasma polymer layer. The AA was used to provide the acid functionality (–COOH), while 1,7-octadiene was used as the diluent to reduce the concentration of acid groups deposited onto the surfaces.

These two chemicals are termed monomers and they were introduced into the chamber using a fine needle valve at various ratios at a combined flow rate of 2 *sccm*. Several ratios of the monomers AA 1,7-octadiene were explored, ranging from 100:0 to 0:100. The plasma was sustained at a power of 2 *W* over a period of 15 *min*. Uncoated Efrofilcon A and Contamac lenses are used as negative controls and Focus Night & Day lens and Ciba Vision were used as positive control lenses.

Each surface was tested for its suitability to promote corneal epithelial cell adhesion, proliferation, retention of stem cells, and differentiation, and it was found that acid-based chemistries promoted better cell adhesion and proliferation.

It was found that the lenses coated with a higher percentage of acid functional groups resulted in a higher number of cells transferred onto the corneal wound bed in rabbit models of LSCD. Immunohistochemistry of the recipient cornea confirmed the presence of autologous, transplanted 5-bromo-2′-deoxyuridine labeled cells. 5-Bromo-2′-deoxyuridine is shown in Figure 5.12.

Hematoxylin staining has also revealed the presence of a stratified epithelium at 26 *d* post-transplantation. Hematoxylin is shown in Figure 5.13.

This study provides the first evidence for *in-vivo* transfer and survival of cells transplanted from a contact lens to the wounded

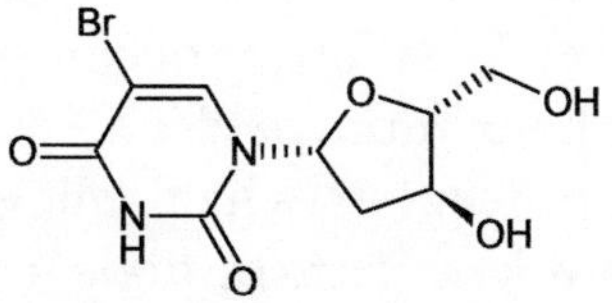

Figure 5.12 5-Bromo-2′-deoxyuridine.

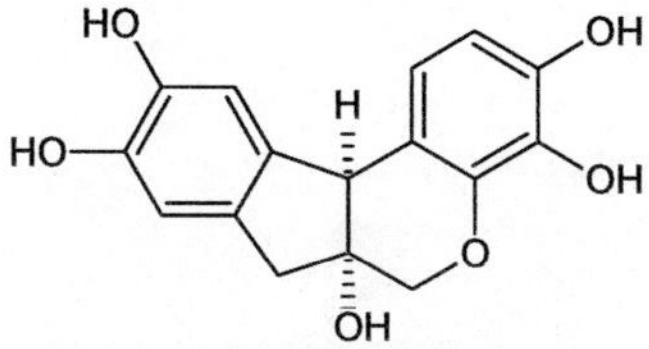

Figure 5.13 Hematoxylin.

corneal surface. It also proposes the possibility of using plasma polymer-coated contact lenses with high acid functional groups as substrates for the culture and transfer of limbal cells in the treatment of LSCD (65).

5.8 Computer Vision Syndrome

As computers become part of our everyday life, more and more people are experiencing a variety of ocular symptoms related to computer use (71). These include eyestrain, tired eyes, irritation, redness, blurred vision, and double vision, collectively referred to as computer vision syndrome. This section describes both the characteristics and treatment modalities that are available at this time. Computer vision syndrome symptoms may be the cause of ocular (ocular surface abnormalities or accommodative spasms) and/or extraocular (ergonomic) etiologies.

However, the major contributor to computer vision syndrome symptoms by far appears to be a dry eye. The visual effects of various display characteristics such as lighting, glare, display quality, refresh rates, and radiation are also discussed as being contributors. Treatment requires a multidirectional approach combining ocular therapy with adjustment of the workstation. Proper lighting, anti-glare filters, ergonomic positioning of computer monitor and regular work breaks may help improve visual comfort. Lubricating eye drops and special computer glasses help relieve ocular surface-related symptoms. More work needs to be done to specifically define the processes that cause computer vision syndrome and to develop and improve effective treatments that successfully address these causes.

The symptoms of computer vision syndrome (CVS) are categorized into 4 main groups (71):

1. Asthenopia,
2. Ocular surface-related,
3. Visual, and
4. Extraocular.

5.8.1 *Tests and Analysis*

The relationship between CVS in computer workers and contact lens use was analyzed according to lens materials (56).

A total of 426 civil-service office workers were analyzed, of whom 22% were contact lens wearers. Workers completed the Computer Vision Syndrome Questionnaire (CVS-Q) and provided information on their contact lenses and exposure to video display terminals at work. CVS was defined as a CVS-Q score of 6 or more. The covariates were age and sex.

Logistic regression was used to calculate the association (crude and adjusted for age and sex) between CVS and individual and work-related factors, and between CVS and contact lens type.

It was found that contact lens wearers are more likely to suffer CVS than non-lens wearers, with a prevalence of 65% vs. 50% (56). Workers who wear contact lenses and are exposed to the computer for more than 6 $h d^{-1}$ are more likely to suffer CVS than non-lens wearers working at the computer for the same amount of time. So, regular contact lens use increases CVS after 6 h of computer work (56).

5.8.2 *Pathophysiology*

Asthenopia is the term to describe eye strain due to any cause, and is the major component of CVS. Ocular surface-related symptoms include dry eyes, red eyes, and irritated eyes. Visual symptoms of CVS include blurring of vision, double vision, difficulty in focusing, and headache. Extraocular symptoms such as neck pain, shoulder pain, and backache are often due to poor ergonomic design and posture.

Symptomatology of CVS is related to exposure of the eyes to a brightly lit screen for prolonged periods, further complicated by poor posture and environmental factors (particularly ambient light). Viewing a monitor screen at a close distance requires accommodation, convergence, and miosis. One must be aware that working on a computer differs vastly from reading a printed text. The text and images on computer screens are composed of small pixels and when there are fewer pixels, the resultant decrease in resolution causes excessive demand on one's visual system. Screen factors, such as brightness, contrast, screen glare, and screen refresh rate, increase stress on the visual apparatus. Low refresh rate causes flickering and is known to contribute to symptoms of CVS (71).

Computer users with myopia and hypermetropia can develop blurring of vision, diplopia, and transient myopia after a day's work. These impairments are transient in most of the workers (72, 73), but may persist in some even after work (74). Dry eyes are a common symptom of CVS among computer users due to corneal drying from reduced blink rate and incomplete blinking (75). The blink rate is significantly reduced while working on computers compared to resting time (76). Small font size and low contrast of suboptimal quality monitors are other factors reducing the blink rate (77). Compared to reading a textbook, one uses a horizontal gaze when reading a computer monitor, resulting in more evaporation of corneal tear film and consequent dryness (78).

5.8.3 *Problems for Radiologists*

In the last century, occupational harm to radiologists was mainly focused on the harmful effects of ionizing radiation (79).

Various guidelines, regulatory frameworks, and progressive equipment improvement were developed in the interest of the health of radiologists and other radiation healthcare workers. As a result, the incidence of radiation work-related injury among radiologists is at a very low level (78).

The daily work pattern of radiologists has evolved dramatically in the last decade. The shift from hard copy viewing to reading from a picture archiving and communication system, means that radiologists have to spend long hours gazing at brightly lit monitors. Typically, a radiologist spends an average of 8–9 *h* per work day in front of the picture archiving and communication system workstation in addition to using brightly lit screens of other digital devices (e.g., smartphones, tablets, personal computers, laptops, television, etc.).

The ocular occupational hazards faced by radiologists have been discussed along with suggestions that may help in minimizing such hazards (78).

5.9 Dry Eye Problems

The main reasons for the discontinuation of contact lens wear are ocular dryness and discomfort. Proteoglycan 4, a mucinous glycoprotein, and hyaluronic acid (HA), a nonsulfated linear glycosaminoglycan, are naturally present in the eye and contribute to ocular hydration and lubrication (80).

The impact of the structure of the recombinant human Proteoglycan HA complex on contact lens properties was investigated, when one agent is grafted and the counterpart is physisorbed on the surface of model conventional or silicone contact lens materials (80). The investigation of the wettability, water retention, antifouling, and boundary lubricant properties of the prepared hydrogels showed that the interactions varied with the configuration of these materials on the hydrogel surface as well as the composition of the underlying substrate used.

5.9.1 *Ions in Tears*

Measurements of electrolytes and some protein concentrations in blood are routinely used to determine the overall health status of patients. In contrast to other medical specialties, far fewer tests are available in ophthalmology, and many diagnoses are based on visual examinations (81).

The present status of testing tear sample for dry eye diseases is limited to either measurement of the rate of tear production or the total electrolyte concentration.

A method to make fluorescent silicone hydrogel contact lens for the estimation of sodium ion concentrations in tears has been described (81).

Three sodium-sensitive fluorophores (SG-C16, SG-LPE and SG-PL) were synthesized by derivatizing the sodium green with 1-hexadecyl amine, 1-oleoyl-2-hydroxy-sn-glycero-3-phosphoethanolamine or poly-l-lysine, respectively. These compounds are shown in Figure 5.14.

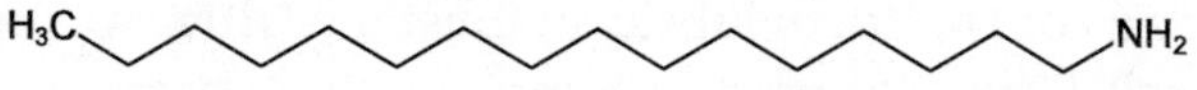

1-Hexadecyl amine

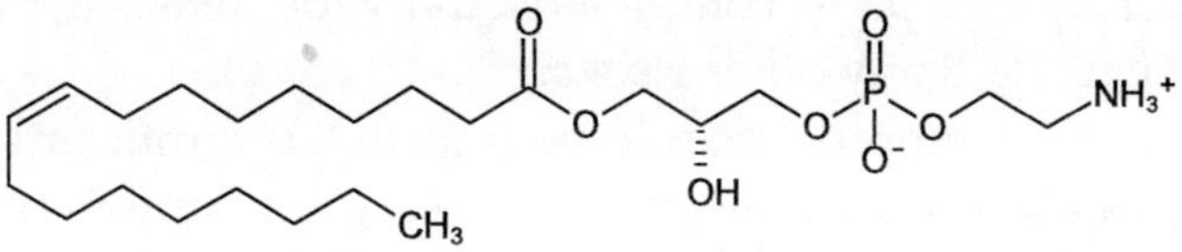

1-Oleoyl-2-hydroxy-sn-glycero-3-phosphoethanolamine

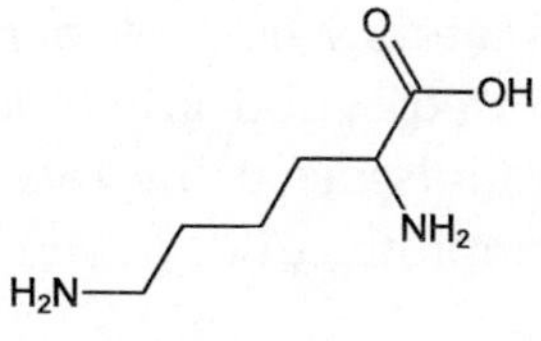

DL-Lysine

Figure 5.14 Compounds for derivatizing.

The probes were bound to a modern silicone hydrogel contact lens, i.e., Biofinity from CooperVision. The so-doped lenses were tested for sodium ion-dependent spectral properties of probes within the contact lens (81).

5.9.2 Treatment Methods

5.9.2.1 Honey Eye Drops

Contact lens-induced dry eye affects approximately 50% of contact lens wearers (82). The effects of Manuka (*Leptospermum* sp.) honey eye drops (Optimel, Melcare, Australia) on dry eye in contact lens wearers were investigated. The safety of the honey eye drops in contact lens wear and contact lens wearers' compliance were also evaluated.

For the study, 24 participants in the age from 20 to 55 years old with contact lens-related dry eye were recruited and randomized into two treatment groups. A total of 20 participants completed the study.

One group used Optimel eye drops twice a day for two weeks followed by a conventional lubricant (Systane Ultra, Alcon) therapy for two weeks. The other group completed the treatments in the reverse order. Before and after each treatment dry eye symptomology, ocular surface inflammation, and tear quantity and quality were assessed. The participants completed a daily log detailing their usage of treatments and any other issues.

The dry eye symptoms could be improved significantly after an Optimel treatment. Patients with more severe symptoms at baseline (BL) showed a greater improvement in their symptoms. No significant differences were observed in the objective signs of dry eye. This was presumably because of the short duration of the treatment (82).

Among the contact wearers who took part in the study, 75% of contact lens wearers reported a good adherence to the Optimel treatment and 95% reported no issues using this product. So, Optimel eye drops reduce the symptoms of dry eye in contact lens wearers and are safe to use (82).

5.9.2.2 Hyaluronic Acid

Contact lenses are widely used for ophthalmic drug delivery, but incorporation of drug or formulation in the contact lenses affects its optical and physical property (83). HA-laden ring implant contact lenses were fabricated with a modified cast-molding method in order to circumvent the changes in critical lens property. HA is shown in Figure 4.41

An attempt was made to improve the ocular residence time of HA by providing a sustained ocular HA delivery through implant contact lenses for the treatment of dry eye syndrome.

The optimization of the HA implant was carried out using 3^2 factorial design by tailoring the amount of crosslinking agent and the thickness of the implant to achieve sustained HA release with constraint on effective ion diffusivity.

The *in-vivo* pharmacokinetic study in rabbit tear fluid showed sustained HA release up to 15 d by fabricating implant (80 μg HA loading) with 78.4 μm thickness (total thickness of lens 100 μm) using 0.925% of crosslinking agent, with an effective ion diffusivity of greater than 1.5×10^{-6} $m^2 min^{-1}$.

An *in-vivo* efficacy study in benzalkonium chloride-induced dry eye syndrome rabbits showed a faster healing with implant contact lenses in comparison to positive control group.

The study demonstrated the promising potential of implantation technology to deliver HA without compromising the optical and physical properties of the contact lens (83).

5.9.2.3 *Diquafosol*

Diquafosol can be used in an ophthalmic solution for the treatment of dry eyes. Issues relating to the use of diquafosol have been presented in a review (84).

Diquafosol tetrasodium can be obtained from 5′-uridylic acid disodium salt and a diphosphoric acid salt (85). Also, a method has been reported of reacting uridine 5′-cyclic triphosphoric acid prepared by a dehydration condensation of uridine 5′-triphosphoric acid with uridine 5′-monophosphoric acid (86).

A therapeutic agent for dry eye has been described (87). It is characterized by being applied to an eye of a dry eye patient wearing soft contact lens, which consists of diquafosol or a salt thereof as an active ingredient. Diquafosol is shown in Figure 5.15.

The concentration of diquafosol is preferably 3% (w/v). In a study, a series of dinucleoside 5′-polyphosphates was synthesized (88). Also, their relative potencies as agonists at some G-protein-coupled receptors were determined. An ophthalmic solution was prepared as follows (87):

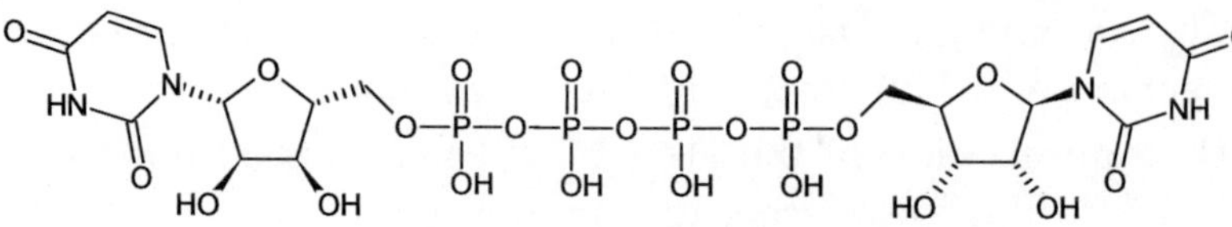

Figure 5.15 Diquafosol.

Preparation 5–2: Diquafosol sodium (3 *g*), sodium hydrogen phosphate hydrate (0.2 *g*), sodium chloride (0.41 *g*), potassium chloride (0.15 *g*) and benzalkonium chloride (0.0075 *g*) were dissolved in water and brought to a final volume of 100 *ml* followed by the addition of a pH adjuster to adjust the pH to 7.5.

5.9.3 *Comparative Study of the Reasons for Dry Eyes*

The reasons for dry eyes were investigated in a comparative study (89). Three groups were collected for the testing:

1. Asymptomatic contact lens wearers,
2. Symptomatic contact lens wearers who become asymptomatic upon lens removal, and
3. Symptomatic contact lens wearers who do not resolve upon lens removal.

The results are shown in Table 5.5.

Table 5.5 Results of dry-eye study (89).

Group property	Number of People	Amount/[%]
Asymptomatic contact lens wearers	37	40
Contact lens-induced dry eye	30	33
Underlying physiological dry eyes	25	27

Visual Analog Scale ratings, OSDI score, and SPEED score were significantly better for the asymptomatic contact lens wearer group but did not distinguish contact lens-induced dry eyes from dry eyes. The dry eye group was significantly worse than the contact lens-induced dry eye group and asymptomatic contact lens wearers, which were similar, in the precorneal noninvasive tear breakup time (8.2 *s* dry eye group vs. 12.3 *s* contact lens-induced dry eye group, and 14.3 *s* asymptomatic contact lens wearer group), anterior displacement of the line of Marx, and superior conjunctival staining (89).

So, many contact lens wearers with dryness symptoms have an underlying dry eye condition and will not respond to treatments aimed at changing lenses or solutions.

5.10 Orthokeratology

Orthokeratology is a clinical technique that uses specially designed rigid contact lenses to reshape the cornea to temporarily reduce or eliminate refractive error (90).

The history of traditional daily wear orthokeratology has been reviewed (90).

Unconfirmed stories suggest that in ancient times, the Chinese slept with small weights or sandbags on their eyelids to reduce myopia. This principle is certainly similar to modern orthokeratology. More than one century ago, in the very early days of glass scleral contact lenses, the French ophthalmologist Eugene Kalt attempted to modify corneal curvature in keratoconic patients by using flat-fitting lenses that applied pressure against the cone (91). It was not until the advent of the corneal lens that the possibility of deliberately manipulating corneal shape with contact lenses to modify refractive error began to be recognized.

Soon after the introduction of PMMA corneal contact lenses in the 1950s, practitioners began to notice unintended changes in corneal curvature and refractive error in some patients, particularly when the lenses were fitted flatter than corneal curvature.

Orthokeratology has undergone drastic changes since first described in the early 1960s (92). The original orthokeratology procedure involved a series of lenses to flatten the central cornea and was plagued by variable results. The introduction of highly oxygen-permeable lens materials that can be worn overnight, corneal topography, and reverse-geometry lens designs revolutionized this procedure (92).

Modern overnight orthokeratology causes rapid, reliable, and reversible reductions in refractive error. With modern designs, patients can wear lenses overnight, remove them in the morning, and see clearly throughout the day without the need for daytime refractive correction (92). Modern reverse-geometry lens designs cause central corneal flattening and mid-peripheral corneal steepening that provides clear foveal vision while simultaneously causing a myopic shift in peripheral retinal defocus.

The reasons for the recent resurgence in interest in the new modality of overnight orthokeratology using reverse-geometry lens designs have been detailed (90).

The time courses of onset and regression of clinical effects of reverse-geometry lens wear have been studied from a number of perspectives. Sridharan and Swarbrick (93) investigated the rate of onset of orthokeratology lens-induced changes over the first eight hours of lens wear. Statistically significant changes in corneal curvature and unaided vision were found after just 10 *min* of open-eye lens wear and these changes progressed significantly over the following hour. For a targeted refractive change of 2.00 *D*, they estimated that 60% of the refractive change had occurred after one hour of lens wear and 80% of the effect after the first occasion of overnight lens wear. The remarkably rapid rates of onset of lens-induced corneal flattening and refractive change with reverse-geometry lenses have since been confirmed by others (94–96).

The clinical efficacy of the common procedure was examined and outcomes from clinical studies in terms of refractive error change and unaided visual acuity were summarized.

The onset of the effects of overnight orthokeratology lens wear was rapid, with most change after the first night of lens wear and stability of refractive change after 7 to 10 *d*.

Mean reductions in myopic refractive error of between 1.75 *D* and 3.33 *D* and individual reductions of up to 5.00 *D* have been reported. There appear to be slight reductions or minimal changes in astigmatism with the use of reverse-geometry lenses and most patients were reported to achieve 6/6 unaided vision or better.

The induction of higher order aberrations, in particular spherical aberration, has been reported and this may affect subjective vision under conditions of low contrast and pupil dilation. Also, the satisfaction of the patients with overnight orthokeratology has been found to be similar to or better than with other popular modalities of contact lens wear (90).

Clinical studies have demonstrated that corneal curvature and refractive error changes continue over the first few days of overnight orthokeratology, until stability is reached after 7 to 10 nights of lens wear, as illustrated in Figure 5.16.

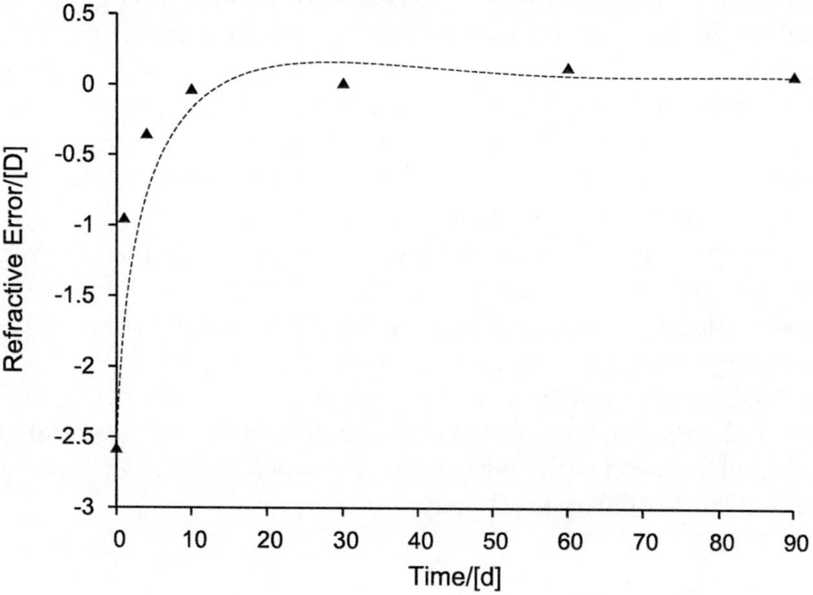

Figure 5.16 Refractive error change with time (90, 97).

Higher refractive error changes typically take longer to achieve than more modest changes (98, 99). There is some evidence that subtle changes in mid-peripheral corneal shape may continue for some weeks to months with continuing overnight lens wear, although their impact on subjective vision is probably minimal.

Available evidence suggests that the corneal changes induced by overnight orthokeratology are fully reversible. The refractive effect in orthokeratology is achieved by central epithelial thinning and this has raised concerns about compromise of the epithelial barrier to microbial infection.

Reports of microbial keratitis in the modality were reviewed and the overall safety of the procedure was also critically examined. Finally, research on stromal contributions to the orthokeratology effect, particularly relating to overnight edema, was summarized (90).

5.10.1 *Myopia*

The peripheral myopic retinal defocus caused by orthokeratology is hypothesized to be responsible for reductions in myopia progression in children fitted with these lenses. The changes in orthokeratology lens design that led to the reverse-geometry orthokeratology lenses that are used today and the optical changes these lenses produce have been reviewed (92). The optical changes reviewed include changes in refractive error and their time course, high- and low-contrast visual acuity changes, changes in higher-order aberrations and visual quality metrics, changes in accommodation, and changes in peripheral defocus caused by orthokeratology.

Also, the use of orthokeratology for myopia control in children has been reviewed, as are hypothesized connections between orthokeratology-induced myopic peripheral defocus and slowed myopia progression in children, and safety and complications associated with lens wear (92). A better understanding of the ocular and optical changes that occur with orthokeratology will be beneficial to both clinicians and patients in making informed decisions regarding the utilization of orthokeratology.

5.10.1.1 *Juvenile Myopia*

The corneal epithelium, which is the most superficial layer of the cornea, not only has a good protective function but is also involved in corneal refractive function. In particular, the central corneal epithelium has an especially important function for corneal refraction (100, 101).

The changes in the corneal thickness profile in juvenile myopia after overnight wear of orthokeratology lenses were investigated (102).

In the study, a total of 53 juveniles (53 right eyes) successfully wore orthokeratology lenses between January 2016 and July 2017 and they were reviewed one day, one week and one month after first wearing the lenses. Epithelial and corneal data were obtained by optical coherence tomography. The changes in uncorrected visual acuity, refractive error, corneal refractive power, and epithelial and corneal thickness were analyzed before and after wearing orthokeratology lenses.

The corneal epithelium was reshaped after 1 *d* of orthokeratology. Furthermore, the myopia degree was reduced, and uncorrected visual acuity reached 0 logMAR at 1 week. The central (2 *mm*) average epithelial thickness was 52.04±2.35 μm, 49.25±2.67 μm, 45.91±2.80 μm, and 47.53±3.44 μm before and after 1 day, 1 week, and 1 month of orthokeratology, respectively (t = 4.497, 9.741, and 7.340, respectively, P<0.001). The central epithelium was thinnest at 1 week, when the average thinning of 6.13±1.67 μm accounted for approximately 11.78%±3.21% of the total epithelium thickness at BL. The epithelial thickness of the reverse curve zone was 51.83±2.49 μm, 57.62±3.01 μm, 59.43±3.19 μm, and 60.22±2.75 μm before and after 1 day, 1 week, and 1 month of orthokeratology, respectively, showing a significant increase over time (t=-4.752, -6.208, and -6.848, respectively, P < 0.001) (102).

In the early stage of orthokeratology, the corneal epithelium was redistributed very quickly. The central epithelium became thin, while the epithelium of the reverse curve zone correspondingly thickened. The refractive power of the cornea was effectively reduced equivalent to the effect of adding a concave glass lens, which ensures uncorrected vision after removal of the lenses (102).

5.10.1.2 Myopia Progression Control

As compared to frame glasses and soft corneal contact lenses, orthokeratology delays the growth rate of the eye axis in children from 32% to 55% (103, 104).

As a safe and efficient treatment for controlling myopia progression, orthokeratology is receiving increasing attention (105, 106).

When following-up with children undergoing orthokeratology, it is necessary to meticulously measure multiple ocular biometric parameters such as axial length, corneal topography and endothelial cell count (107). As compared to stable corneal structure in adults, the corneal shape of a child's eye can easily deform in addition to having poorer fixation and shorter cooperation. So, the repeatability and reproducibility of ocular biometric measurements in children tend to be lower than in adults.

However, precision of measurements by ocular instruments in children and the influence of wearing orthokeratology contact lenses on the precision of such measurements have been rarely reported (107).

An optical biometer, i.e., OA-2000 (Tomey, Nagoya, Japan), uses swept-source optical coherence tomography (SS-OCT) technology to measure the optical distance between ocular structures (108). Details are given in Section 3.17.

It provides measurements of the axial length, keratometry, anterior chamber depth, corneal thickness, lens thickness, pupil diameter and corneal diameter. The optical biometer IOLMaster (Carl Zeiss Meditec AG, Jena, Germany), which introduced the partial coherence interferometry technology, has been reported to show high precision of measurements in normal and cataract eyes, and is regarded as the gold standard for non-contact biometry (109, 110).

In contrast to the IOLMaster, the new SS-OCT biometer has an automatic correction function and a continuous measurement model. So, the SS-OCT biometer was reported to have a high repeatability and reproducibility in measuring normal subjects and cataract patients (111, 112).

The SS-OCT optical biometer and partial coherence interferometry optical biometer were used to measure ocular biometric parameters of children before and after orthokeratology in order to evaluate the intra-operator repeatability and inter-operator reproducibility of the SS-OCT biometer, as well as the agreement between the two instruments. Also, whether or not orthokeratology influences the precision and agreement measurements of the SS-OCT biometer was first investigated.

In a prospective study, 51 eyes of 51 normal children (24 males and 27 females) were examined (107). The age range of subjects was 8 *y* to 16 *y* (mean: 11.98±2.15 *y*). The range of spherical equivalent was −0.75 *D* to −5.125 *D*.

The new SS-OCT biometer showed a remarkable intra-operator repeatability for axial length, mean keratometry, central corneal thickness, anterior chamber depth, lens thickness and corneal diameter measurements, both pre- and post-orthokeratology (107).

5.10.1.3 Accommodative Response

The effects of two months of an orthokeratology treatment in the accommodative response of young adult myopes were evaluated

(113).

Twenty eyes (21.8±1.8 *y*) were fitted with the Paragon CRT® 100 LENS to treat myopia between -1.00 and -2.00 *D*. Low- and high-contrast visual acuity, central objective refraction, light disturbance, and objective accommodative response were measured at BL before lens wear and after 1, 15, 30, and 60 nights of orthokeratology. This was done, using the Grand Seiko WAM-5500 open-field autorefractometer coupled with a Badal system (114, 115).

Refractive error correction was achieved during the first 50 days of orthokeratology lens wear, with minimal changes afterwards. Light disturbance analysis showed a transient increase followed by a reduction to baseline levels over the first 30 nights of treatment.

The accommodative response was lower than expected for all target vergences in all visits (BL: 0.61 *D* at 1.00 *D* to 0.96 *D* at 5.00 *D*; 60 N: 0.36 *D* at 1.00 *D* to 0.79 *D* at 5.00 *D*). On average, the accommodative lag decreases over time with orthokeratology lens wear. However, these differences were not statistically significant ($p > 0.050$, repeated measures ANOVA and Friedman test).

The Friedman test is a non-parametric statistical test developed by Milton Friedman (116, 117). Similar to the parametric repeated measures ANOVA, it is used to detect differences in treatments across multiple test attempts. The procedure involves ranking each row (or block) together, then considering the values of ranks by columns (116).

The tests showed that overnight orthokeratology treatment does not affect objectively measuring the accommodative response of young, low myopic eyes after two months of treatment stabilization *D* (113).

References

1. N. Efron, *Contact Lenses A-Z*, Butterworth-Heinemann, 2nd edition, 2002.
2. E.S. Bennett and V.A. Henry, *Clinical Manual of Contact Lenses*, Lippincott Williams & Wilkins, 5th edition, 2019.
3. R. Sinha and V.K. Dada, *Textbook of Contact Lenses*, Jaypee Brothers, Medical Publishers Pvt. Limited, 5th edition, 2017.

4. Wikipedia contributors, Eye disease — Wikipedia, the free encyclopedia, https://en.wikipedia.org/w/index.php?title=Eye_disease&oldid=995468825, 2020. [Online; accessed 21-December-2020].
5. C.H. Dohlman, (Ed.), *Corneal Edema*, Vol. 8-3 of *International Ophthalmology Clinics*, Little, Brown & Co., 1968.
6. J.E. Levenson and ALCON Laboratories, *Corneal Edema: Cause and Treatment*, Clinical signs in ophthalmology, Mosby-Year Book, 1993.
7. A. Guzman-Aranguez, B. Fonseca, G. Carracedo, A. Martin-Gil, A. Martinez-Aguila, and J. Pintor, Dry eye treatment based on contact lens drug delivery: A review, *Eye & Contact Lens*, Vol. 42, p. 280, 2016.
8. S. La Porta Weber, R. Becco de Souza, J. Àvaro Pereira Gomes, and A.L. Hofling-Lima, The use of the esclera scleral contact lens in the treatment of moderate to severe dry eye disease, *American Journal of Ophthalmology*, Vol. 163, p. 167, 2016.
9. T. Kojima, Contact lens-associated dry eye disease: Recent advances worldwide and in Japan, *Investigative Ophthalmology & Visual Science*, Vol. 59, p. DES102, 2018.
10. S. Sharma, P. Garg, and G.N. Rao, Patient characteristics, diagnosis, and treatment of non-contact lens related Acanthamoeba keratitis, *British Journal of Ophthalmology*, Vol. 84, p. 1103, 2000.
11. L. Keay, K. Edwards, T. Naduvilath, K. Forde, and F. Stapleton, Factors affecting the morbidity of contact lens–related microbial keratitis: A population study, *Investigative Ophthalmology & Visual Science*, Vol. 47, p. 4302, 2006.
12. E.B. Papas, J.B. Ciolino, D. Jacobs, W.L. Miller, H. Pult, A. Sahin, S. Srinivasan, J. Tauber, J.S. Wolffsohn, and J.D. Nelson, The TFOS international workshop on contact lens discomfort: Report of the management and therapy subcommittee, *Investigative Ophthalmology & Visual Science*, Vol. 54, p. TFOS183, 2013.
13. S.C. Grant, A.O. Hernandez-Pons, and J.M. Rinehart, Contact lens use in the treatment of an ophthalmologic condition, US Patent 9 086 580, assigned to Osio Corp., July 21, 2015.
14. J.D. Bartlett, J.F. Howes, N.R. Ghormley, J.F. Amos, R. Laibovitz, and B. Horwitz, Safety and efficacy of loteprednol etabonate for treatment of papillae in contact lens-associated giant papillary conjunctivitis, *Current Eye Research*, Vol. 12, p. 313, 1993.
15. V.M. Finnemore and J.E. Korb, Corneal edema with polymethylmethacrylate versus gas-permeable rigid polymer contact lenses of identical design, *Journal of the American Optometric Association*, Vol. 51, p. 271, 1980.
16. D. Fonn, B.A. Holden, P. Roth, G. Gooley, and J. Kenefick, Comparative physiologic performance of polymethyl methacrylate

and gas-permeable contact lenses, *Archives of Ophthalmology*, Vol. 102, p. 760, 05 1984.

17. H.A. Krebs and K. Henseleit, Untersuchungen über die Harnstoffbildung im Tierkörper, *Klinische Wochenschrift*, Vol. 11, p. 757, 1932.
18. M.D. Rohde and J.W. Huff, Contact lens-induced edema in vitro amelioration by lactate dehydrogenase inhibitors, *Current Eye Research*, Vol. 5, p. 751, 1986.
19. D.F. Sweeney and B.A. Holden, The closed-eye swelling response of the cornea to Polycon and Menicon 02 gas-permeable hard lenses, *The Australian Journal of Optometry*, Vol. 66, p. 186, 1983.
20. E.B. Hendiger, M. Padzik, I. Sifaoui, M. Reyes-Batlle, A. López-Arencibia, D. Zyskowska, M. Grodzik, A. Pietruczuk-Padzik, J. Hendiger, G. Oledzka, L. Chomicz, J.E. Piñero, and J. Lorenzo-Morales, Silver nanoparticles conjugated with contact lens solutions may reduce the risk of Acanthamoeba keratitis, *Pathogens*, Vol. 10, 2021.
21. Wikipedia contributors, Presbyopia — Wikipedia, the free encyclopedia, https://en.wikipedia.org/w/index.php?title=Presbyopia&oldid=951036142, 2020. [Online; accessed 14-June-2020].
22. E. Bauman, Material effect on multifocal contact lens fitting of lenses of the same optical design with the same fitting guide, *Contact Lens and Anterior Eye*, Vol. 41, p. S60, 2018. BCLA Conference Abstracts 2015 – 2018.
23. M. Merchea, D. Evans, S. Kannarr, J. Miller, M. Kaplan, and L. Nixon, Assessing a modified fitting approach for improved multifocal contact lens fitting, *Contact Lens and Anterior Eye*, Vol. 42, p. 540, 2019.
24. Wikipedia contributors, Near-sightedness — Wikipedia, the free encyclopedia, https://en.wikipedia.org/w/index.php?title=Near-sightedness&oldid=960835040, 2020. [Online; accessed 14-June-2020].
25. S.-M. Saw, G. Gazzard, E.C. Shih-Yen, and W.-H. Chua, Myopia and associated pathological complications, *Ophthalmic and Physiological Optics*, Vol. 25, p. 381, 2005.
26. Q. Ji, Y.-S. Yoo, H. Alam, and G. Yoon, Through-focus optical characteristics of monofocal and bifocal soft contact lenses across the peripheral visual field, *Ophthalmic and Physiological Optics*, Vol. 38, p. 326, 2018.
27. O. Pärssinen and A.L. Lyyra, Myopia and myopic progression among schoolchildren: A three-year follow-up study, *Investigative Ophthalmology & Visual Science*, Vol. 34, p. 2794, August 1993.
28. S.-M. Saw, M.-Z. Zhang, R.-Z. Hong, Z.-F. Fu, M.-H. Pang, and D.T.H. Tan, Near-work activity, night-lights, and myopia in the

Singapore-China study, *Archives of Ophthalmology*, Vol. 120, p. 620, 05 2002.

29. L. Remón, P. Pérez-Merino, R.J. Macedo-de Araújo, A.I. Amorim-de Sousa, and J.M. González-Méijome, Bifocal and multifocal contact lenses for Presbyopia and Myopia control, *Journal of Ophthalmology*, Vol. 2020, p. 8067657, 2020.
30. N. Kara-José, C. Coral-Ghanem, and C.E. Joslin, Complications associated with contact lens use in *Contact Lenses in Ophthalmic Practice*, chapter 22, pp. 243–266. Springer, New York, NY, 2004.
31. C.H.L. Lim, F. Stapleton, and J.S. Mehta, Review of contact lens-related complications, *Eye & Contact Lens*, Vol. 44, p. S1, 2018.
32. B.J. Mondino, S.M. Salamon, and G.W. Zaidman, Allergic and toxic reactions in soft contact lens wearers, *Survey of Ophthalmology*, Vol. 26, p. 337, 1982.
33. M.V. Blanco and D.L. Maurer, Soft contact lens preserving solutions, US Patent 4 029 817, assigned to Allergan Pharmaceuticals (Irvine, CA), June 14, 1977.
34. B. Chávez-Munguía, M. OmañA-Molina, M. González-Lázaro, A. González-Robles, P. Bonilla, and A. Matínez-Palomo, Ultrastructural study of encystation and excystation in Acanthamoeba castellanii, *Journal of Eukaryotic Microbiology*, Vol. 52, p. 153, 2005.
35. F. Marciano-Cabral, R. Puffenbarger, and G.A. Cabral, The increasing importance of Acanthamoeba infections, *Journal of Eukaryotic Microbiology*, Vol. 47, p. 29, 2000.
36. N.A. Turner, A.D. Russell, J.R. Furr, and D. Lloyd, Emergence of resistance to biocides during differentiation of Acanthamoeba castellanii, *Journal of Antimicrobial Chemotherapy*, Vol. 46, p. 27, 07 2000.
37. M. Omaña-Molina, D. Hernandez-Martinez, R. Sanchez-Rocha, U. Cardenas-Lemus, C. Salinas-Lara, A.R. Mendez-Cruz, L. Colin-Barenque, P. Aley-Medina, J. Espinosa-Villanueva, L. Moreno-Fierros, and J. Lorenzo-Morales, In vivo CNS infection model of Acanthamoeba genotype T4: The early stages of infection lack presence of host inflammatory response and are a slow and contact-dependent process, *Parasitology Research*, Vol. 116, p. 725, 2017.
38. J. Lorenzo-Morales, C.M. Martín-Navarro, A. López-Arencibia, F. Arnalich-Montiel, J.E. Piñero, and B. Valladares, Acanthamoeba keratitis: An emerging disease gathering importance worldwide?, *Trends in Parasitology*, Vol. 29, p. 181, 2013.
39. S.T. Awwad, W.M. Petroll, J.P. McCulley, and H.D. Cavanagh, Updates in Acanthamoeba keratitis, *Eye & Contact Lens*, Vol. 33, p. 1, 2007.

40. Y.A. Khan, R.T. Kashiwabuchi, S.A. Martins, J.M. Castro-Combs, S. Kalyani, P. Stanley, D. Flikier, and A. Behrens, Riboflavin and ultraviolet light a therapy as an adjuvant treatment for medically refractive Acanthamoeba keratitis: Report of 3 cases, *Ophthalmology*, Vol. 118, p. 324, 2011.
41. M. Mohammadpour, F. Rahimi, and M. Khorrami-Nejad, Total necrosis of cornea, iris and crystalline lens with exposure of vitreous hyaloid face in the context of recalcitrant Acanthamoeba keratitis, *Journal of Current Ophthalmology*, Vol. 30, p. 377, 2018.
42. A. Fernández-Ferreiro, M. Santiago-Varela, M. Gil-Martínez, M. González-Barcia, A. Luaces-Rodríguez, V. Díaz-Tome, M. Pardo, J.B. Méndez, A. Pineiro-Ces, M.T. Rodríguez-Ares, M.J. Lamas, and F.J. Otero-Espinar, In vitro evaluation of the ophthalmic toxicity profile of chlorhexidine and propamidine isethionate eye drops, *Journal of Ocular Pharmacology and Therapeutics*, Vol. 33, p. 202, 2017.
43. A. Shapiro, Alcohol-based wide spectrum disinfectant comprising nonoxynol-9, US Patent 7 560 422, assigned to ALDA Pharmaceuticals Corp., July 14, 2009.
44. D.J. McCanna, S.E. Maier, D.J. Heiler, S.P. Spooner, and E. Xia, Compositions comprising polyquaterniums in combination with polymeric biguanides for disinfecting contact lenses, US Patent 6 153 568, assigned to Bausch & Lomb Incorporated (Rochester, NY), November 28, 2000.
45. F.X. Smith, Ophthalmic and contact lens solutions containing simple saccharides as preservative enhancers, US Patent 9 492 582, assigned to FXS Ventures LLC, November 15, 2016.
46. Wikipedia contributors, Carbohydrate — Wikipedia, the free encyclopedia, https://en.wikipedia.org/w/index.php?title=Carbohydrate&oldid=988130406, 2020. [Online; accessed 28-November-2020].
47. F.X. Smith and K.S. Crawford, Ophthalmic and contact lens solutions containing peptides as preservative, US Patent 7 939 501, assigned to Bio-Concept Laboratories Inc., May 10, 2011.
48. T.E. Creighton, *Proteins: Structures and Molecular Properties*, pp. 179–182. W.H. Freeman & Co., New York, 1984.
49. J.D. Dickinson, F.S. Fowkes, and T.J. Rose, Manufacture of polymeric diguanides, US Patent 3 428 576, assigned to Imperial Chemical Industries Ltd., February 18, 1969.
50. G. Rembarz, H. Brandner, and H. Finger, Reaktionen mit Natriumdicyanimid, *Journal für Praktische Chemie*, Vol. 26, p. 314, 1964.
51. Y. Zhang, J. Jiang, and Y. Chen, Synthesis and antimicrobial activity of polymeric guanidine and biguanidine salts, *Polymer*, Vol. 40, p. 6189, 1999.

52. Z. Zhu, L. Jin, F. Yu, F. Wang, Z. Weng, J. Liu, Z. Han, and X. Wang, ZnO/CPAN modified contact lens with antibacterial and harmful light reduction capabilities, *Advanced Healthcare Materials*, Vol. n/a, p. 2100259, 2021.
53. K. Dumbleton, N. Keir, A. Moezzi, Y. Feng, L. Jones, and D. Fonn, Objective and subjective responses in patients refitted to daily-wear silicone hydrogel contact lenses, *Optometry and Vision Science*, Vol. 83, p. 758, 2006.
54. S.M. Dillehay and M.B. Miller, Performance of Lotrafilcon B silicone hydrogel contact lenses in experienced low-Dk/t daily lens wearers, *Eye & Contact Lens*, Vol. 33, p. 272, 2007.
55. L. Szczotka-Flynn and R. Chalmers, Incidence and epidemiologic associations of corneal infiltrates with silicone hydrogel contact lenses, *Eye & Contact Lens*, Vol. 39, p. 48, 2013.
56. A. Tauste, E. Ronda, M.-J. Molina, and M. Seguí, Effect of contact lens use on computer vision syndrome, *Ophthalmic and Physiological Optics*, Vol. 36, p. 112, 2016.
57. S.-w. Cheung, P. Cho, B. Chan, C. Choy, and V. Ng, A comparative study of biweekly disposable contact lenses: Silicone hydrogel versus hydrogel, *Clinical and Experimental Optometry*, Vol. 90, p. 124, 2007.
58. F. Alba-Bueno, Àngel Beltran-Masgoret, C. Sanjuan, M. Biarnés, and J. Marín, Corneal shape changes induced by first and second generation silicone hydrogel contact lenses in daily wear, *Contact Lens and Anterior Eye*, Vol. 32, p. 8, 2009.
59. M.C. Lin and T.N. Yeh, Mechanical complications induced by silicone hydrogel contact lenses, *Eye & Contact Lens*, Vol. 39, p. 115, 2013.
60. D.F. Sweeney, Have silicone hydrogel lenses eliminated hypoxia?, *Eye & Contact Lens*, Vol. 39, p. 53, 2013.
61. M.S. Yung, M. Boost, P. Cho, and M. Yap, Microbial contamination of contact lenses and lens care accessories of soft contact lens wearers (university students) in Hong Kong, *Ophthalmic and Physiological Optics*, Vol. 27, p. 11, 2007.
62. P. Cho, S.Y. Cheng, W.Y. Chan, and W.K. Yip, Soft contact lens cleaning: Rub or no-rub?, *Ophthalmic and Physiological Optics*, Vol. 29, p. 49, 2009.
63. K.A. Dumbleton, C.A. Woods, L.W. Jones, and D. Fonn, The relationship between compliance with lens replacement and contact lens-related problems in silicone hydrogel wearers, *Contact Lens and Anterior Eye*, Vol. 34, p. 216, 2011.
64. D.M. Robertson, The effects of silicone hydrogel lens wear on the corneal epithelium and risk for microbial keratitis, *Eye & Contact Lens*, Vol. 39, p. 67, January 2013.

65. K.D. Brown, S. Low, I. Mariappan, K.M. Abberton, R. Short, H. Zhang, S. Maddileti, V. Sangwan, D. Steele, and M. Daniell, Plasma polymer-coated contact lenses for the culture and transfer of corneal epithelial cells in the treatment of limbal stem cell deficiency, *Tissue Engineering Part A*, Vol. 20, p. 646, 2014.
66. M.V. Riley, Anion-sensitive ATPase in rabbit corneal endothelium and its relation to corneal hydration, *Experimental Eye Research*, Vol. 25, p. 483, 1977.
67. G. Cotsarelis, S.-Z. Cheng, G. Dong, T.-T. Sun, and R.M. Lavker, Existence of slow-cycling limbal epithelial basal cells that can be preferentially stimulated to proliferate: Implications on epithelial stem cells, *Cell*, Vol. 57, p. 201, 1989.
68. J.J. Chen and S.C. Tseng, Corneal epithelial wound healing in partial limbal deficiency, *Investigative Ophthalmology & Visual Science*, Vol. 31, p. 1301, July 1990.
69. K. Watanabe, K. Nishida, M. Yamato, T. Umemoto, T. Sumide, K. Yamamoto, N. Maeda, H. Watanabe, T. Okano, and Y. Tano, Human limbal epithelium contains side population cells expressing the ATP-binding cassette transporter ABCG2, *FEBS Letters*, Vol. 565, p. 6, 2004.
70. F. Majo, A. Rochat, M. Nicolas, G.A. Jaoudé, and Y. Barrandon, Oligopotent stem cells are distributed throughout the mammalian ocular surface, *Nature*, Vol. 456, p. 250, 2008.
71. C. Blehm, S. Vishnu, A. Khattak, S. Mitra, and R.W. Yee, Computer vision syndrome: A review, *Survey of Ophthalmology*, Vol. 50, p. 253, 2005.
72. P.T. Yeow and S.P. Taylor, Effects of long-term visual display terminal usage on visual functions, *Optometry and Vision Science: Official Publication of the American Academy of Optometry*, Vol. 68, p. 930, December 1991.
73. S. Gur, S. Ron, and A. Heicklen-Klein, Objective evaluation of visual fatigue in VDU workers, *Occupational Medicine*, Vol. 44, p. 201, 10 1994.
74. S. Gur and S. Ron, Does work with visual display units impair visual activities after work?, *Documenta Ophthalmologica*, Vol. 79, p. 253, 1992.
75. M. Rosenfield, Computer vision syndrome: A review of ocular causes and potential treatments, *Ophthalmic and Physiological Optics*, Vol. 31, p. 502, 2011.
76. K. Tsubota and K. Nakamori, Dry eyes and video display terminals, *New England Journal of Medicine*, Vol. 328, p. 584, 1993.
77. S. Gowrisankaran, J.E. Sheedy, and J.R. Hayes, Eyelid squint response to asthenopia-inducing conditions, *Optometry and Vision Science*, Vol. 84, p. 611, 2007.

78. A. Chawla, T.C. Lim, S.N. Shikhare, P.L. Munk, and W.C.G. Peh, Computer vision syndrome: Darkness under the shadow of light, *Canadian Association of Radiologists Journal*, Vol. 70, p. 5, 2019.
79. C.M. Barrett, Radiation hazards in the practice of radiology, *Radiology*, Vol. 63, p. 400, 1954.
80. M. Korogiannaki, M. Samsom, A. Matheson, K. Soliman, T.A. Schmidt, and H. Sheardown, Investigating the synergistic interactions of surface immobilized and free natural ocular lubricants for contact lens applications: A comparative study between hyaluronic acid and proteoglycan 4 (lubricin), *Langmuir*, Vol. 37, p. 1062, 2021.
81. R. Badugu, H. Szmacinski, E.A. Reece, B.H. Jeng, and J.R. Lakowicz, Sodium-sensitive contact lens for diagnostics of ocular pathologies, *Sensors and Actuators B: Chemical*, Vol. 331, p. 129434, 2021.
82. D. Wong, J.M. Albietz, H. Tran, C. Du Toit, A.H. Li, T. Yun, J. Han, and K.L. Schmid, Treatment of contact lens related dry eye with antibacterial honey, *Contact Lens and Anterior Eye*, Vol. 40, p. 389, 2017.
83. F.A. Maulvi, A.A. Shaikh, D.H. Lakdawala, A.R. Desai, M.M. Pandya, S.S. Singhania, R.J. Vaidya, K.M. Ranch, B.A. Vyas, and D.O. Shah, Design and optimization of a novel implantation technology in contact lenses for the treatment of dry eye syndrome: In vitro and in vivo evaluation, *Acta Biomaterialia*, Vol. 53, p. 211, 2017.
84. G.M. Keating, Diquafosol ophthalmic solution 3%: A review of its use in dry eye, *Drugs*, Vol. 75, p. 911, 2015.
85. P. Xu, H. Wang, P. Shen, P. Peng, Y. Tu, Y. Sun, J. Wang, C. Xu, Z. Qiu, R. Ge, Z. Li, and J. Bian, Practical and efficient approach to the preparation of Diquafosol Tetrasodium, *Organic Process Research & Development*, Vol. 24, p. 1477, 2020.
86. K. Yamada, Method for producing P1,P4-di(uridine 5′-)tetraphosphate, US Patent Application 20 160 194 347, assigned to Yamasa Corp., July 07, 2016.
87. Y. Oshita, H. Nakazawa, I. Matsuoka, and A. Kamimura, Therapeutic agent for dry eye characterized by being applied to eye of dry eye patient wearing soft contact lens, US Patent Application 20 200 254 000, assigned to Santen Pharmaceutical Co. Ltd., August 13, 2020.
88. W. Pendergast, B.R. Yerxa, J.G. Douglass, S.R. Shaver, R.W. Dougherty, C.C. Redick, I.F. Sims, and J.L. Rideout, Synthesis and P2Y receptor activity of a series of uridine dinucleoside 5′-polyphosphates, *Bioorganic & Medicinal Chemistry Letters*, Vol. 11, p. 157, 2001.
89. K. Molina, A.D. Graham, T. Yeh, M. Lerma, W. Li, V. Tse, and M.C. Lin, Not all dry eye in contact lens wear is contact lens–induced, *Eye & Contact Lens*, Vol. 46, p. 214, 2020.

90. H.A. Swarbrick, Orthokeratology review and update, *Clinical and Experimental Optometry*, Vol. 89, p. 124, 2006.
91. R.M. Pearson, Kalt, keratoconus, and the contact lens, *Optometry and Vision Science*, Vol. 66, p. 643, 1989.
92. A.N. Nti and D.A. Berntsen, Optical changes and visual performance with orthokeratology, *Clinical and Experimental Optometry*, Vol. 103, p. 44, 2020.
93. R. Sridharan and H. Swarbrick, Corneal response to short-term orthokeratology lens wear, *Optometry and Vision Science*, Vol. 80, p. 200, 2003.
94. N. Tahhan, E. Papas, R. Du Toit, J. Stern, A. Kalliris, R. Wong, and B. Holden, Corneal topographic change after short periods of reverse geometry rigid gas permeable lens wear, *Investigative Ophthalmology & Visual Science*, Vol. 43, p. 972, 2002.
95. J.M. Jackson, T. Bildstein, J. Anderson, B. Leak, and K. Buresh, Short–term corneal changes with corneal refractive therapy (CRT), *Investigative Ophthalmology & Visual Science*, Vol. 45, p. 1547, 2004.
96. Y. Kamei, K. Cassar, J. Shen, and P.S. Soni, Short–term corneal changes in closed eye condition with orthokeratology lenses, *Investigative Ophthalmology & Visual Science*, Vol. 46, p. 2060, 2005.
97. A. Alharbi and H.A. Swarbrick, The effects of overnight orthokeratology lens wear on corneal thickness, *Investigative Ophthalmology & Visual Science*, Vol. 44, p. 2518, 2003.
98. L. Fan, J. Jun, Q. Jia, J. Wangqing, M. Xinjie, and S. Yi, Clinical study of orthokeratology in young myopic adolescents, *International Contact Lens Clinic*, Vol. 26, p. 113, 1999.
99. H. Owens, L.F. Garner, J.P. Craig, and G. Gamble, Posterior corneal changes with orthokeratology, *Optometry and Vision Science*, Vol. 81, p. 421, 2004.
100. J. Wang, D. Fonn, T.L. Simpson, L. Sorbara, R. Kort, and L. Jones, Topographical thickness of the epithelium and total cornea after overnight wear of reverse-geometry rigid contact lenses for myopia reduction, *Investigative Ophthalmology & Visual Science*, Vol. 44, p. 4742, 2003.
101. S. Haque, L. Jones, and T. Simpson, Thickness mapping of the cornea and epithelium using optical coherence tomography, *Optometry and Vision Science*, Vol. 85, p. E963, 2008.
102. J. Zhang, J. Li, X. Li, F. Li, and T. Wang, Redistribution of the corneal epithelium after overnight wear of orthokeratology contact lenses for myopia reduction, *Contact Lens and Anterior Eye*, Vol. 43, p. 232, 2020.
103. T. Kakita, T. Hiraoka, and T. Oshika, Influence of overnight orthokeratology on axial elongation in childhood myopia, *Investigative Ophthalmology & Visual Science*, Vol. 52, p. 2170, 2011.

104. J. Santodomingo-Rubido, C. Villa-Collar, B. Gilmartin, and R. Gutiérrez-Ortega, Myopia control with orthokeratology contact lenses in Spain: Refractive and biometric changes, *Investigative Ophthalmology & Visual Science*, Vol. 53, p. 5060, 07 2012.
105. S.W. Cheung, P. Cho, W.S. Chui, and G.C. Woo, Refractive error and visual acuity changes in orthokeratology patients, *Optometry and Vision Science*, Vol. 84, p. 410, 2007.
106. K.-S. Na, Y.-S. Yoo, H.S. Hwang, J.W. Mok, H.S. Kim, and C.-K. Joo, The influence of overnight orthokeratology on ocular surface and meibomian glands in children and adolescents, *Eye & Contact Lens*, Vol. 42, p. 68, 2016.
107. B. Shu, F. Bao, G. Savini, W. Lu, R. Tu, H. Chen, B. Song, Q. Wang, and J. Huang, Effect of orthokeratology on precision and agreement assessment of a new swept-source optical coherence tomography biometer, *Eye and Vision*, Vol. 7, p. 13, 2020.
108. S. Goebels, M. Pattmöller, T. Eppig, A. Cayless, B. Seitz, and A. Langenbucher, Comparison of 3 biometry devices in cataract patients, *Journal of Cataract & Refractive Surgery*, Vol. 41, p. 2387, 2015.
109. H.J. Shammas and S. Chan, Precision of biometry, keratometry, and refractive measurements with a partial coherence interferometry–keratometry device, *Journal of Cataract & Refractive Surgery*, Vol. 36, p. 1474, 2010.
110. P. Kunavisarut, P. Poopattanakul, C. Intarated, and K. Pathanapitoon, Accuracy and reliability of IOL master and A-scan immersion biometry in silicone oil-filled eyes, *Eye*, Vol. 26, p. 1344, 2012.
111. J. Huang, G. Savini, K.J. Hoffer, H. Chen, W. Lu, Q. Hu, F. Bao, and Q. Wang, Repeatability and interobserver reproducibility of a new optical biometer based on swept-source optical coherence tomography and comparison with IOLMaster, *British Journal of Ophthalmology*, Vol. 101, p. 493, 2017.
112. C. McAlinden, Q. Wang, R. Gao, W. Zhao, A. Yu, Y. Li, Y. Guo, and J. Huang, Axial length measurement failure rates with biometers using swept-source optical coherence tomography compared to partial-coherence interferometry and optical low-coherence interferometry, *American Journal of Ophthalmology*, Vol. 173, p. 64, 2017.
113. A.F. Pereira-da Mota, J. Costa, A. Amorim-de Sousa, J.M. González-Méijome, and A. Queirós, The impact of overnight orthokeratology on accommodative response in myopic subjects, *Journal of Clinical Medicine*, Vol. 9, p. 3687, November 2020.
114. J.-A. Badal and C. Lafon, Tratamiento médico de las cataratas incipientes, *Archivos de Oftalmología Hispano-Americanos*, Vol. 8, p. 208, 1908.
115. J.-A. Badal and L.P. Marqués, Las auto-mutilaciones oculares, *Archivos de Oftalmología Hispano-Americanos*, Vol. 9, p. 145, 1909.

116. Wikipedia contributors, Friedman test — Wikipedia, the free encyclopedia, https://en.wikipedia.org/w/index.php?title=Friedman_test&oldid=991650361, 2020. [Online; accessed 1-December-2020].
117. M. Friedman, A comparison of alternative tests of significance for the problem of *m* rankings, *The Annals of Mathematical Statistics*, Vol. 11, p. 86, 03 1940.

Index

Acronyms

GP
Gas-permeable, 149
GPC
Gel permeation chromatography, 52
HA
Hyaluronic acid, 46, 239, 331, 390
HEMA
2-Hydroxyethyl methacrylate, 48, 172, 238, 274
HPMC
Hydroxypropyl methylcellulose, 274
IPN
Interpenetrating network, 124
LASIK
Laser-assisted *in-situ* keratomileusis, 134
LED
Light-emitting diode, 98
LSCD
Limbal stem cell deficiency, 385
MA
Methacrylic acid, 37, 300
MALDI-TOF
Matrix-assisted laser desorption/ionization time-of-flight mass spectrometry, 244
MPC
2-Methacryloyloxyethyl phosphorylcholine, 121
NIPAAm
N-Isopropylacrylamide, 274
NVP
N-Vinyl-2-pyrrolidone, 99, 274
OSDi
Ocular Surface Disease Index, 249
PAN
Poly(acrylonitrile), 197
PCBDA
Poly(carboxylbetaine-*co*-dopamine methacrylamide), 195
PDMS
Poly(dimethyl siloxane), 275
PEG
Poly(ethylene glycol), 111, 238, 295
PEO
Poly(ethylene oxide), 231
PETG
Poly(ethylene terephthalate glycol), 218

Chemicals

Boldface numbers refer to Figures

General Index